Netter's Atlas of Human Neuroscience

Netter's Atlas of Human Neuroscience

David L. Felten, MD, PhD
University of California, Irvine
College of Medicine

Ralph Józefowicz, MD
University of Rochester

Illustrations by Frank H. Netter, MD

Contributing Illustrators

John A. Craig, MD

Carlos A. G. Machado, MD

James A. Perkins, MS, MFA

Icon Learning Systems · Teterboro, New Jersey

Published by Icon Learning Systems LLC, a subsidiary of MediMedia USA, Inc.
Copyright © 2003 MediMedia, Inc.

FIRST EDITION

ISBN 1929007-16-7
Library of Congress Catalog No.: 2003106966

Printed in the U.S.A.
First Printing, 2003
Second Printing, 2004

NOTICE

Every effort has been taken to confirm the accuracy of the information presented and to describe generally accepted practices. Neither the publisher nor the authors can be held responsible for errors or for any consequences arising from the use of the information contained herein, and make no warranty, expressed or implied, with respect to the contents of the publication.

Executive Editor: Paul Kelly
Editorial Director: Greg Otis
Managing Editor: Jennifer Surich
Director of Print Production: Mary Ellen Curry
Production Manager: Stephanie Klein
Graphic Artist: Colleen Quinn
Media Project Editor: Karen Oswald

Binding and Printing by Banta Book Group
Color Corrections by Page Imaging
Digital Separations by Page Imaging
Composition and Layout by Graphic Arts Center/Indianapolis

DEDICATION

In memory of Walle J.H. Nauta, MD, PhD, Institute Professor of Neuroscience at MIT
A distinguished, brilliant, pioneering neuroscientist
An outstanding and inspirational teacher
A kind, supportive, insightful, and gracious mentor
An incredible role model and human being

and

To my wife, Mary Maida Felten, PhD
A wonderful wife, partner, and friend
My inspiration and motivation
A superb researcher, teacher, and CEO
A woman who has it all: brains, beauty, kindness, and accomplishment

David L. Felten

To the medical students and residents we have taught over the years at the University of Rochester

Ralph F. Józefowicz

PREFACE

Netter's Atlas of Human Neuroscience combines the richness and beauty of Dr. Frank Netter's illustrations depicting both regional and systemic neuroscience with updated information and beautiful new illustrations to reflect our growing understanding of many regions and systems of the brain, the spinal cord, and the periphery. This *Atlas* also includes new cross-sections through the spinal cord and the brain stem, as well as coronal and horizontal sections correlated with MRIs. We have chosen to let the illustrations provide the focal point for learning, rather than offer long, detailed written explanations that could constitute a full textbook in itself. We have provided succinct figure legends to point out some of the major functional aspects of each illustration, particularly as these aspects relate to problems that a clinician may encounter in assessing a patient with neurological symptoms. The figure legends, combined with the excellent illustrations, provide a thorough understanding of the basic components, organization, and functional aspects of the region or system under consideration.

In order to provide an optimal learning experience for students of neuroscience, we have organized this *Atlas* in three parts: I. Overview of the Nervous System, II. Regional Neuroscience, and III. Systemic Neuroscience. This organization affords the reader the benefit of looking at some of these complex neural structures and systems in two or three different contexts, or from two or three different points of view, sometimes as part of an overview, sometimes with a regional emphasis, and sometimes with a view toward understanding the functioning of a specific system spanning the neuraxis. Thoughtful repetition from novel perspectives is a useful tool in acquiring a comfortable working knowledge of the nervous system that will serve clinicians well in evaluating and treating patients with neurological problems and that will provide neuroscience researchers and educators with a broader and more comprehensive understanding of the nervous system.

With some information, such as that on upper and lower motor neurons and their control, detailed factual information must be acquired and understood as a preliminary step toward understanding clinical aspects of motor disorders; with such an understanding, the clinical aspects fall nicely into place. We introduce core information

and provide regional and functional contexts for the information, as appropriate, to encourage true understanding rather than rote memorization. In a discipline as complex as the neurosciences, the acquisition of a true understanding of the major regions and hierarchies of the nervous system is essential for developing a working competence in basic and clinical neuroscience.

This *Atlas* illustrates basic human neuroscience, not clinical conditions and disorders, such as multiple sclerosis, Alzheimer's disease, strokes, spinal cord and brain injuries, the agnosias, aphasias, and apraxias, or other major conditions. These topics are more appropriate for a future volume.

Part I. Overview of the Nervous System

We begin with an introductory overview of neurons and their properties, gross features of the nervous system, and an understanding of the supporting tissues and systems such as the vasculature, the meninges, and the cerebrospinal fluid because we believe that it is necessary to understand this body of information before delving into the details of regional and systemic neuroscience. Thus, Part I. Overview of the Nervous System first presents the unique characteristics and properties of the cellular foundations of the nervous system, including neurons and their structural, neurotransmitter, and electrical properties, and the supporting cells, the glia. Specific examples of primary sensory neurons, lower motor neurons, and autonomic preganglionic and postganglionic neurons provide preparatory examples of the inputs and outputs of the nervous system, essential for understanding both regional and systemic neuroscience.

The next portion of the Overview introduces the major structural features of the nervous system, including the principal subdivisions and their functional roles, in a manner that is consistent with introductory laboratory examination of the human nervous system. Thus, students are introduced to lateral, midsagittal, basal, and some cross-sectional views of the forebrain, with the intention of obtaining a "big picture" view. This is followed by a similar introduction to the brain stem and cerebellum and the spinal cord. It is during this introductory overview that students should become familiar with the telencephalon, the diencephalon, the brain stem, the spinal cord, and the peripheral nervous system and acquire an understanding of the major associations and relationships among these components.

Subsequent sections of the Overview introduce the meninges, the ventricles and cerebrospinal fluid, and the vasculature, all components of the extensive supportive and protective infrastructure of the nervous system. Because the vasculature of the brain and spinal cord is a very important part of neurological assessment and understanding, we thoroughly introduce it in the Overview and follow this with additional reference and explanation of more specific details in Part II. Regional Neuroscience and Part III. Systemic Neuroscience. Finally, the Overview presents developmental neuroscience, showing how the mature nervous system develops and how some of the important functional relationships reflect associations that began during neural development.

Part II. Regional Neuroscience

Part II. Regional Neuroscience begins in the peripheral nervous system (PNS) and moves rostrally. This approach permits students to gain a thorough understanding of the inputs and outputs of the central nervous system (CNS), the brain and spinal cord, before attempting to understand more rostral regions that are involved in processing of inputs to, and regulation of outputs of, the CNS.

The introduction to the PNS establishes a thorough understanding of primary sensory inputs and motor and autonomic outputs of the CNS. Conceptually, some of the most important illustrations in the *Atlas* are those that outline (1) secondary sensory channels—the reflex, cerebellar, and lemniscal channels that further process primary sensory input to the CNS, (2) motor hierarchies, focused first on the lower motor neurons (LMNs) that supply skeletal muscle fibers, regulation of these LMNs by brain stem and cortical upper motor neurons (UMNs), and the coordination and modulation of UMN regulation by the cerebellum and the basal ganglia, and (3) preganglionic autonomic connections to peripheral targets through autonomic ganglia, and the central circuits from the brain stem, the hypothalamus, and the limbic structures that regulate and coordinate both autonomic and neuroendocrine outflow. A thorough understanding of these hierarchies—as presented in the introduction to the PNS—is the foundation for the rest of the *Atlas*.

The section on the PNS next offers a systematic collection of illustrations of roots, plexuses, and peripheral somatic nerves, which provides a smooth transition between the central and the peripheral aspects of neuroscience. The illustrations of the major peripheral nerves are conducive to acquiring a better understanding of neuropathies, which are so frequently encountered in medical practice. We have tried to bring together the basics of peripheral nerve anatomy, function, and clinical deficits in as simple and succinct a fashion as possible in the figure legends for the peripheral nerves.

The section on the PNS next outlines the organization and the major distribution networks of the autonomic nervous system. These illustrations are important for many reasons, including understanding autonomic disorders and the effects of a host of pharmacological agents that influence the autonomic nervous system and its associated adrenergic and cholinergic receptors. In addition, we are becoming increasingly aware that major life stressors and life style factors play an important role in the onset, progression, and outcome of atherosclerosis and cardiovascular disease (including cerebrovascular disease), cancer, diabetes, chronic pulmonary disease, and even neurodegenerative diseases and that these factors exert their physiological effect in large part through neural outflow via the autonomic nervous system and via hypothalamo-pituitary-neuroendocrine outflow and that they have an impact on cytokines, hormones, inflammatory mediators, and a variety of immune responses. The updates to our understanding of peripheral autonomic mechanisms include the depiction of autonomic interactions with cells of the immune system and with metabolic cells such as hepatocytes and fat cells.

The brain stem is usually the "terra incognita" of neuroscience courses and can be an exercise in memorization and minutiae if not properly organized. This *Atlas* provides the organization for rather straightforward understanding of the brain stem, despite its complexities and intricacies. The brain stem has six major components: (1) sensory nuclei and their pathways—including secondary sensory nuclei and pathways for incoming sensory information to the brain stem (trigeminal, auditory, vestibular, taste, visual), as well as somatosensory nuclei and channels, (2) LMNs for the cranial nuclei, and descending UMN channels that control

LMNs in both the brain stem and the spinal cord, (3) parasympathetic preganglionic neurons, and descending autonomic pathways and associated nuclei that regulate the outflow of both the sympathetic and the parasympathetic components of the autonomic nervous system, (4) cranial nerve nuclei and their axons, which directly overlap with, and are included in, the first three components, (5) the cerebellum and its afferent and efferent connections, and (6) the reticular formation. The cranial nerves and their nuclei are vital components for understanding both the brain stem and the localization of lesions in the context of the neurological history and examination, and they are the appropriate vehicle for understanding the first three components of the brain stem, noted above. The Netter illustrations are lucid, thorough, and readily understandable foundations for this process.

In addition to the Netter illustrations, we have added cross-sections through the spinal cord and the brain stem. These cross-sections will allow *Netter's Atlas of Human Neuroscience* to be used as a laboratory and basic sciences guide for students, eliminating the need for a separate, detailed photographic atlas. In addition, an excellent set of forebrain horizontal and coronal sections, correlated with MRI images, is provided. These cross-sections, coronals, and horizontals emphasize the functionally important structures and avoid the use of endless labels and minutiae that get in the way of true understanding and obscure the "big picture." Also added to this section on the brain stem are new illustrations of the reticular formation, a complex region of the CNS that cuts across all systems and is involved in widely varied neural activities.

The spinal cord, brain stem, and forebrain components of the Regional Neuroscience section focus on localizing and regional information important for understanding the consequences of lesions at specific sites. In the forebrain section, we emphasize the thalamus and the hypothalamus in the section on the diencephalon; we include the subthalamus with the basal ganglia and the epithalamus with the hypothalamus and the limbic system. Although the telencephalon has four major functional components—cerebral cortex, basal ganglia, limbic forebrain system, and olfactory system—we particularly emphasize the cerebral cortex anatomy and connections in the Regional Neuroscience section. The details of basal ganglia anatomy, limbic

forebrain structures and their connections, and the olfactory system are provided Part III, Systemic Neuroscience. We also have updated the forebrain section with an overview of the chemically specific systems of the brain, specifically the noradrenergic, serotonergic, dopaminergic, and cholinergic systems, which provide extensive innervation to widespread CNS regions and which are so frequently targeted with neurological and psychiatric drugs.

Part III. Systemic Neuroscience
Part III. Systemic Neuroscience provides a more detailed understanding of the peripheral and central mechanisms of the sensory systems, the motor systems, the autonomic-hypothalamic-limbic systems, and some higher functions. The foundations for understanding the secondary sensory and higher-order processing of sensory pathways begin with the illustrations in the introduction to the PNS in Part II. The systemic sensory components include the somatosensory, trigeminal sensory, taste, auditory, vestibular, and visual systems. To reflect current understanding, several modifications to Dr. Netter's artwork have been made, as well as new art created by John Craig, MD and Jim Perkins, MS, MFA, particularly in the sections on the somatosensory system and the visual system. Although we focus extensively on the lemniscal pathways for sensory processing and conscious interpretation of incoming sensory information, appropriate diagrams and connections for reflex and cerebellar pathways are included when appropriate (for example, with the vestibular system).

The systemic motor components include LMNs, UMNs, the cerebellum, and the basal ganglia—of course, with the acknowledgment that the cerebellum and the basal ganglia are involved in coordinating and modulating central circuits more widespread than just motor systems. For the UMN pathways, each system is illustrated, with emphasis on the functional role. The cerebellar connections included in this section emphasize the relationships between specific zones of the cerebellum (vermis, paravermis, lateral hemispheres) with appropriate deep nuclei (fastigial, globose and emboliform, dentate) and the UMN systems with which they connect (reticulospinal and vestibulospinal, rubrospinal, corticospinal). Similarly, the basal ganglia connections show interconnections with the cortex through the thalamus, including modulation of the cells of origin of the corticospinal system and other cortical outflow. However, other basal ganglia loops are also included: even though basal ganglia disorders have become known for their motor involvement, and are often called "movement disorders," we now know that many other loops exist, linking other regions of the thalamus and the cortex with the basal ganglia, for cognitive as well as emotional behavioral influences.

The autonomic-hypothalamic-limbic section includes detailed updates and understanding of this important set of interconnected circuitry through the hypothalamus and limbic system that ultimately regulates many behaviors, neuroendocrine outflow, and visceral activities of the autonomic nervous system. We begin with the understanding that many of the connections of the hypothalamus and limbic system focus on autonomic and neuroendocrine outflow. In the last decade, the role of the hypothalamus as a focal point for converging influences from forebrain sources, brain stem sources,

and circulating mediators has become better elucidated. This is reflected in several new illustrations. The sections on limbic forebrain structures (hippocampal formation, amygdaloid nuclei, septum, cingulate cortex) have been redone and expanded, reflecting both the newly discovered complexities of the circuitry and the focus on converging influences, particularly through the hypothalamus and autonomic outflow of the CNS.

It is our hope that the three parts of this *Atlas*— Overview of the Nervous System, Regional Neuroscience, and Systemic Neuroscience—will provide students with a comfortable working knowledge of the basic components, organization, and functional aspects of the nervous system and that this foundation will serve them well for interpreting neurological examinations, understanding most neurological diseases and disorders, and evaluating and treating patients with neurological problems.

Frank H. Netter, MD

Frank H. Netter was born in 1906 in New York City. He studied art at the Art Student's League and the National Academy of Design before entering medical school at New York University, where he received his M.D. degree in 1931. During his student years, Dr. Netter's notebook sketches attracted the attention of the medical faculty and other physicians, allowing him to augment his income by illustrating articles and textbooks. He continued illustrating as a sideline after establishing a surgical practice in 1933, but he ultimately opted to give up his practice in favor of a full-time commitment to art. After service in the United States Army during World War II, Dr. Netter began his long collaboration with the CIBA Pharmaceutical Company (now Novartis Pharmaceuticals). This 45-year partnership resulted in the production of the extraordinary collection of medical art so familiar to physicians and other medical professionals worldwide.

Icon Learning Systems acquired the Netter Collection in July 2000 and continues to update Dr. Netter's original paintings and to add newly commissioned paintings by artists trained in the style of Dr. Netter.

Dr. Netter's works are among the finest examples of the use of illustration in the teaching of medical concepts. The 13-book Netter Collection of Medical Illustrations, which includes the greater part of the more than 20,000 paintings created by Dr. Netter, became and remains one of the most famous medical works ever published. The Netter Atlas of Human Anatomy, first published in 1989, presents the anatomical paintings from the Netter Collection. Now translated into 11 languages, it is the anatomy atlas of choice among medical and health professions students the world over.

The Netter illustrations are appreciated not only for their aesthetic qualities, but more importantly, for their intellectual content. As Dr. Netter wrote in 1949, ". . . clarification of a subject is the aim and goal of illustration. No matter how beautifully painted, how delicately and subtly rendered a subject may be, it is of little value as a medical illustration if it does not serve to make clear some medical point." Dr. Netter's planning, conception, point of view, and approach are what inform his paintings and what makes them so intellectually valuable.

Frank H. Netter, MD, physician and artist, died in 1991.

ABOUT THE AUTHORS

David L. Felten, MD, PhD, is Professor of Anatomy and Neurobiology, and Executive Director of the Susan Samueli Center for Complementary Medicine at the University of California, Irvine. He was previously the Kilian J. and Caroline F. Schmitt Professor and Chair of the Department of Neurobiology and Anatomy, and Director of the Markey Charitable Trust Institute for Neurobiology at the University of Rochester School of Medicine. Dr. Felten carried out pioneering studies of autonomic innervation of lymphoid organs, and neural-immune signaling that underlies the mechanistic foundations for many aspects of integrative medicine. He is the recipient of numerous awards, including a prestigious John D. and Catherine T. MacArthur Foundation Prize Fellowship, two simultaneous NIH Merit awards from the NIA and NIMH, several other fellowships, and a multitude of teaching awards. He has served for many years on the National Board of Medical Examiners, including as Chairman of the Neurosciences Committee. Dr. Felten is a co-editor (with Robert Ader and Nicholas Cohen) of *Psychoneuroimmunology,* 3rd edition (Academic Press, 2001), the principal text in this field, and the author of more than 200 peer-reviewed journal articles. He is a founding co-editor of the journal, *Brain, Behavior, and Immunity.* He is the co-founder and Chief Scientific and Medical Advisor of Sumavera Medical Innovations, an IP holding company for developing novel medical products. Dr. Felten received his BS from MIT in 1969 and his MD (1973) and his PhD (1974) from the University of Pennsylvania.

Ralph F. Józefowicz, MD, is Professor of Neurology and Medicine and Associate Chair for Education in the Department of Neurology at the University of Rochester. He is also Director of the second-year medical student "Mind, Brain and Behavior" course, the third-year Neurology Clerkship, and the Neurology Residency Program at the University of Rochester. He is the recipient of the Robert J. Glaser Alpha Omega Alpha Distinguished Teacher Award from the Association of American Medical Colleges in 2002, the Gold Medal Award for Excellence in Medical Student Education from the Alumni Association of the University of Rochester School of Medicine and Dentistry in 1998, the Distinguished Teacher Award from the American Neurological Association in 1998, and the Fulbright Scholar Award for Lecturing in Neural Sciences, Neuromuscular Diseases and Clinical Neurology from the Jagiellonian University Collegium Medicum in Krakow, Poland, in 1993. Dr. Józefowicz received his bachelor's degree in Biology, with honors, from the Johns Hopkins University in 1975 and his medical degree from Columbia University College of Physicians and Surgeons in 1979. A member of both Phi Beta Kappa and Alpha Omega Alpha, he completed residencies in Internal Medicine and in Neurology and a fellowship in Neuromuscular Diseases at the University of Rochester School of Medicine and Dentistry, New York.

ACKNOWLEDGMENTS

For decades, Dr. Frank Netter's beautiful and informative artwork has provided the visual basis for understanding anatomy, physiology, and relationships of great importance in medicine. Generations of physicians and healthcare professionals have learned "from the master" and have carried Dr. Netter's legacy forward through their own knowledge and contributions to patient care. Dr. Netter's artwork cannot be compared to anything else, because it stands in a class of its own. *The Netter Collection Volume I* on the nervous system has been a flagship volume for students of neuroscience for many decades. We are honored to provide the framework, organization, and new information for this updated edition of *Netter's Atlas of Human Neuroscience*. The opportunity to make a lasting contribution to the next generations of students is perhaps the greatest honor anyone could receive.

I also gratefully acknowledge Walle J.H. Nauta, MD, PhD, whose inspirational teaching of the nervous system contributed to the organizational framework for this *Atlas*. Professor Nauta always emphasized the value of an overview; the plates in the beginning of Part II on the conceptual organization of the sensory, motor, and autonomic systems especially reflect his approach. I am particularly honored to contribute to this updated *Atlas* because I first learned neurosciences as an undergraduate in Professor Nauta's laboratory at MIT, using *The Netter Collection Volume I* by Dr. Frank Netter and the masterful insights and explanations from Professor Nauta. It is our hope that continuing generations of students can benefit from the legacy of this great scientist.

I thank the outstanding artists, Jim Perkins, MS, MFA, and John Craig, MD, for their clear and beautiful contributions to this *Atlas*. Jim Perkins took some of my almost incomprehensible modifications of original Netter plates, and seamlessly incorporated them into those illustrations. He also took my "stick figures" and confusing, crowded, hand-drawn brain circuitry and made them come to life. John Craig provided the brain stem cross-sections and the horizontal and coronal sections, as well as several other illustrations. In the Netter tradition, he painted them to show the structures and relationships with beauty, and to clarify rather than intimidate.

Special thanks go to the superb group of professionals at Icon Learning Systems, who made this long and challenging task an energizing and enjoyable experience. Paul Kelly, Executive Editor, kept our vision focused on "the view from 30,000 feet" and kept us on course with our overall goal. Kate Kelly, Developmental Editor, took my rambling and often convoluted explanations and helped to turn them into succinct and clarifying figure legends. Jennifer Surich, Managing Editor, provided great direction in laying out the plates and coming up with an organization scheme that made sense. Stephanie Klein, Manager of Production Editing, provided outstanding direction for the final layout of the *Atlas* and helped pull all of the unfinished components together. We particularly thank the Icon staff for their patience and guidance and their meticulous attention to both the details and the overall organization.

Special thanks also go to John Hansen, PhD, Consulting Editor for the *Atlas of Human Anatomy*, and author (with Bruce Koeppen, MD, PhD) of *Netter's Atlas of Human Physiology*. A long-standing friend and colleague, he provided valuable advice and suggestions throughout the project, and reinforced our adherence to the "view from 30,000 feet." I also would like to acknowledge my friend, colleague, and co-author on this *Atlas*, Ralph Józefowicz, MD. We co-directed the Medical Neurosciences course at the University of Rochester School of Medicine for 15 years, and taught each other everything we could to better educate our students. Their success is our greatest reward. We have had a wonderful collaboration for more than two decades, and I thank him for the great insights he provides, and the example he sets as a truly gifted, dedicated, and outstanding teacher and clinician.

And finally, to my wife, Mary, thank you for encouraging me to take on this challenging project, for your unwavering support, and for your patience with the long hours and the mountains of papers and folders you encountered along the way. Your love and support are deeply appreciated.

David L. Felten

CONTENTS

I. OVERVIEW OF THE NERVOUS SYSTEM

SECTION A. NEURONS AND THEIR PROPERTIES

A.1. STRUCTURE

A.2. NEUROTRANSMISSION

A.3. ELECTRICAL PROPERTIES

SECTION B. BRAIN

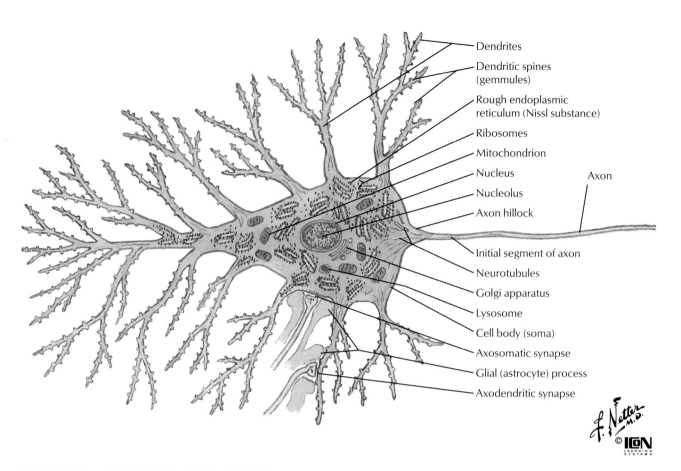

Dendrites
Dendritic spines (gemmules)
Rough endoplasmic reticulum (Nissl substance)
Ribosomes
Mitochondrion
Nucleus
Nucleolus
Axon hillock
Axon
Initial segment of axon
Neurotubules
Golgi apparatus
Lysosome
Cell body (soma)
Axosomatic synapse
Glial (astrocyte) process
Axodendritic synapse

FIGURE I.1: NEURONAL STRUCTURE

Neuronal structure reflects the functional characteristics of each neuron. Incoming information arrives at a neuron mainly through axonal terminations on the cell body and dendrites. These synapses are isolated and protected by astrocytic processes. The dendrites usually provide the greatest surface area of the neuron. Some protrusions from dendritic branches (dendritic spines) are sites of specific axodendritic synapses. Each neuronal type has a characteristic dendritic branching pattern (dendritic tree, or arborizations). The neuronal cell body varies from a few micrometers to more than 100 μm in diameter. The neuronal cytoplasm contains extensive rough endoplasmic reticulum (rough ER), which reflects the massive amount of protein synthesis necessary to maintain the neuron and its processes. The Golgi apparatus is involved in packaging potential signal molecules for transport and release. Large numbers of mitochondria are needed to meet the huge energy demands of neurons, particularly to maintain ion pumps and membrane potentials. Each neuron has a single (or occasionally no) axon. The cell body tapers to the axon at the axon hillock, and the initial segment of the axon containing the Na^+ channels is the first site where axon potentials are initiated. The axon extends for a variable (up to 1 m or more) distance from the cell body. Axons larger than 1 to 2 μm in diameter are insulated by myelin sheaths provided by oligodendroglia in the CNS or by Schwann cells in the PNS. An axon may branch into more than 500,000 axon terminals and may terminate in a highly localized and circumscribed zone (e.g., somatosensory projections for fine discriminative touch), or it may distribute to many disparate brain regions (e.g., noradrenergic axonal projections of the locus coeruleus). Axons of macroneurons (Golgi type I neurons) terminate at a distance from the cell body and dendritic tree. Axons of microneurons (Golgi type II neurons, local circuit neurons, or interneurons) terminate locally, close to the cell body and dendritic tree. Because each neuron type has its own specialization, there is no "typical" neuron, although pyramidal cells or lower motor neurons often are used to portray the "typical" neuron.

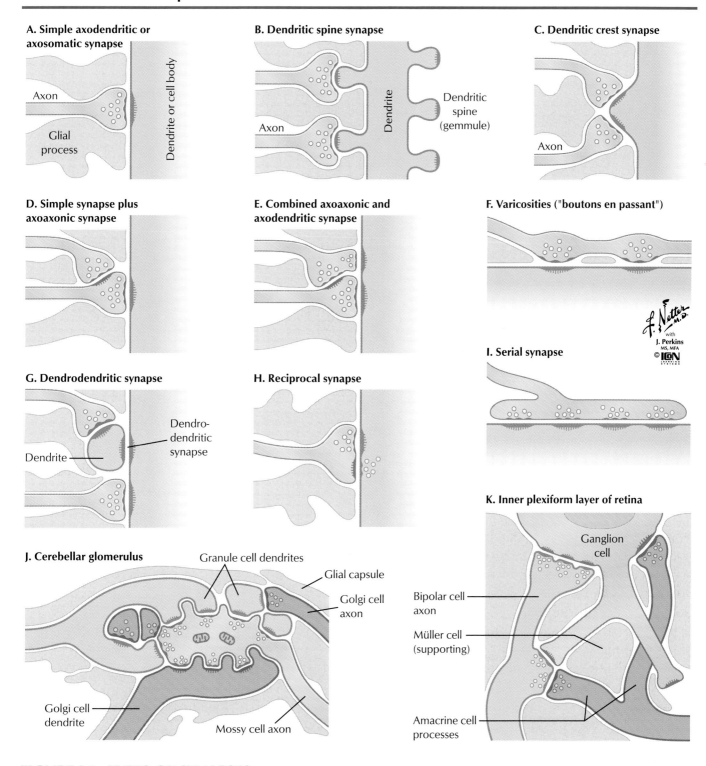

A. Simple axodendritic or axosomatic synapse

Axon

Glial process

Dendrite or cell body

B. Dendritic spine synapse

Axon

Dendrite

Dendritic spine (gemmule)

C. Dendritic crest synapse

Axon

D. Simple synapse plus axoaxonic synapse

E. Combined axoaxonic and axodendritic synapse

F. Varicosities ("boutons en passant")

I. Serial synapse

G. Dendrodendritic synapse

Dendrite

Dendrodendritic synapse

H. Reciprocal synapse

K. Inner plexiform layer of retina

Ganglion cell

Bipolar cell axon

Müller cell (supporting)

Amacrine cell processes

J. Cerebellar glomerulus

Granule cell dendrites

Glial capsule

Golgi cell axon

Golgi cell dendrite

Mossy cell axon

FIGURE I.2: TYPES OF SYNAPSES

A synapse is a site where an arriving action potential, through excitation-secretion coupling involving Ca^{2+} influx, triggers the release of one or more neurotransmitters into the synaptic cleft (typically 20 μm). The neurotransmitter acts on receptors on the target neuronal membrane, altering the membrane potential from its resting state. These post-synaptic potentials are called "graded" potentials. Most synapses carrying information toward a target neuron terminate as axodendritic or axosomatic synapses. Specialized synapses, such as reciprocal synapses, or complex arrays of synaptic interactions provide specific regulatory control over the excitability of their target neurons. Dendrodendritic synapses aid in the coordinated firing of groups of related neurons (such as phrenic nucleus neurons causing contraction of the diaphragm).

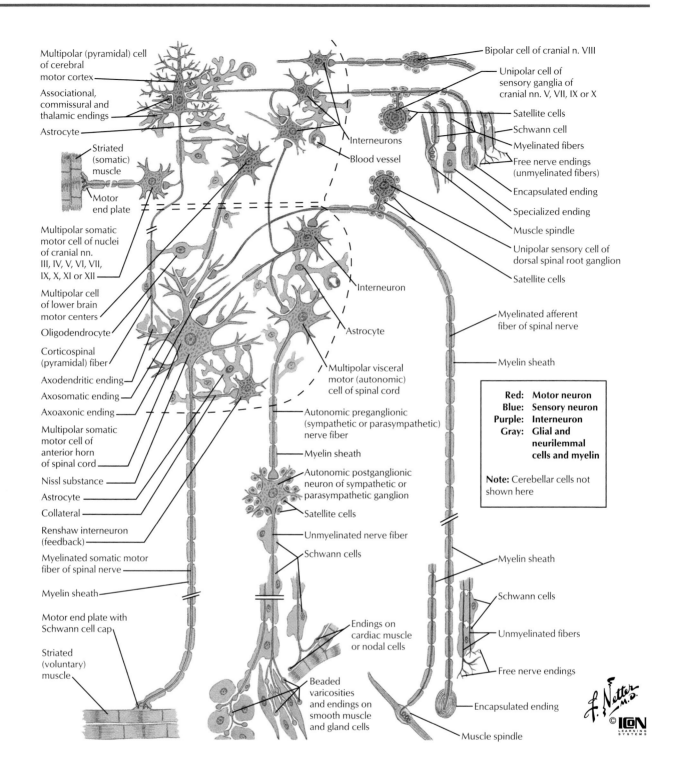

FIGURE I.3: NEURONAL CELL TYPES

Local interneurons and projection neurons demonstrate characteristic size, dendritic arborizations, and axonal projections. In the CNS, glial cells (astrocytes, microglia, oligodendroglia) provide support, protection, and maintenance of neurons. Schwann cells and satellite cells provide these functions in the PNS. The primary sensory neurons (blue) provide sensory transduction of incoming energy or stimuli into electrical signals that are conveyed into the CNS. The neuronal outflow from the CNS is motor (red) to skeletal muscle fibers via neuromuscular junctions, or autonomic preganglionic (red) to autonomic ganglia, whose neurons innervate cardiac muscle, smooth muscle, secretory glands, metabolic cells, or cells of the immune system.

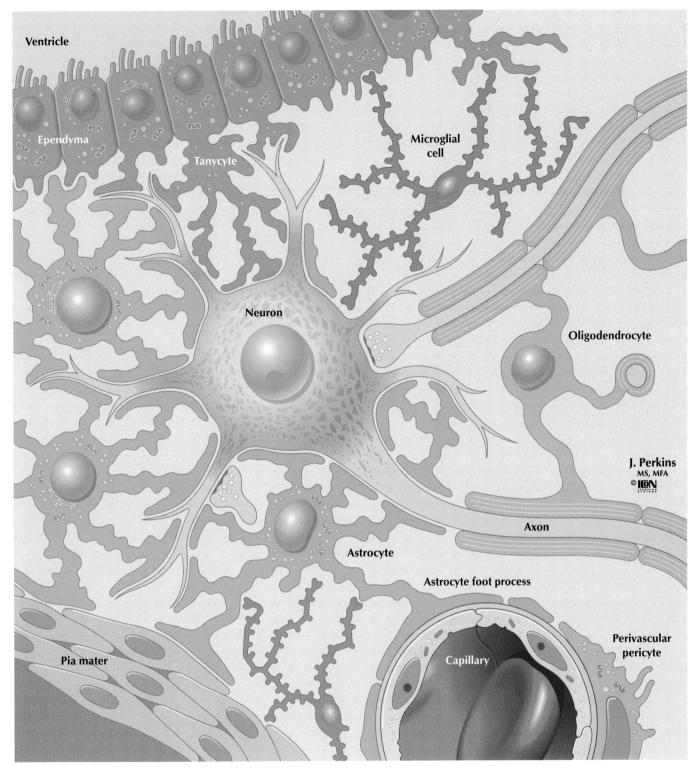

Ventricle

Ependyma

Tanycyte

Microglial cell

Neuron

Oligodendrocyte

J. Perkins
MS, MFA
©ION

Axon

Astrocyte

Astrocyte foot process

Pia mater

Capillary

Perivascular pericyte

FIGURE I.4: GLIAL CELL TYPES

Astrocytes provide structural isolation of neurons and their synapses, and they provide ionic (K$^+$) sequestration, trophic support, and support for growth and signaling functions to neurons. Oligodendroglia provide myelination of axons in the CNS. Microglia are scavenger cells that participate in phagocytosis, inflammatory responses, cytokine and growth factor secretion, and some immune reactivity in the CNS. Perivascular cells participate in similar activities at sites near the blood vessels. Schwann cells provide myelination, ensheathment, trophic support, and actions for growth and repair for peripheral neurons. Activated T lymphocytes can enter and traverse the CNS for immune surveillance for a period of approximately 24 hours.

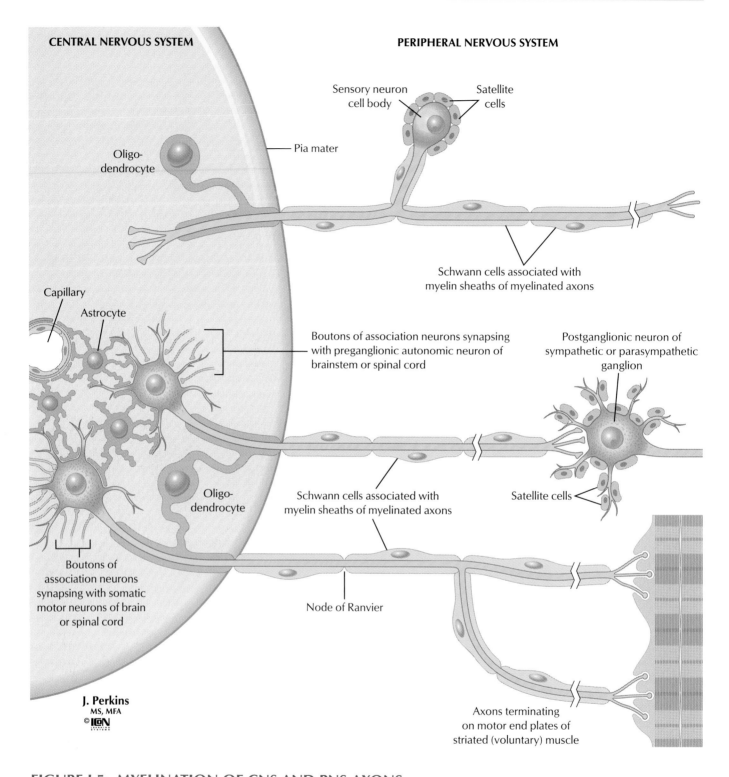

CENTRAL NERVOUS SYSTEM

PERIPHERAL NERVOUS SYSTEM

Oligo-
dendrocyte

Pia mater

Sensory neuron
cell body

Satellite
cells

Schwann cells associated with
myelin sheaths of myelinated axons

Capillary

Astrocyte

Boutons of association neurons synapsing
with preganglionic autonomic neuron of
brainstem or spinal cord

Postganglionic neuron of
sympathetic or parasympathetic
ganglion

Oligo-
dendrocyte

Schwann cells associated with
myelin sheaths of myelinated axons

Satellite cells

Boutons of
association neurons
synapsing with somatic
motor neurons of brain
or spinal cord

Node of Ranvier

J. Perkins
MS, MFA
©I©N

Axons terminating
on motor end plates of
striated (voluntary) muscle

FIGURE I.5: MYELINATION OF CNS AND PNS AXONS

Central myelination of axons is provided by oligo-dendroglia. Each oligodendroglial cell myelinates a single segment of several separate central axons. In the PNS, sensory, motor, and preganglionic autonomic axons are myelinated by Schwann cells. A Schwann cell myelinates only a single segment of one axon. Unmyelinated sensory and autonomic postganglionic axons are ensheathed by a Schwann cell, which provides a single enwrapping arm of cytoplasm around each of several such axons. The space between adjacent myelin segments (a node of Ranvier), the site where the axon membrane contains sodium channels, and allows the reinitiation of action potentials in the course of propagation, a process called saltatory conduction.

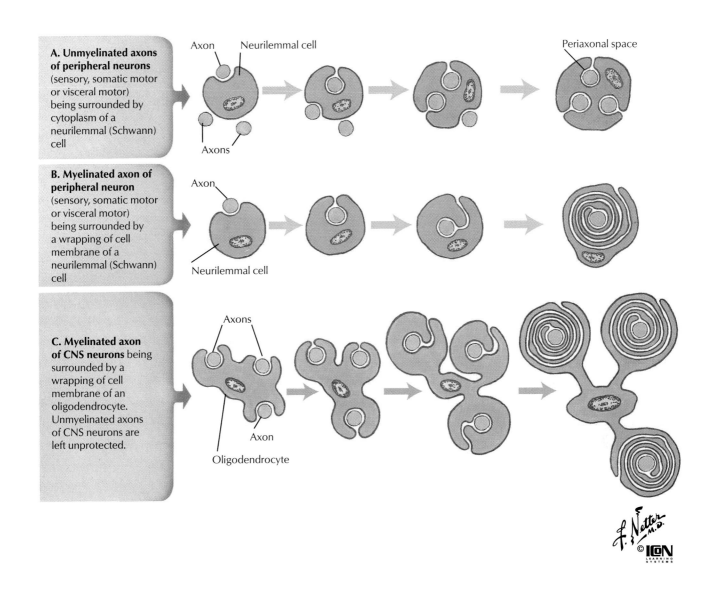

A. Unmyelinated axons of peripheral neurons (sensory, somatic motor or visceral motor) being surrounded by cytoplasm of a neurilemmal (Schwann) cell

Axon   Neurilemmal cell

Axons

Periaxonal space

B. Myelinated axon of peripheral neuron (sensory, somatic motor or visceral motor) being surrounded by a wrapping of cell membrane of a neurilemmal (Schwann) cell

Axon

Neurilemmal cell

C. Myelinated axon of CNS neurons being surrounded by a wrapping of cell membrane of an oligodendrocyte. Unmyelinated axons of CNS neurons are left unprotected.

Axons

Axon

Oligodendrocyte

FIGURE I.6: DEVELOPMENT OF MYELINATION AND AXON ENSHEATHMENT

Myelination is a cooperative interaction between the neuron and its myelinating support cell. Unmyelinated peripheral axons are invested with a single layer of Schwann cell cytoplasm. When a peripheral axon of at least 1 μm in diameter triggers myelination, a Schwann cell wraps many layers of tightly packed cell membrane around a single segment of that axon. The oligodendroglial cell extends several arms of cytoplasm, which then wrap multiple layers of tightly packed membrane around a single segment of each of several axons.

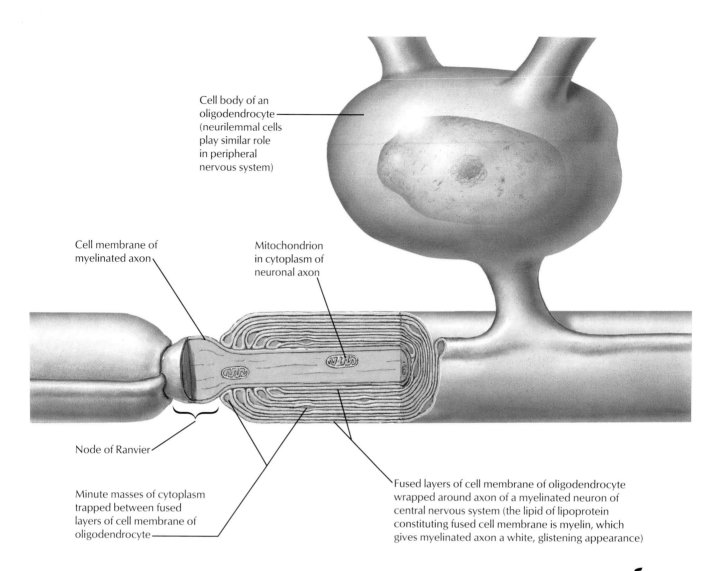

Cell body of an oligodendrocyte (neurilemmal cells play similar role in peripheral nervous system)

Cell membrane of myelinated axon

Mitochondrion in cytoplasm of neuronal axon

Node of Ranvier

Minute masses of cytoplasm trapped between fused layers of cell membrane of oligodendrocyte

Fused layers of cell membrane of oligodendrocyte wrapped around axon of a myelinated neuron of central nervous system (the lipid of lipoprotein constituting fused cell membrane is myelin, which gives myelinated axon a white, glistening appearance)

FIGURE I.7: HIGH MAGNIFICATION VIEW OF A CENTRAL MYELIN SHEATH

Fused layers of oligodendroglial cell membrane wrap around a segment of a central axon, preventing ionic flow across the cell membrane for the entire myelinated segment. The node between 2 adjacent segments is bare axon membrane, which contains Na$^+$ channels. These nodes are sites where action potentials are reinitiated in the conduction of propagated action potentials. Illustration after Bunge, Bunge, and Riis.

Schematic of synaptic endings

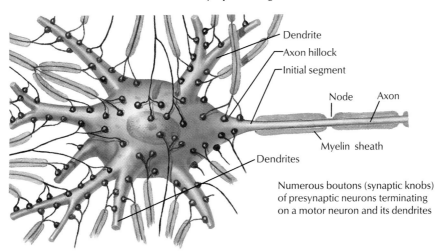

Dendrite
Axon hillock
Initial segment
Node   Axon
Myelin sheath
Dendrites

Numerous boutons (synaptic knobs)
of presynaptic neurons terminating
on a motor neuron and its dendrites

Enlarged section of bouton

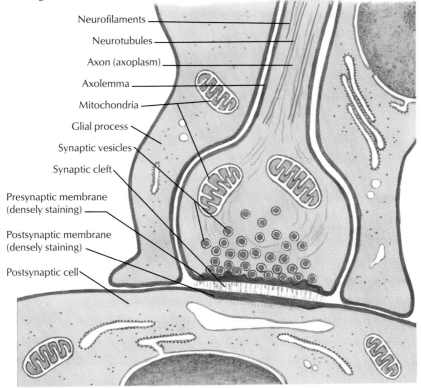

Neurofilaments
Neurotubules
Axon (axoplasm)
Axolemma
Mitochondria
Glial process
Synaptic vesicles
Synaptic cleft
Presynaptic membrane
(densely staining)
Postsynaptic membrane
(densely staining)
Postsynaptic cell

FIGURE I.8: SYNAPTIC MORPHOLOGY

Synapses are sites where neurons communicate with each other and with effector or target cells. The upper figure shows a typical neuron that receives many synaptic contacts on its cell body and associated dendrites. Incoming axons lose their myelin sheaths, exhibit extensive branching, and terminate as synaptic boutons (terminals) on the target (in this example, motor) neuron. The lower figure shows an enlarged axosomatic terminal. Chemical neurotransmitters are packaged in synaptic vesicles. When an action potential invades the terminal region, depolarization triggers

Ca^{2+} influx, and many synaptic vesicles fuse with the presynaptic membrane, releasing packets of neurotransmitter into the synaptic cleft. The neurotransmitter binds to receptors on the postsynaptic membrane, which results in graded excitatory or inhibitory postsynaptic potentials, or in neuromodulatory effects on intracellular signaling systems, in the target cell. Some nerve terminals possess presynaptic receptors for their released neurotransmitter. Activation of these receptors regulates neurotransmitter release.

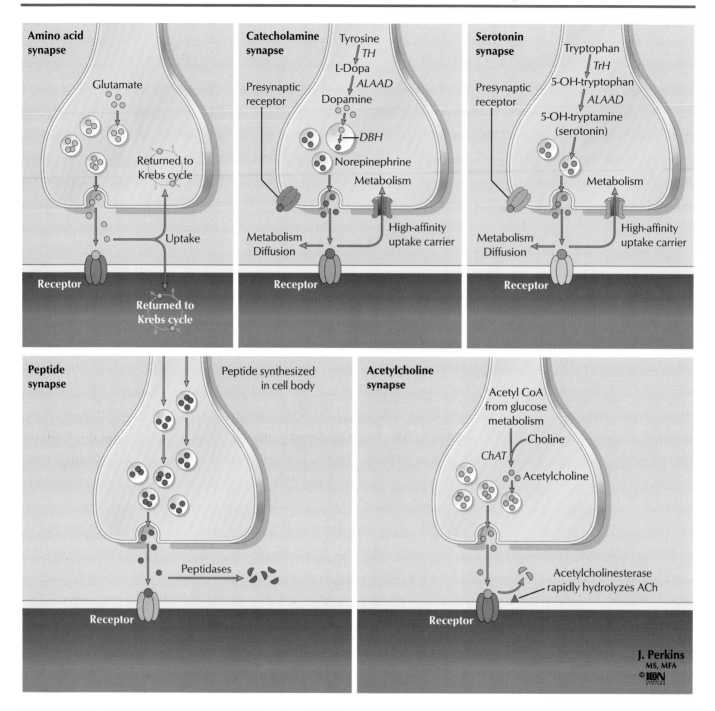

FIGURE I.9: CHEMICAL NEUROTRANSMISSION: AMINO ACID SYNAPSES

Amino acids are compartmentalized in synaptic vesicles for release as neurotransmitters. The amino acid glutamate (depicted in the diagram) is the most abundant excitatory neurotransmitter in the CNS. Following release from the synaptic vesicle, some glutamate binds to postsynaptic receptors. Released glutamate is inactivated by uptake into both the pre- and the postsynaptic neurons, where the amino acid is incorporated into the Krebs cycle or reutilized for a variety of functions.

CATECHOLAMINE SYNAPSES

Catecholamines (CAs) are synthesized from the dietary amino acid tyrosine, taken up competitively into the brain by a carrier system. Tyrosine is synthesized to L-dopa by tyrosine hydroxylase (TH), a rate-limiting synthetic enzyme. Additional conversion to dopamine (DA) occurs in the cytoplasm via aromatic L-amino acid decarboxylase (ALAAD). DA is stored in synaptic vesicles for subsequent release. In noradrenergic nerve terminals, dopamine beta hydroxylase (DBH) further hydroxylates DA to norepinephrine in the synaptic vesicles. In adrenergic nerve terminals, norepinephrine is methylated to epinephrine by phenylethanolamine N-methyl transferase (PNMT). Following release, the CA neurotransmitter binds to appropriate receptors (DA, alpha and beta adrenergic receptors) on the postsynaptic membrane, altering postsynaptic excitability and/or second messengers. CAs also can activate presynaptic receptors, modulating the excitability of the presynaptic terminal. CAs are inactivated mainly by presynaptic reuptake (high affinity uptake carrier) and by metabolism (MAO deamination and COMT methylation) and diffusion.

SEROTONIN SYNAPSES

Serotonin is synthesized from the dietary amino acid tryptophan, taken up competitively into the brain by a carrier system. Tryptophan is synthesized to 5-hydroxytryptophan by tryptophan hydroxylase (TrH), a rate-limiting synthetic enzyme. Conversion of 5-hydroxytryptophan to 5-hydroxytryptamine (5-HT, serotonin) by the decarboxylase ALAAD occurs in the cytoplasm. Serotonin is stored in synaptic vesicles. Following release, it can bind to receptors on the postsynaptic membrane, altering postsynaptic excitability and/or second messenger activation. Serotonin can act on presynaptic receptors (5-HT receptors), modulating excitability of the presynaptic terminal. Serotonin is inactivated mainly by presynaptic reuptake (high affinity uptake carrier) and also by metabolism and diffusion.

PEPTIDERGIC SYNAPSES

Neuropeptides are synthesized from prohormones, large peptides synthesized in the cell body from an mRNA template. The larger precursor peptide is cleaved posttranslationally to active neuropeptides, which are packaged in synaptic vesicles and transported anterogradely by the process of axoplasmic transport. These vesicles are stored in the nerve terminals until released by appropriate excitation-secretion coupling induced by an action potential. The neuropeptide binds to receptors on the postsynaptic membrane. In the CNS, there is often an anatomical mismatch between the localization of peptidergic nerve terminals and the localization of cells possessing membrane receptors responsive to that neuropeptide, suggesting that the amount of release and the extent of diffusion are important factors in neuropeptide neurotransmission. Released neuropeptides are inactivated by peptidases.

CHOLINERGIC SYNAPSES

Acetylcholine (ACh) is synthesized from dietary choline and acetyl CoA, derived from the metabolism of glucose, via the enzyme choline acetyltransferase (ChAT). ACh is stored in synaptic vesicles; following release, it binds to cholinergic receptors (nicotinic or muscarinic) on the postsynaptic membrane, influencing the excitability of the postsynaptic cell. Enzymatic hydrolysis (cleavage) by acetylcholine esterase (AChE) rapidly inactivates ACh.

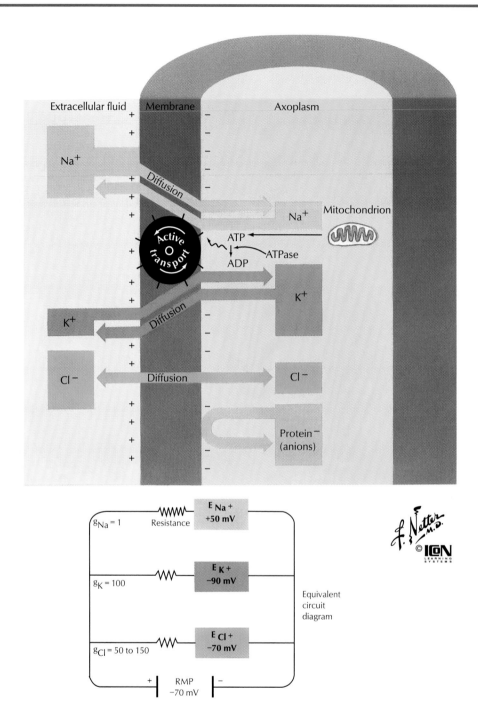

FIGURE I.10: NEURONAL RESTING POTENTIAL

Cations (+) and anions (−) are distributed unevenly across the neuronal cell membrane because the membrane is differentially permeable to these ions. The membrane's permeability to ions changes with depolarization (toward 0) or hyperpolarization (away from 0). Ion distribution depends on the forces of charge separation and diffusion. The typical neuronal resting potential is approximately −90 mV with respect to the nextracellular fluid. The extracellular concentrations of Na^+ and Cl^- of 145 and 105 mEq/L are high compared to the intracellular concentrations of 15 and 8 mEq/L. The extracellular concentration of K^+ of 3.5 mEq/L is low compared to the intracellular concentration of 130 mEq/L. The resting potential of neurons is close to the equilibrium potential for K^+ (as if the membrane were permeable only to K^+). Na^+ is actively pumped out of the cell, in exchange for inward pumping of K^+, by the Na^+-K^+-ATPase membrane pump. Equivalent circuit diagrams for K^+ and for Cl^-, calculated using the Nernst equation, are illustrated above.

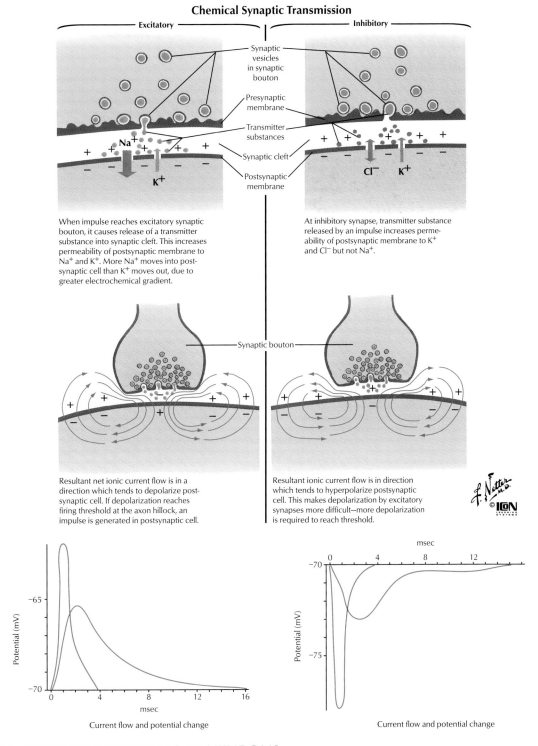

Chemical Synaptic Transmission

Excitatory | Inhibitory

Synaptic vesicles in synaptic bouton

Presynaptic membrane

Transmitter substances

Synaptic cleft

Postsynaptic membrane

When impulse reaches excitatory synaptic bouton, it causes release of a transmitter substance into synaptic cleft. This increases permeability of postsynaptic membrane to Na+ and K+. More Na+ moves into post-synaptic cell than K+ moves out, due to greater electrochemical gradient.

At inhibitory synapse, transmitter substance released by an impulse increases perme-ability of postsynaptic membrane to K+ and Cl– but not Na+.

Synaptic bouton

Resultant net ionic current flow is in a direction which tends to depolarize post-synaptic cell. If depolarization reaches firing threshold at the axon hillock, an impulse is generated in postsynaptic cell.

Resultant ionic current flow is in direction which tends to hyperpolarize postsynaptic cell. This makes depolarization by excitatory synapses more difficult—more depolarization is required to reach threshold.

Current flow and potential change

Current flow and potential change

FIGURE I.11: GRADED POTENTIALS IN NEURONS

Excitatory and inhibitory neurotransmission are processes by which released neurotransmitter, acting on postsynaptic membrane receptors, elicits a local or regional perturbation in the membrane potential: (1) toward 0 (depolarization, excitatory postsynaptic potential [EPSP]) via an inward flow of Na^+ caused by increased permeability of the membrane to positive ions or (2) away from 0 (hyperpolarization, inhibitory postsynaptic potential

[IPSP]) via an inward flow of Cl^- and a compensatory outward flow of K^+ caused by increased membrane permeability to Cl^-. The resultant EPSPs and IPSPs exert local influences that dissipate over time and distance but contribute to the overall excitability and ion distribution in the neuron. If sufficient excitatory influences bring about depolarization of the initial segment of the axon above threshold, an action potential is fired.

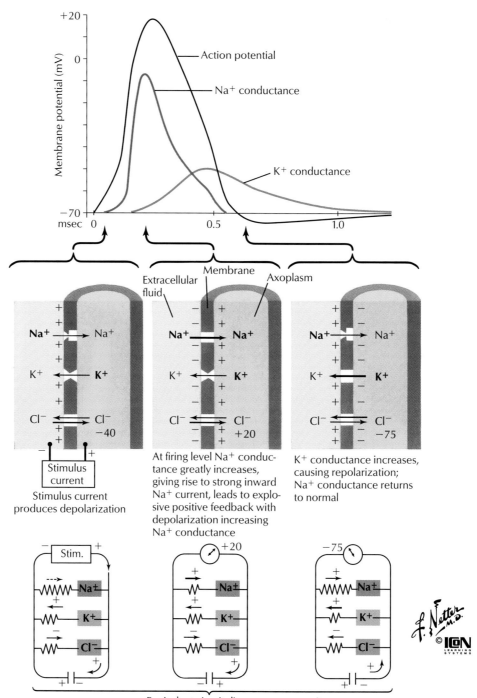

FIGURE I.12: ACTION POTENTIALS

Action potentials (APs) are all-or-none, nondecremental, electrical potentials that allow an electrical signal to travel long distances (a meter or more) and trigger neurotransmitter release through electrochemical coupling (excitation-secretion coupling). APs are usually initiated at the initial segment of axons when temporal and spatial summation of EPSPs cause sufficient excitation (depolarization) to open Na^+ channels, allowing the

membrane to reach threshold. Threshold is the point at which Na^+ influx through these Na^+ channels cannot be countered by efflux of K^+. When threshold is reached, an AP is fired. As the axon rapidly depolarizes during the rising phase of the AP, the axonal membrane increases its K^+ conductance, which then allows influx of K^+ to counter the rapid depolarization and bring the membrane potential back toward its resting level.

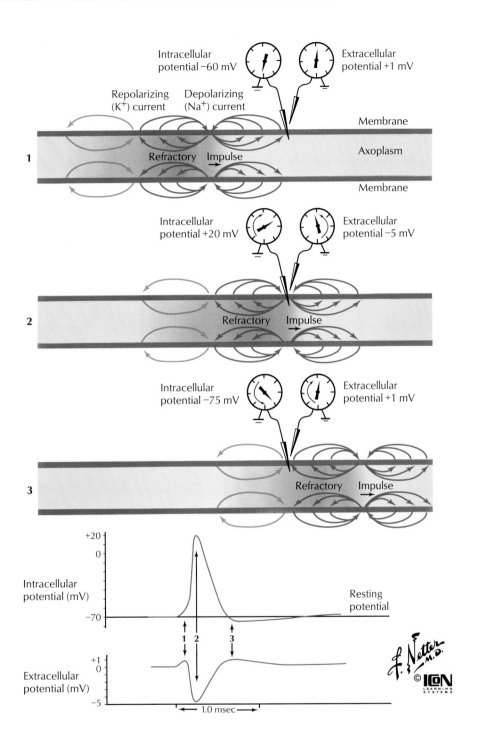

FIGURE I.13: PROPAGATION OF THE ACTION POTENTIAL

When an AP is initiated at a specific site on the axonal membrane (usually the initial segment), the inward flow of Na$^+$ alters the extracellular ion environment, causing a local flow of charge from adjacent regions of the axon. This induces a depolarized state in the adjacent node of Ranvier or patch of axonal membrane, bringing that region to threshold and resulting in the reinitiation of the AP. The presence of myelination along axonal segments results in the reinitiation of the AP at the next node, thus hastening the velocity of conduction of the AP. The resultant appearance of the AP skipping from node to node down the axon is called saltatory conduction.

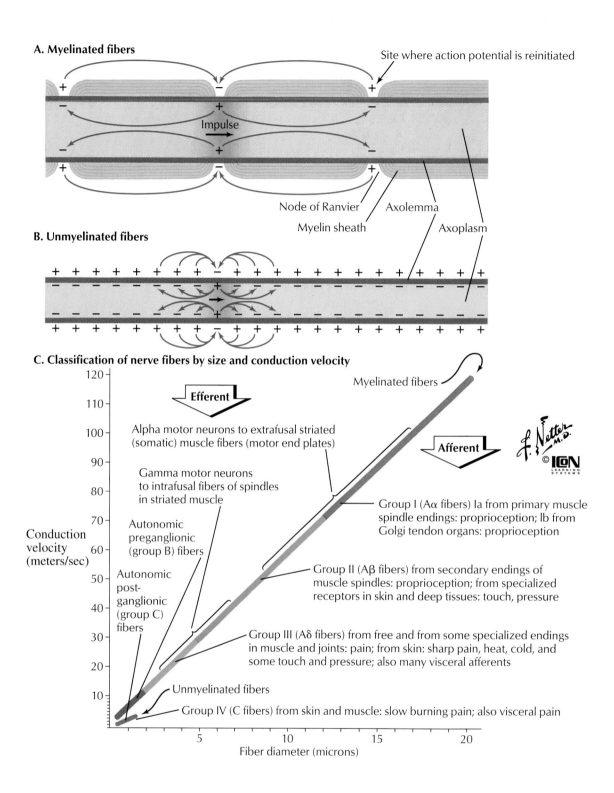

A. Myelinated fibers

Site where action potential is reinitiated

Impulse

Node of Ranvier   Axolemma

Myelin sheath   Axoplasm

B. Unmyelinated fibers

C. Classification of nerve fibers by size and conduction velocity

Myelinated fibers

Efferent

Alpha motor neurons to extrafusal striated (somatic) muscle fibers (motor end plates)

Afferent

Gamma motor neurons to intrafusal fibers of spindles in striated muscle

Group I (Aα fibers) Ia from primary muscle spindle endings: proprioception; Ib from Golgi tendon organs: proprioception

Autonomic preganglionic (group B) fibers

Autonomic post-ganglionic (group C) fibers

Group II (Aβ fibers) from secondary endings of muscle spindles: proprioception; from specialized receptors in skin and deep tissues: touch, pressure

Group III (Aδ fibers) from free and from some specialized endings in muscle and joints: pain; from skin: sharp pain, heat, cold, and some touch and pressure; also many visceral afferents

Unmyelinated fibers

Group IV (C fibers) from skin and muscle: slow burning pain; also visceral pain

Conduction velocity (meters/sec)

Fiber diameter (microns)

FIGURE I.14: CONDUCTION VELOCITY

The AP travels down the axon by depolarizing adjacent patches of membrane (panel B), leading to the AP's reinitiation. The speed of propagation increases with larger axonal diameter and in the presence of a myelin sheath (panel C). In myelinated axons, the AP is propagated from node to node, a process called saltatory conduction (panel A).

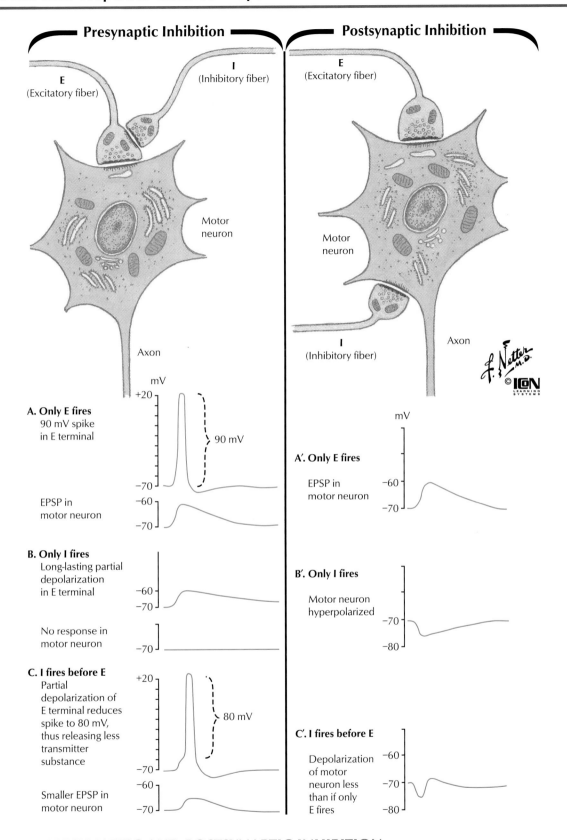

FIGURE I.15: PRESYNAPTIC AND POSTSYNAPTIC INHIBITION

Inhibitory synapses modulate neuronal excitability. Presynaptic inhibition (left) and postsynaptic inhibition (right) are shown in relation to a motor neuron. Postsynaptic inhibition causes local hyperpolarization at the postsynaptic site. Presynaptic inhibition involves the depolarization of an excitatory axon terminal, which decreases the amount of Ca^{++} influx that occurs with depolarization of that excitatory terminal, thus reducing the resultant EPSP.

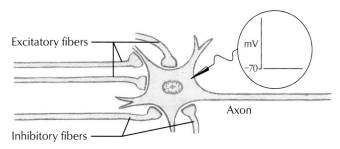

A. Resting state: motor nerve cell shown with synaptic boutons of excitatory and inhibitory nerve fibers ending close to it

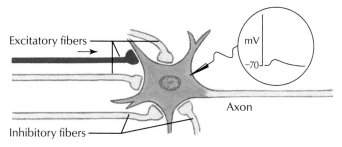

B. Partial depolarization: impulse from one excitatory fiber has caused partial (below firing threshold) depolarization of motor neuron

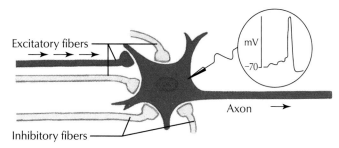

C. Temporal excitatory summation: a series of impulses in one excitatory fiber together produce a suprathreshold depolarization that triggers an action potential

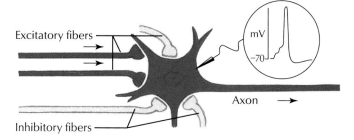

D. Spatial excitatory summation: impulses in two excitatory fibers cause two synaptic depolarizations that together reach firing threshold triggering an action potential

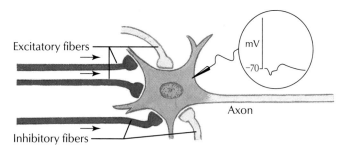

E. Spatial excitatory summation with inhibition: impulses from two excitatory fibers reach motor neuron but impulses from inhibitory fiber prevent depolarization from reaching threshold

■ Axon(s) activated in each scenario

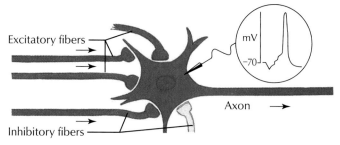

E. (continued): motor neuron now receives additional excitatory impulses and reaches firing threshold despite a simultaneous inhibitory impulse; additional inhibitory impulses might still prevent firing

FIGURE I.16: SPATIAL AND TEMPORAL SUMMATION

Neurons receive multiple excitatory and inhibitory inputs. Temporal summation occurs when a series of subthreshold EPSPs in one excitatory fiber produces an AP in the postsynaptic cell (panel C). This occurs because the EPSPs are superimposed on each other temporally before the local region of membrane has completely returned to its resting state. Spatial summation occurs when subthreshold EPSPs from 2 or more synapses trigger an AP because of synergistic interactions (panel D). Both temporal and spatial summation can be modulated by simultaneous inhibitory input (panel E). Inhibitory and excitatory neurons use a wide variety of neurotransmitters, whose actions depend on the ion channels opened by the ligand-receptor interaction.

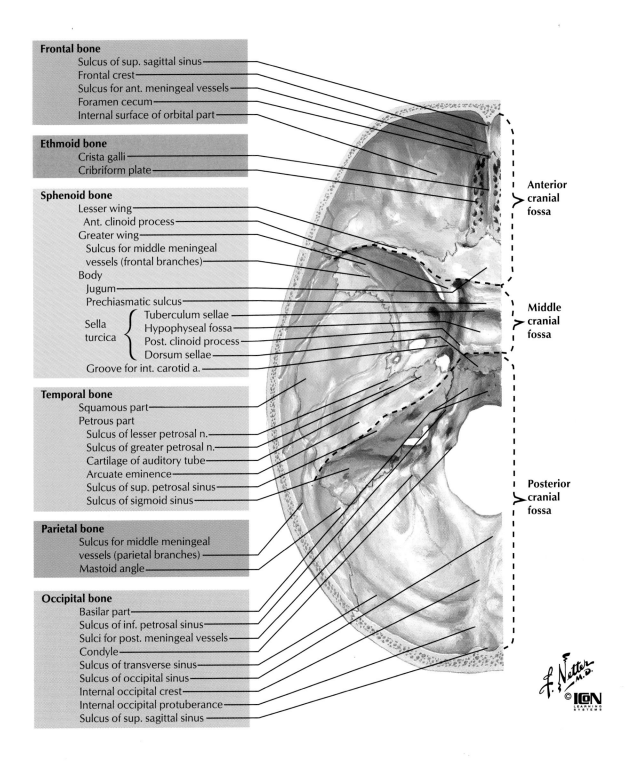

Frontal bone
Sulcus of sup. sagittal sinus
Frontal crest
Sulcus for ant. meningeal vessels
Foramen cecum
Internal surface of orbital part

Ethmoid bone
Crista galli
Cribriform plate

Sphenoid bone
Lesser wing
Ant. clinoid process
Greater wing
Sulcus for middle meningeal
vessels (frontal branches)
Body
Jugum
Prechiasmatic sulcus
Sella   Tuberculum sellae
turcica   Hypophyseal fossa
           Post. clinoid process
           Dorsum sellae
Groove for int. carotid a.

Temporal bone
Squamous part
Petrous part
Sulcus of lesser petrosal n.
Sulcus of greater petrosal n.
Cartilage of auditory tube
Arcuate eminence
Sulcus of sup. petrosal sinus
Sulcus of sigmoid sinus

Parietal bone
Sulcus for middle meningeal
vessels (parietal branches)
Mastoid angle

Occipital bone
Basilar part
Sulcus of inf. petrosal sinus
Sulci for post. meningeal vessels
Condyle
Sulcus of transverse sinus
Sulcus of occipital sinus
Internal occipital crest
Internal occipital protuberance
Sulcus of sup. sagittal sinus

Anterior
cranial
fossa

Middle
cranial
fossa

Posterior
cranial
fossa

FIGURE I.17: INTERIOR VIEW OF THE BASE OF THE ADULT SKULL

The anterior, middle, and posterior cranial fossae house the anterior frontal lobe, the temporal lobe, and the cerebellum and brain stem, respectively. The fossae are separated from each other by bony structures and dural membranes. Swelling or mass lesions can selectively exert pressure within the individual fossae. The perforated cribriform plate allows the olfactory nerves to penetrate into the olfactory bulb, a site where head trauma can result in the tearing of the penetrating olfactory nerve fibers.

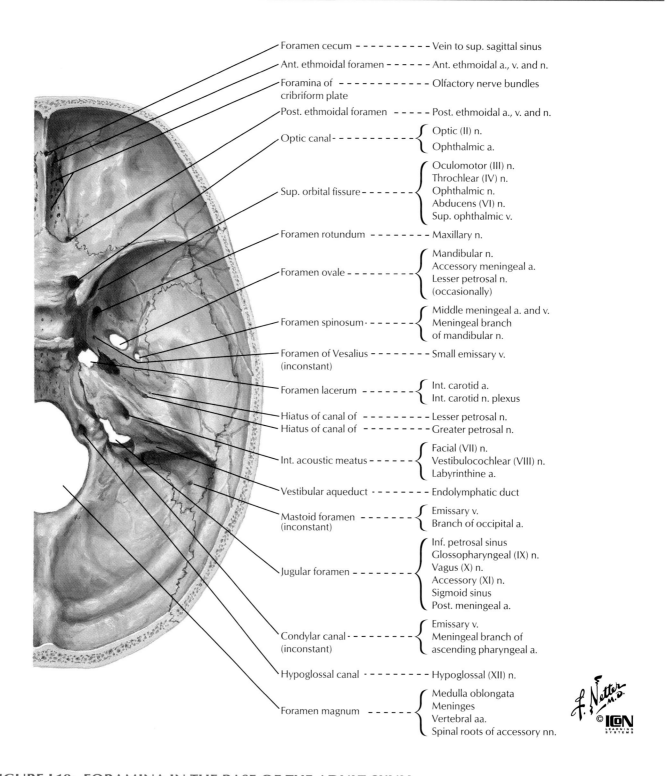

Foramen cecum - - - - - - - - Vein to sup. sagittal sinus

Ant. ethmoidal foramen - - - - - Ant. ethmoidal a., v. and n.

Foramina of - - - - - - - - - - Olfactory nerve bundles
cribriform plate

Post. ethmoidal foramen - - - - Post. ethmoidal a., v. and n.

Optic canal - - - - - - - - - {
Optic (II) n.
Ophthalmic a.

Sup. orbital fissure - - - - - - {
Oculomotor (III) n.
Throchlear (IV) n.
Ophthalmic n.
Abducens (VI) n.
Sup. ophthalmic v.

Foramen rotundum - - - - - - - Maxillary n.

Foramen ovale - - - - - - - - {
Mandibular n.
Accessory meningeal a.
Lesser petrosal n.
(occasionally)

Foramen spinosum - - - - - - {
Middle meningeal a. and v.
Meningeal branch
of mandibular n.

Foramen of Vesalius - - - - - - - Small emissary v.
(inconstant)

Foramen lacerum - - - - - - - {
Int. carotid a.
Int. carotid n. plexus

Hiatus of canal of - - - - - - - - Lesser petrosal n.
Hiatus of canal of - - - - - - - - Greater petrosal n.

Int. acoustic meatus - - - - - {
Facial (VII) n.
Vestibulocochlear (VIII) n.
Labyrinthine a.

Vestibular aqueduct - - - - - - - Endolymphatic duct

Mastoid foramen - - - - - - - {
Emissary v.
Branch of occipital a.
(inconstant)

Jugular foramen - - - - - - - {
Inf. petrosal sinus
Glossopharyngeal (IX) n.
Vagus (X) n.
Accessory (XI) n.
Sigmoid sinus
Post. meningeal a.

Condylar canal - - - - - - - {
Emissary v.
Meningeal branch of
ascending pharyngeal a.
(inconstant)

Hypoglossal canal - - - - - - - Hypoglossal (XII) n.

Foramen magnum - - - - - - {
Medulla oblongata
Meninges
Vertebral aa.
Spinal roots of accessory nn.

FIGURE I.18: FORAMINA IN THE BASE OF THE ADULT SKULL

This illustration of the foramina in the base of the skull lists the major nerves and blood vessels that course through each opening. Pressure, traction, or masses can damage structures traversing in these tightly confined spaces.

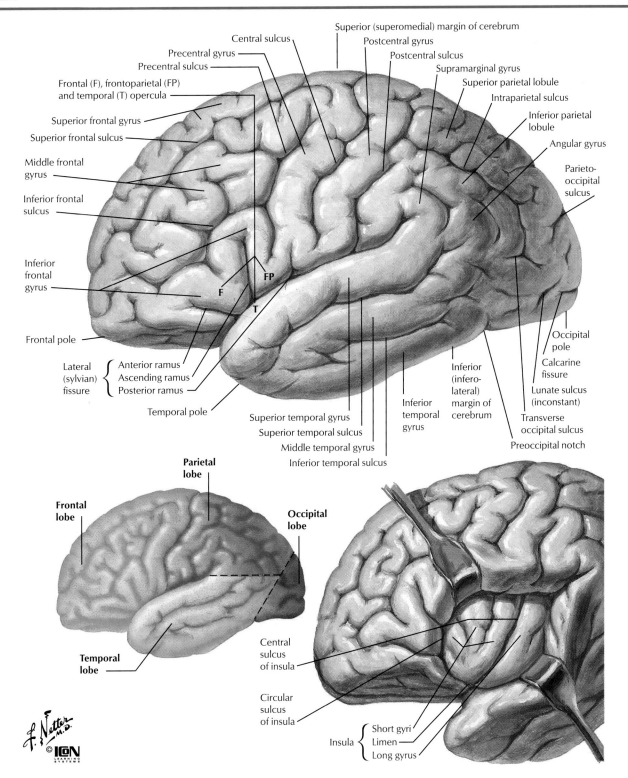

FIGURE I.19: SURFACE ANATOMY OF THE FOREBRAIN: LATERAL VIEW

The convolutions of the cerebral cortex allow a large expanse of cortex to be compactly folded into a small volume, an adaptation particularly prominent in primates. Major dependable landmarks (lateral fissure, central sulcus, parieto-occipital fissure) separate the forebrain into lobes. The lateral (sylvian) fissure separates the temporal lobe below from the parietal and frontal lobes above, and the central sulcus separates the parietal and the frontal lobes. Several of the named gyri are associated with specific functional activities, such as the precentral gyrus (motor cortex) and the postcentral gyrus (primary sensory cortex). The insula, the fifth lobe of the cerebral cortex, is deep to the outer cortex and can be seen by opening the lateral fissure.

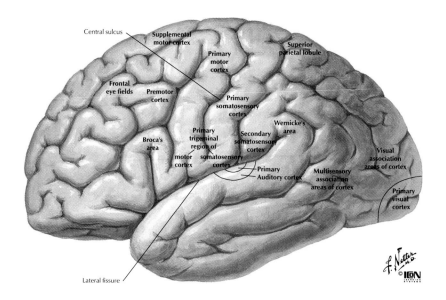

FIGURE I.20: LATERAL VIEW OF THE FOREBRAIN: FUNCTIONAL REGIONS

Some circumscribed regions of the cerebral hemi-sphere are associated with specific functional activities, including the motor cortex and the supplemental and premotor cortices, the frontal eye fields, and the primary and association sensory cortices. Part of the auditory cortex is visible at the inferior edge of the lateral fissure (the transverse temporal gyrus of Heschl). The visual cortex is seen at the occipital pole. Language areas of the left hemisphere include Broca's area (expressive language) and Wernicke's area (receptive language). Damage to these cortical regions results in loss of specific functional capabilities. There is some overlap but not absolute concordance between functional areas and the named gyri (e.g., motor cortex and precentral gyrus).

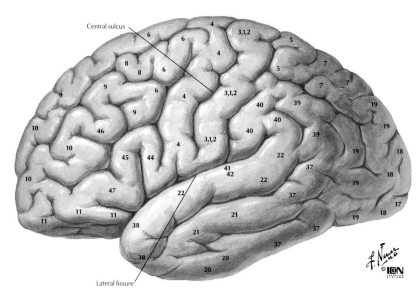

FIGURE I.21: LATERAL VIEW OF THE FOREBRAIN: BRODMANN AREAS

Brodmann areas of the cerebral cortex reflect unique architectural characteristics of the thickness and layering of the cerebral cortex from histological observations originally made by Korbinian Brodmann in 1909. This numbering of cortical areas is still used as a shorthand for describing func-tional areas or regions of the cortex, particularly those related to sensory functions. Some overlap exists between functional areas. For example, the motor cortex is area 4, the primary sensory cortex includes areas 3, 1, and 2, and the primary visual cortex is area 17.

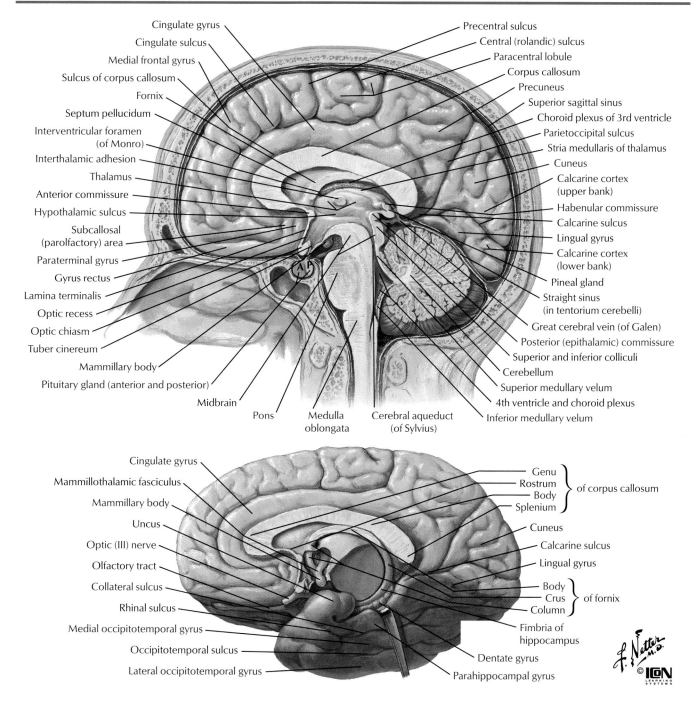

Cingulate gyrus
Cingulate sulcus
Medial frontal gyrus
Sulcus of corpus callosum
Fornix
Septum pellucidum
Interventricular foramen (of Monro)
Interthalamic adhesion
Thalamus
Anterior commissure
Hypothalamic sulcus
Subcallosal (parolfactory) area
Paraterminal gyrus
Gyrus rectus
Lamina terminalis
Optic recess
Optic chiasm
Tuber cinereum
Mammillary body
Pituitary gland (anterior and posterior)
Midbrain
Pons
Medulla oblongata
Cerebral aqueduct (of Sylvius)

Precentral sulcus
Central (rolandic) sulcus
Paracentral lobule
Corpus callosum
Precuneus
Superior sagittal sinus
Choroid plexus of 3rd ventricle
Parietoccipital sulcus
Stria medullaris of thalamus
Cuneus
Calcarine cortex (upper bank)
Habenular commissure
Calcarine sulcus
Lingual gyrus
Calcarine cortex (lower bank)
Pineal gland
Straight sinus (in tentorium cerebelli)
Great cerebral vein (of Galen)
Posterior (epithalamic) commissure
Superior and inferior colliculi
Cerebellum
Superior medullary velum
4th ventricle and choroid plexus
Inferior medullary velum

Cingulate gyrus
Mammillothalamic fasciculus
Mammillary body
Uncus
Optic (III) nerve
Olfactory tract
Collateral sulcus
Rhinal sulcus
Medial occipitotemporal gyrus
Occipitotemporal sulcus
Lateral occipitotemporal gyrus

Genu
Rostrum
Body
Splenium
} of corpus callosum
Cuneus
Calcarine sulcus
Lingual gyrus
Body
Crus
Column
} of fornix
Fimbria of hippocampus
Dentate gyrus
Parahippocampal gyrus

FIGURE I.22: ANATOMY OF THE MEDIAL (MIDSAGITTAL) SURFACE OF THE BRAIN

The entire neuraxis from the spinomedullary junction through the brain stem, diencephalon, and telencephalon is visible. The corpus callosum, a major commissural fiber bundle interconnecting the 2 hemispheres, is a landmark separating the cerebral cortex above from the thalamus, fornix, and subcortical forebrain below. The ventricular system—including the interventricular foramen, the third ventricle (diencephalon), the cerebral aqueduct (midbrain), and the fourth ventricle (pons and medulla)—provides internal and external (subarachnoid [SA] space) fluid protection to the brain.

The thalamus serves as a gateway to the cortex. The proximity of the hypothalamus to the median eminence (tuber cinereum) and the pituitary gland reflects the important role of the hypothalamus in regulating neuroendocrine function. The C-shaped course of the fornix, from the hippocampal formation in the temporal lobe to the septum and the hypothalamus, is shown below. The midsagittal cut through the brain stem reveals the midbrain colliculi, sometimes called the visual (superior) and auditory (inferior) tecta.

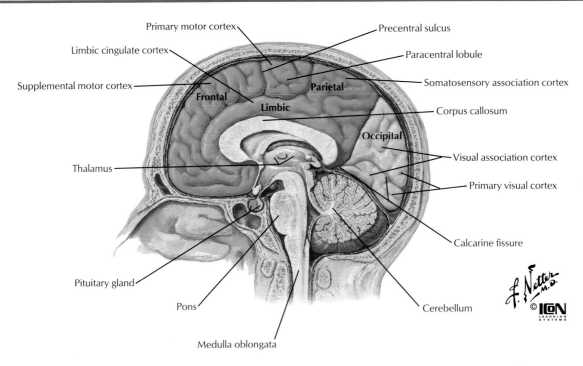

FIGURE I.23: MEDIAL SURFACE OF THE BRAIN: LOBES AND FUNCTIONAL AREAS

The cingulate cortex is labeled the limbic lobe, reflecting its association with other limbic forebrain structures and hypothalamic control of the autonomic nervous system. Functional areas of the cortex, particularly those involved with vision, are best seen on a midsagittal view. The sensory and motor cortices associated with the lower extremities are located medially and are supplied by the anterior cerebral artery. This region is selectively vulnerable to vascular or mass lesions, resulting in contralateral motor and sensory deficits of the lower extremity.

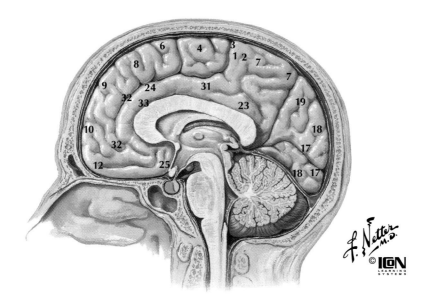

FIGURE I.24: MEDIAL SURFACE OF THE BRAIN: BRODMANN AREAS

The Brodmann areas of the cerebral cortex are labeled on this midsagittal view. The major regions are the primary (17) and associative (18, 19) visual cortices and the continuation of area 4 (motor) and areas 3, 1, and 2 (primary sensory) onto the paracentral lobule in the midline.

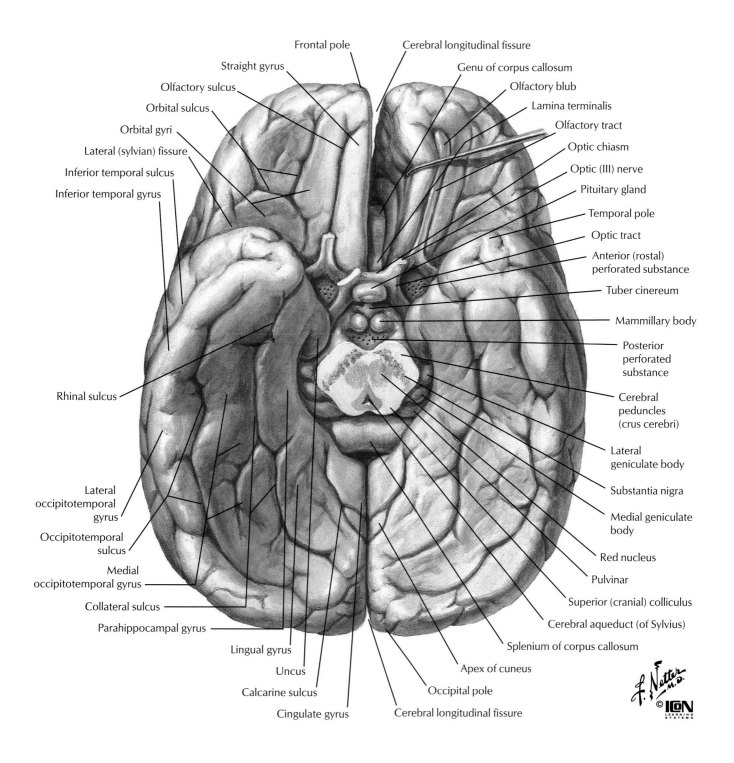

Frontal pole
Straight gyrus
Olfactory sulcus
Orbital sulcus
Orbital gyri
Lateral (sylvian) fissure
Inferior temporal sulcus
Inferior temporal gyrus

Cerebral longitudinal fissure
Genu of corpus callosum
Olfactory blub
Lamina terminalis
Olfactory tract
Optic chiasm
Optic (III) nerve
Pituitary gland
Temporal pole
Optic tract
Anterior (rostal) perforated substance
Tuber cinereum
Mammillary body
Posterior perforated substance
Cerebral peduncles (crus cerebri)
Lateral geniculate body
Substantia nigra
Medial geniculate body
Red nucleus
Pulvinar
Superior (cranial) colliculus
Cerebral aqueduct (of Sylvius)
Splenium of corpus callosum
Apex of cuneus
Occipital pole
Cerebral longitudinal fissure

Rhinal sulcus
Lateral occipitotemporal gyrus
Occipitotemporal sulcus
Medial occipitotemporal gyrus
Collateral sulcus
Parahippocampal gyrus
Lingual gyrus
Uncus
Calcarine sulcus
Cingulate gyrus

FIGURE I.25: ANATOMY OF THE BASAL SURFACE OF THE BRAIN: WITH THE BRAIN STEM AND CEREBELLUM REMOVED

Removal of the brain stem and cerebellum with a cut through the midbrain exposes the underlying cerebral cortex, the base of the diencephalon, and the basal forebrain. Basal hypothalamic landmarks, from caudal to rostral, include the mammillary bodies, the tuber cinereum, the pituitary gland, and the optic chiasm. The proximity of the pituitary gland to the optic chiasm is important because bitemporal hemianopia can result from optic chiasm fiber damage, a possible early indication of a pituitary tumor.

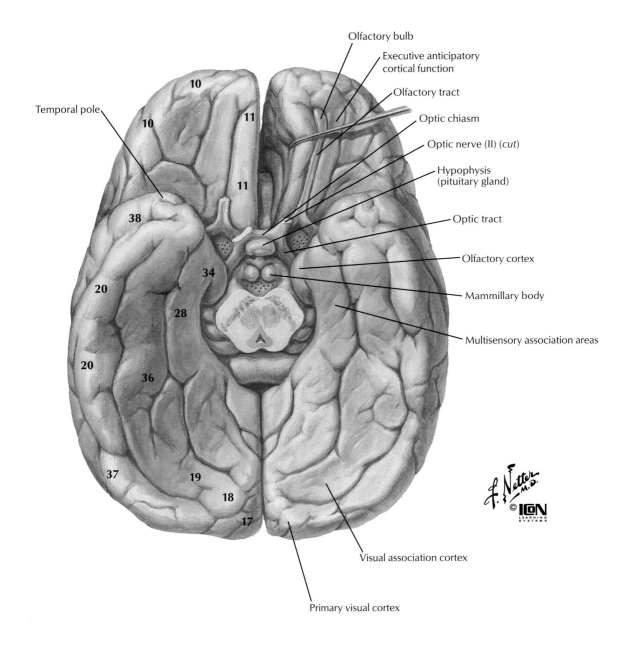

FIGURE I.26: BASAL SURFACE OF THE BRAIN: FUNCTIONAL AREAS AND BRODMANN AREAS

This view provides information about the medial temporal lobe on the left side of the brain, especially the cortical regions associated with the hippocampal formation, the amygdaloid nuclei, and the olfactory system. On the right side of the brain, the Brodmann areas are noted.

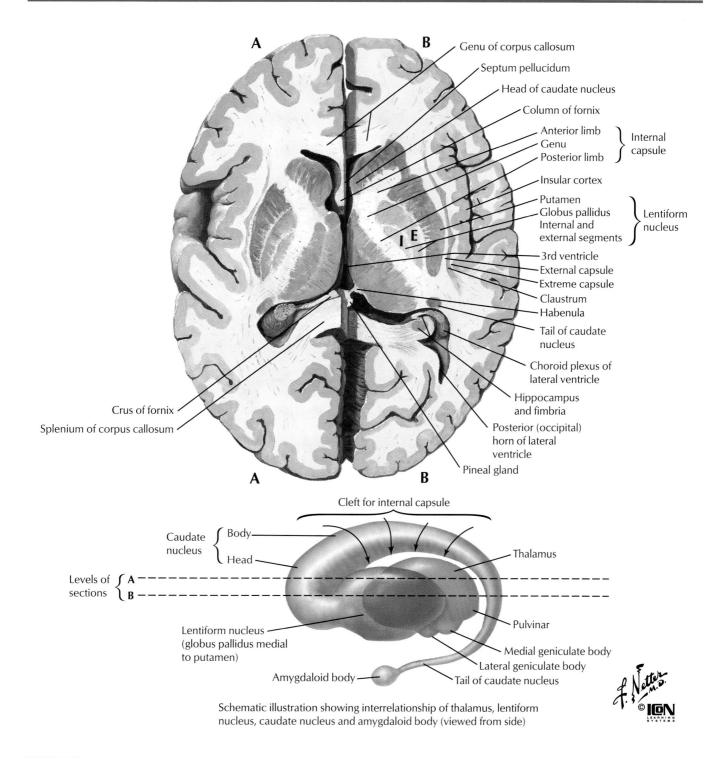

Schematic illustration showing interrelationship of thalamus, lentiform nucleus, caudate nucleus and amygdaloid body (viewed from side)

FIGURE I.27: HORIZONTAL BRAIN SECTIONS SHOWING THE BASAL GANGLIA

Two levels of horizontal sections through the forebrain reveal the major anatomical features and relationships of the basal ganglia, the internal capsule, and the thalamus (bottom illustration). The C-shaped caudate nucleus sweeps from the frontal lobe into the temporal lobe. In the internal capsule, the anterior and posterior limbs and the genu contain major connections into and out of the cerebral cortex. The relationships of the basal ganglia, the internal capsule, and the thalamus are important for understanding imaging studies and the involvement of specific functional systems in vascular lesions or strokes. The external capsule, the claustrum, the extreme capsule, and the insular cortex, labeled from medial to lateral, are landmarks used in imaging studies. The fornix is sectioned in the crus and the column.

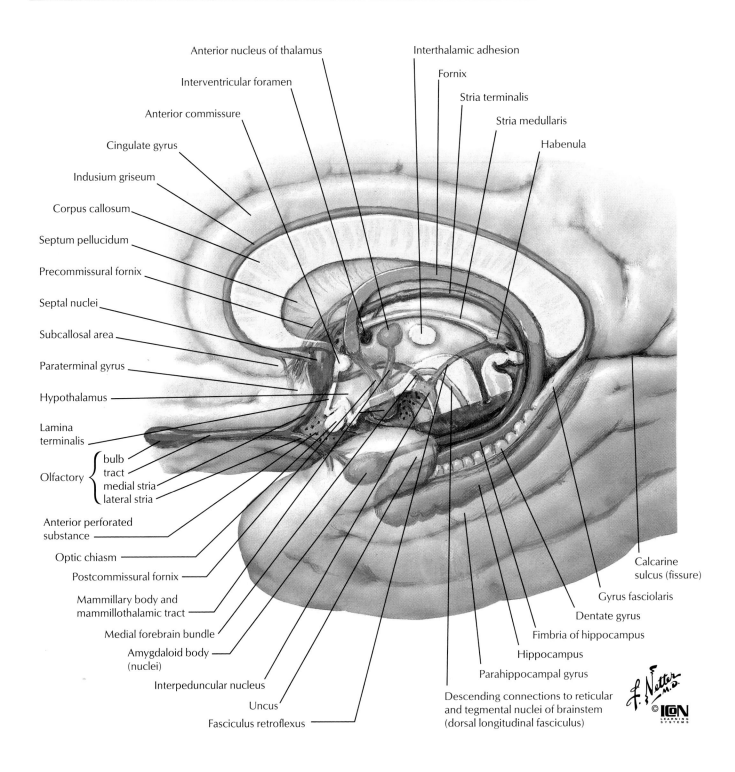

Anterior nucleus of thalamus

Interventricular foramen

Anterior commissure

Cingulate gyrus

Indusium griseum

Corpus callosum

Septum pellucidum

Precommissural fornix

Septal nuclei

Subcallosal area

Paraterminal gyrus

Hypothalamus

Lamina terminalis

Olfactory { bulb / tract / medial stria / lateral stria

Anterior perforated substance

Optic chiasm

Postcommissural fornix

Mammillary body and mammillothalamic tract

Medial forebrain bundle

Amygdaloid body (nuclei)

Interpeduncular nucleus

Uncus

Fasciculus retroflexus

Interthalamic adhesion

Fornix

Stria terminalis

Stria medullaris

Habenula

Calcarine sulcus (fissure)

Gyrus fasciolaris

Dentate gyrus

Fimbria of hippocampus

Hippocampus

Parahippocampal gyrus

Descending connections to reticular and tegmental nuclei of brainstem (dorsal longitudinal fasciculus)

FIGURE I.28: MAJOR LIMBIC FOREBRAIN STRUCTURES

Many of the structures and their pathways in the limbic system form a ring (limbus) around the diencephalon. They are involved in emotional behavior and interpretation of external and internal stimuli. The hippocampal formation and its pathways, the fornix, curve into the anterior pole of the diencephalon. The amygdaloid nuclei give rise to the stria terminalis, a C-shaped projection to the hypothalamic and basal forebrain structures. The olfactory tract communicates directly with the cortex and other forebrain structures, bypassing the thalamus. Connections from the septal nuclei to the habenula (stria terminalis) interconnect the limbic forebrain with the brain stem. The amygdaloid nuclei and the hippocampal formation (shaded) are deep to the cortex.

Anatomy of the Corpus Callosum

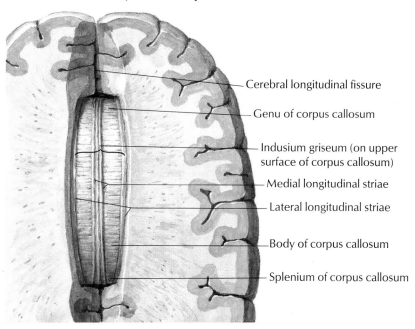

Cerebral longitudinal fissure

Genu of corpus callosum

Indusium griseum (on upper
surface of corpus callosum)

Medial longitudinal striae

Lateral longitudinal striae

Body of corpus callosum

Splenium of corpus callosum

FIGURE I.29: CORPUS CALLOSUM: HORIZONTAL VIEW

The corpus callosum, the major fiber commissure between the hemispheres, is a conspicuous landmark in imaging studies. It is viewed from above after dissection of the tissue just dorsal to its upper surface. Horizontal cuts taken deeper (more ventral) will section the genu anteriorly and the splenium posteriorly (see Figure I.27).

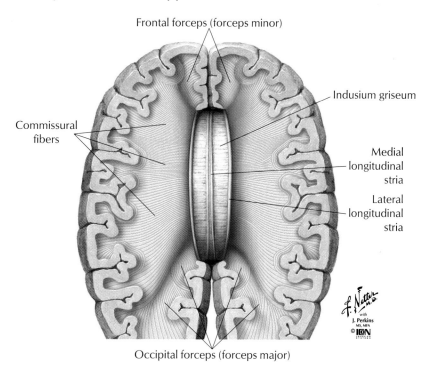

Frontal forceps (forceps minor)

Indusium griseum

Commissural fibers

Medial longitudinal stria

Lateral longitudinal stria

Occipital forceps (forceps major)

FIGURE I.30: CORPUS CALLOSUM: SCHEMATIC VIEW OF THE LATERAL EXTENT OF MAJOR COMPONENTS

Many of the commissural fibers of the corpus callosum, particularly the "forceps" of fibers interconnecting the frontal and the occipital areas, curve rostrally and caudally after crossing the midline. These interconnections allow communication to take place between the hemispheres, which is essential for coordinating the activity of these 2 "separate" hemispheres.

Dissection of the Hippocampal Formation and Fornix

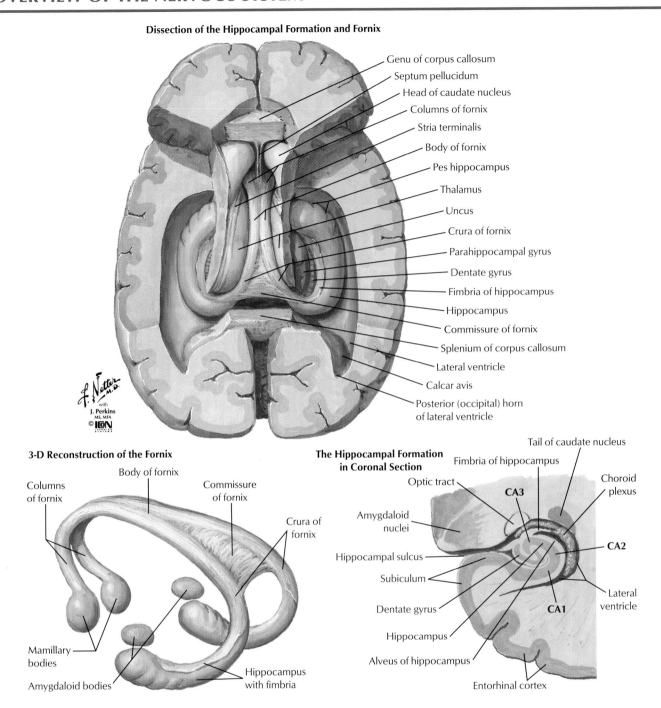

3-D Reconstruction of the Fornix

The Hippocampal Formation in Coronal Section

FIGURE I.31: HIPPOCAMPAL FORMATION AND FORNIX

The cortex, white matter, and corpus callosum have been removed, the lateral ventricles have been opened, and the head of the caudate and the thalamus have been dissected away close to the midline, allowing a downward view of the full extent of the hippocampal formation, including the dentate gyrus, and the associated fornix. This view reveals the relationship between the hippocampus proper and the dentate gyrus. The 2 limbs of the fornix sweep upward medially, eventually running side by side at their most dorsal position beneath the corpus callosum. The full extent of this arching,

C-shaped bundle is seen in the lower left diagram. The hippocampal formation occupies a large portion of the temporal pole of the lateral ventricle. The dentate gyrus is adjacent to subcomponents of the cornu Ammonis (CA) regions of the hippocampus proper (the CA1 and CA3 regions), the subiculum and the entorhinal cortex. CA1 pyramidal neurons in the CA1 region are sensitive to ischemic damage, and their counterparts in the CA3 region are sensitive to damage from high levels of corticosteroids (cortisol).

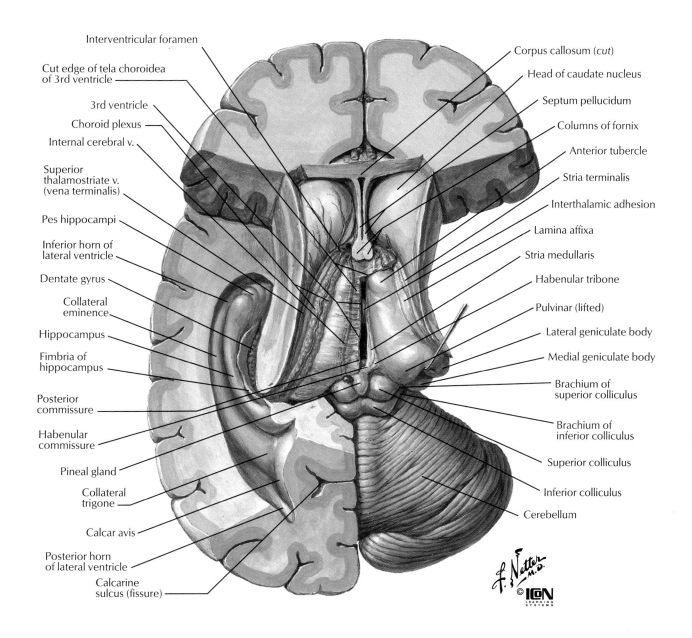

Interventricular foramen

Cut edge of tela choroidea of 3rd ventricle

3rd ventricle

Choroid plexus

Internal cerebral v.

Superior thalamostriate v. (vena terminalis)

Pes hippocampi

Inferior horn of lateral ventricle

Dentate gyrus

Collateral eminence

Hippocampus

Fimbria of hippocampus

Posterior commissure

Habenular commissure

Pineal gland

Collateral trigone

Calcar avis

Posterior horn of lateral ventricle

Calcarine sulcus (fissure)

Corpus callosum (*cut*)

Head of caudate nucleus

Septum pellucidum

Columns of fornix

Anterior tubercle

Stria terminalis

Interthalamic adhesion

Lamina affixa

Stria medullaris

Habenular tribone

Pulvinar (lifted)

Lateral geniculate body

Medial geniculate body

Brachium of superior colliculus

Brachium of inferior colliculus

Superior colliculus

Inferior colliculus

Cerebellum

FIGURE I.32: THALAMIC ANATOMY

The thalamus is viewed from above. The entire right side of the brain, just lateral to the thalamus, has been removed, the head of the caudate nucleus has been sectioned, the corpus callosum and all tissue dorsal to the thalamus have been removed, and the third ventricle has been opened from its dorsal surface. The pineal gland is present in the midline, just caudal to the third ventricle; it produces melatonin, a hormone that helps regulate circadian rhythms, sleep, and immune responses.

The superior and inferior colliculi are shown, depicting the dorsal surface of the midbrain. On the left, the temporal horn of the lateral ventricle, with the hippocampal formation, has been exposed to show the relationship of these structures to the thalamus. The terminal vein and the choroid plexus accompany the stria terminalis along the lateral margin of the thalamus. The stria medullaris runs along the medial surface of the dorsal thalamus.

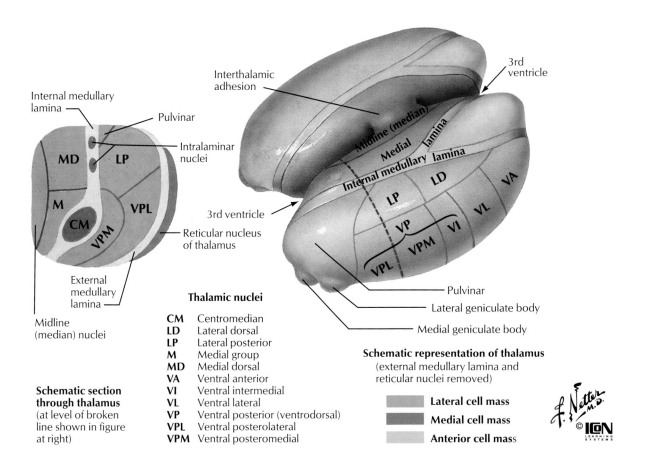

Internal medullary lamina
Pulvinar
Intralaminar nuclei
Interthalamic adhesion
3rd ventricle
MD
LP
Midline (median)
Medial
Internal medullary lamina
LD
VA
LP
M
VPL
VP
VL
CM
VI
VPM
VPM
VPL
3rd ventricle
Reticular nucleus of thalamus
Pulvinar
External medullary lamina
Lateral geniculate body
Midline (median) nuclei
Medial geniculate body

Thalamic nuclei

CM	Centromedian
LD	Lateral dorsal
LP	Lateral posterior
M	Medial group
MD	Medial dorsal
VA	Ventral anterior
VI	Ventral intermedial
VL	Ventral lateral
VP	Ventral posterior (ventrodorsal)
VPL	Ventral posterolateral
VPM	Ventral posteromedial

Schematic section through thalamus
(at level of broken line shown in figure at right)

Schematic representation of thalamus
(external medullary lamina and reticular nuclei removed)

Lateral cell mass
Medial cell mass
Anterior cell mass

FIGURE I.33: THALAMIC NUCLEI

These figures illustrate the subdivision of the thalamus into nuclear groups (medial, lateral, and anterior), separated by medullary (white matter) laminae. Many of these nuclei are "specific" thalamic nuclei that are reciprocally connected with discrete regions of the cerebral cortex. Some of the nuclei, such as those embedded in the internal medullary lamina (intralaminar nuclei such as centromedian and parafascicular nuclei), and the outer, lateral shell nucleus (reticular nucleus of the thalamus) have very diffuse, "nonspecific" associations with the cerebral cortex.

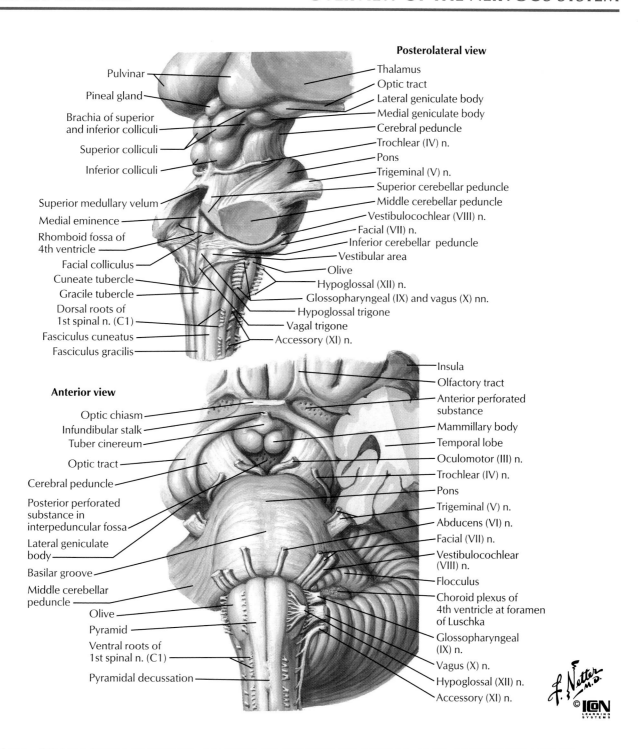

Posterolateral view

Pulvinar
Pineal gland
Brachia of superior and inferior colliculi
Superior colliculi
Inferior colliculi
Superior medullary velum
Medial eminence
Rhomboid fossa of 4th ventricle
Facial colliculus
Cuneate tubercle
Gracile tubercle
Dorsal roots of 1st spinal n. (C1)
Fasciculus cuneatus
Fasciculus gracilis

Thalamus
Optic tract
Lateral geniculate body
Medial geniculate body
Cerebral peduncle
Trochlear (IV) n.
Pons
Trigeminal (V) n.
Superior cerebellar peduncle
Middle cerebellar peduncle
Vestibulocochlear (VIII) n.
Facial (VII) n.
Inferior cerebellar peduncle
Vestibular area
Olive
Hypoglossal (XII) n.
Glossopharyngeal (IX) and vagus (X) nn.
Hypoglossal trigone
Vagal trigone
Accessory (XI) n.

Anterior view

Optic chiasm
Infundibular stalk
Tuber cinereum
Optic tract
Cerebral peduncle
Posterior perforated substance in interpeduncular fossa
Lateral geniculate body
Basilar groove
Middle cerebellar peduncle
Olive
Pyramid
Ventral roots of 1st spinal n. (C1)
Pyramidal decussation

Insula
Olfactory tract
Anterior perforated substance
Mammillary body
Temporal lobe
Oculomotor (III) n.
Trochlear (IV) n.
Pons
Trigeminal (V) n.
Abducens (VI) n.
Facial (VII) n.
Vestibulocochlear (VIII) n.
Flocculus
Choroid plexus of 4th ventricle at foramen of Luschka
Glossopharyngeal (IX) n.
Vagus (X) n.
Hypoglossal (XII) n.
Accessory (XI) n.

FIGURE I.34: BRAIN STEM SURFACE ANATOMY: POSTEROLATERAL AND ANTERIOR VIEWS

(Top) The entire telencephalon, most of the diencephalon, and the cerebellum are removed to show the dorsal surface of the brain stem. The 3 cerebellar peduncles (superior, middle, inferior) are sectioned, and the cerebellum is removed. The dorsal roots and the cranial nerves provide input to the spinal cord and provide input and output to the brain stem, respectively. The fourth nerve (trochlear) is the only cranial nerve to exit dorsally from the brain stem. The tubercles and trigones on the floor of the fourth ventricle are named for nuclei just beneath them. (Bottom) The left temporal lobe is dissected to show the anterior (ventral) surface of the brain stem. The cerebral peduncles, caudal extensions of the posterior limb of the internal capsule, carry corticospinal and corticobulbar fibers from the internal capsule to the spinal cord and the brain stem, respectively. The decussation of the pyramids marks the boundary between the caudal medulla and the cervical spinal cord.

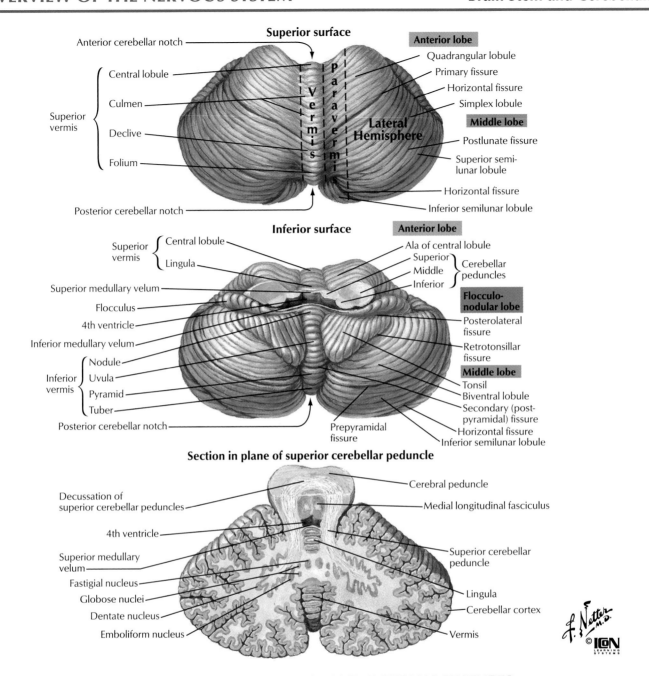

FIGURE I.35: CEREBELLAR ANATOMY: EXTERNAL AND INTERNAL FEATURES

(Top) The top 2 diagrams show the superior (dorsal) and inferior (ventral) surfaces of the cerebellum. The ventral surface of the cerebellum is the roof of the fourth ventricle. The anterior, middle, and flocculonodular lobes of the cerebellum are traditional anatomical subdivisions with well-described syndromes from lesions. The vermis, paravermis, and lateral hemispheres are cerebellar cortical zones with specific projection relationships with deep cerebellar nuclei (vermis with fastigial nucleus and lateral vestibular nucleus, paravermis with globose and emboliform nuclei, lateral hemispheres with dentate nucleus), connecting with specific upper motor neuronal systems regulating specific types of motor activities. (Bottom) The major internal subdivisions of the cerebellum are shown. The cerebellar cortex (3-layered), the outer zone, is infolded to form numerous folia. The white matter, carrying afferents and efferents associated with the cerebellar cortex, is deep to the folia. The deep cerebellar nuclei are deep to the white matter. These cell groups receive most of the output from the cerebellar cortex via Purkinje cell axon projections and receive collaterals from mossy fiber and climbing fiber inputs to the cerebellum. The cerebellar peduncles are interior to the deep nuclei; these massive fiber bundles interconnect the cerebellum with the brain stem and the thalamus.

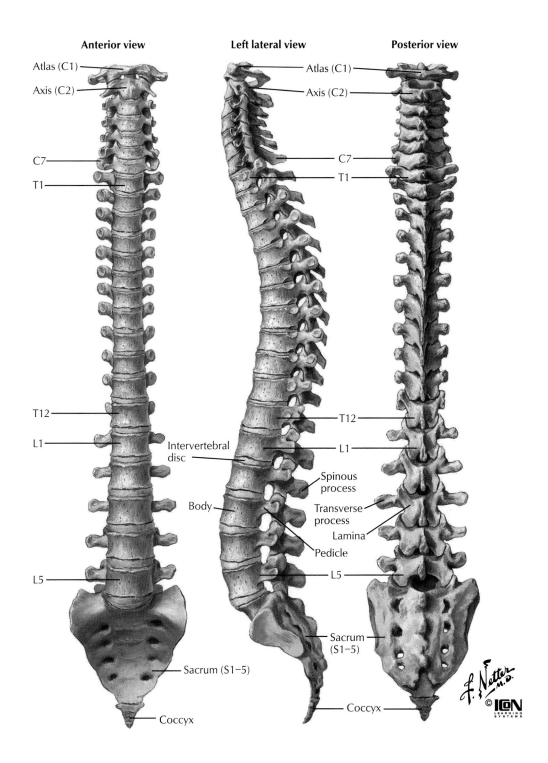

Anterior view   Left lateral view   Posterior view

Atlas (C1)
Axis (C2)
C7
T1
T12
L1
Intervertebral disc
Body
Spinous process
Transverse process
Lamina
Pedicle
L5
Sacrum (S1–5)
Coccyx
Atlas (C1)
Axis (C2)

FIGURE I.36: SPINAL COLUMN: BONY ANATOMY

Anterior, lateral, and posterior views of the bony spinal column show the relationships of the intervertebral discs with the vertebral body. The discs' proximity to the intervertebral foramina provides an anatomical substrate for understanding the possible impingement of a herniated nucleus pulposus on spinal roots. Such impingement can cause excruciating, radiating pain if dorsal roots are involved and loss of motor control of affected muscles if ventral roots are involved. In the adult, the spinal cord extends caudally only as far as the L1 vertebral body, leaving the lumbar cistern (subarachnoid [SA] space) accessible for withdrawal of CSF.

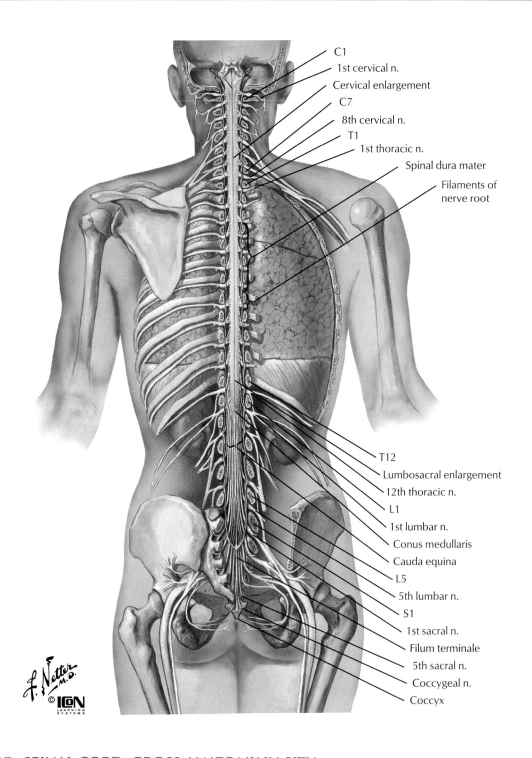

C1
1st cervical n.
Cervical enlargement
C7
8th cervical n.
T1
1st thoracic n.
Spinal dura mater
Filaments of nerve root

T12
Lumbosacral enlargement
12th thoracic n.
L1
1st lumbar n.
Conus medullaris
Cauda equina
L5
5th lumbar n.
S1
1st sacral n.
Filum terminale
5th sacral n.
Coccygeal n.
Coccyx

FIGURE I.37: SPINAL CORD: GROSS ANATOMY IN SITU

The posterior portion of the vertebrae is removed to show the posterior (dorsal) surface of the spinal cord. Cervical and lumbosacral enlargements reflect innervation of the limbs. The spinal cord extends rostrally through the foramen magnum, continuous with the medulla. The conus medullaris is located under the L1 vertebral body. The longitudinal growth of the spinal column exceeds that of the spinal cord, causing the spinal cord to end consider- ably more rostral in an adult than it does in a new- born. The associated nerve roots traverse a consid- erable distance through the SA space of the lumbar cistern to reach the appropriate intervertebral foramina of exit. In the lumbar cistern, this collec- tion of nerve roots is the cauda equina (horse's tail). The lumbar cistern is a large reservoir from which CSF can be withdrawn. The filum terminale anchors the spinal cord caudally to the coccyx.

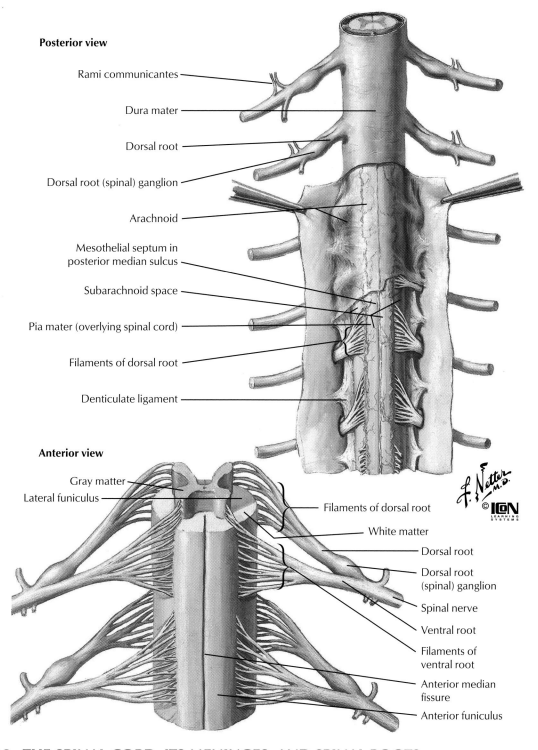

Posterior view

- Rami communicantes
- Dura mater
- Dorsal root
- Dorsal root (spinal) ganglion
- Arachnoid
- Mesothelial septum in posterior median sulcus
- Subarachnoid space
- Pia mater (overlying spinal cord)
- Filaments of dorsal root
- Denticulate ligament

Anterior view

- Gray matter
- Lateral funiculus
- Filaments of dorsal root
- White matter
- Dorsal root
- Dorsal root (spinal) ganglion
- Spinal nerve
- Ventral root
- Filaments of ventral root
- Anterior median fissure
- Anterior funiculus

FIGURE I.38: THE SPINAL CORD, ITS MENINGES, AND SPINAL ROOTS

The upper illustration shows both intact and reflected meninges. The pia adheres to every contour of the spinal cord surface. The arachnoid extends over these contours and adheres to the overlying dura, a very tough, fibrous, protective membrane. These meninges extend outward to the nerve roots. The denticulate ligaments are fibrous structures that help anchor the spinal cord in place.

The posterior spinal arteries supply the dorsal spinal cord with blood and run just medial to the dorsal root entry zone. The lower illustration shows the spinal cord with the meninges stripped away. Both the dorsal and the ventral roots consist of a convergence of rootlets that provide a continuous dorsal and ventral array of rootlets throughout the spinal cord.

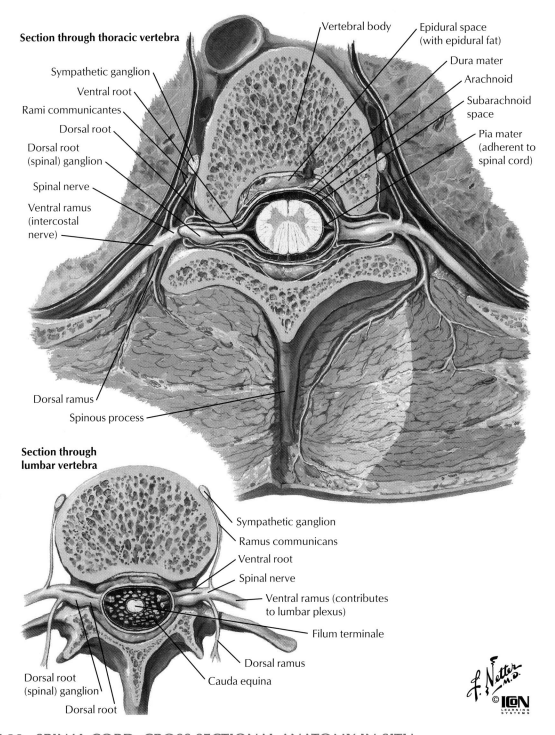

Section through thoracic vertebra

Vertebral body

Epidural space (with epidural fat)

Dura mater

Arachnoid

Subarachnoid space

Pia mater (adherent to spinal cord)

Sympathetic ganglion

Ventral root

Rami communicantes

Dorsal root

Dorsal root (spinal) ganglion

Spinal nerve

Ventral ramus (intercostal nerve)

Dorsal ramus

Spinous process

Section through lumbar vertebra

Sympathetic ganglion

Ramus communicans

Ventral root

Spinal nerve

Ventral ramus (contributes to lumbar plexus)

Filum terminale

Dorsal ramus

Cauda equina

Dorsal root (spinal) ganglion

Dorsal root

FIGURE I.39: SPINAL CORD: CROSS-SECTIONAL ANATOMY IN SITU

(Top) The spinal cord in the spinal canal is surrounded by meninges. Dorsal and ventral roots course through the intervertebral foramina. The epidural space, with its associated fat, is sometimes used for infusion of anesthetics. Arteries and veins are associated with the spinal nerves and nerve roots. Some segmental arteries provide anastomotic channels for blood flow from the aorta to augment flow from the anterior and posterior spinal arterial systems, which cannot sustain the entire spinal cord. The sympathetic chain ganglia (paravertebral), important for fight-or-flight responses, lie adjacent to the vertebral body (ventrally). The dorsal and ventral rami of the spinal nerves distribute to specific regions. The spinous process extends dorsally, where it can be palpated by physical exam. (Bottom) The SA space of a lumbar vertebra, containing the filum terminale and the roots of the cauda equina, is shown.

Sections through spinal cord at various levels

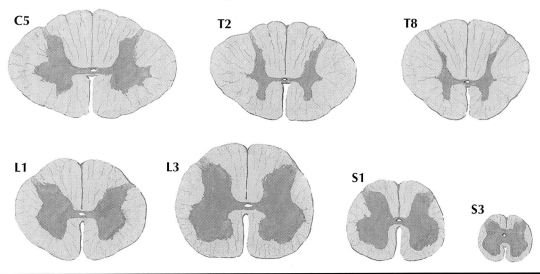

Principal fiber tracts of spinal cord (composite)

- Ascending pathways
- Descending pathways
- Fibers passing in both directions

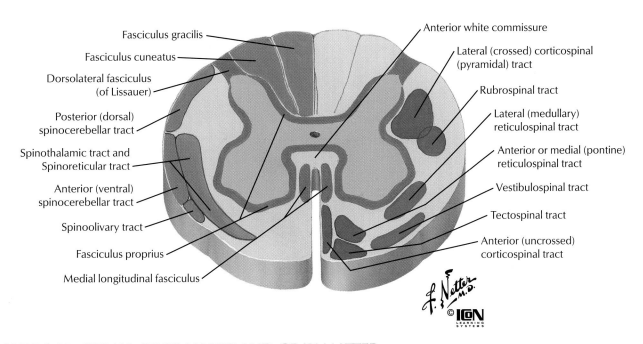

Fasciculus gracilis

Fasciculus cuneatus

Dorsolateral fasciculus (of Lissauer)

Posterior (dorsal) spinocerebellar tract

Spinothalamic tract and Spinoreticular tract

Anterior (ventral) spinocerebellar tract

Spinoolivary tract

Fasciculus proprius

Medial longitudinal fasciculus

Anterior white commissure

Lateral (crossed) corticospinal (pyramidal) tract

Rubrospinal tract

Lateral (medullary) reticulospinal tract

Anterior or medial (pontine) reticulospinal tract

Vestibulospinal tract

Tectospinal tract

Anterior (uncrossed) corticospinal tract

FIGURE I.40: SPINAL CORD WHITE AND GRAY MATTER

(Top) Seven spinal cord levels are shown, depicting the relative size and the variability in the amount of gray matter at each level. Levels associated with the limbs have greater amounts of gray matter. White matter increases in absolute amount from caudal to rostral, reflecting the level-by-level addition of ascending tracts and the termination of descending tracts. (Bottom) The gray matter consists of dorsal and ventral horns and, in the T1 to L2 segments, an intermediolateral cell column (lateral horn) where preganglionic sympathetic neurons reside. The white matter is subdivided into dorsal, lateral, and ventral funiculi, each containing multiple tracts (fasciculi, bundles). The tracts conveying pain and temperature information travel rostrally in the anterolateral funiculus, the spinothalamic/spinoreticular system. Fine discriminative sensation is conveyed through the dorsal funiculus. Dorsal root entry zones and ventral root exit zones are present at each cross-sectional level.

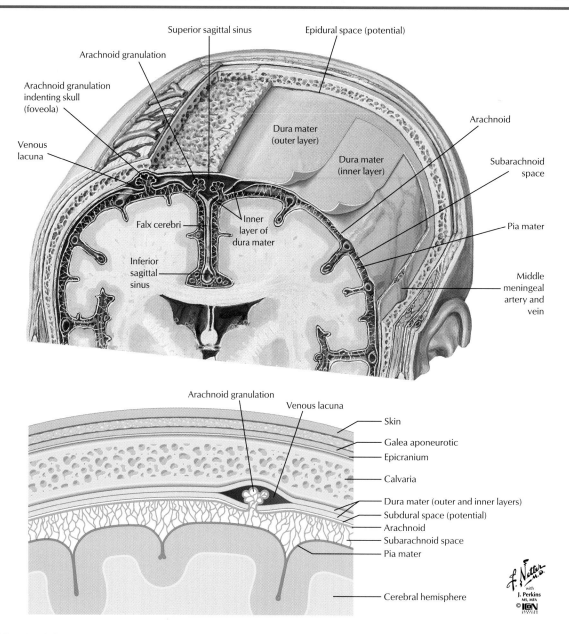

FIGURE I.41: SCHEMATIC OF THE MENINGES AND THEIR RELATIONSHIP TO THE BRAIN

The meninges provide protection and support for neural tissue in the CNS. The innermost membrane, the pia mater adheres to every contour of neural tissue, into sulci, folia, and other infoldings. It adheres tightly to glial endfoot processes of astrocytes. The arachnoid mater, a fine, lacy membrane external to the pia, extends across the neural sulci and foldings. The subarachnoid (SA) space (between the arachnoid and the pia), into which the CSF flows, provides buoyancy and protection to the brain. Arteries and veins run through the SA space to and from the CNS. The rupture of an arterial aneurysm of cerebral arteries results in an SA hemorrhage. The dura mater, usually adherent to the inner arachnoid, is a tough protective outer membrane. It splits into 2 layers in some locations

to provide channels for venous blood, the venous (dural) sinuses. The arachnoid granulations, one-way valves, extend from the SA space into the venous sinuses, especially the superior sagittal sinus, allowing CSF to drain into the venous blood, back to the heart. Blockage (e.g., acute purulent meningitis) can result in increased intracranial pressure. Bridging veins drain into the dural sinuses. These veins are subject to tearing as they enter the sinus as a result of trauma, especially if there is some atrophy in the brain, permitting venous blood to accumulate in the subdural space as it dissects the inner dura from the arachnoid. This subdural hematoma can be life-threatening from increased intracranial pressure, edema, and the accumulation of blood from the hematoma itself.

Ventricles of Brain

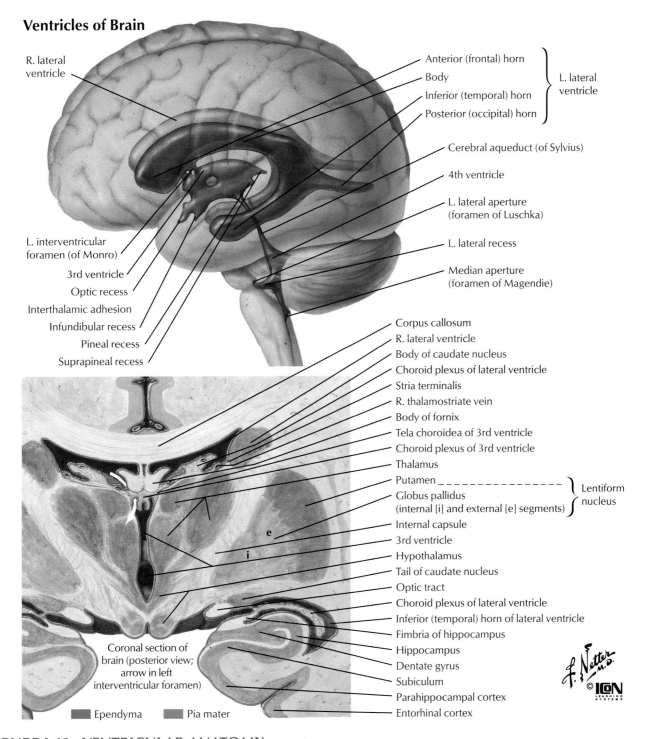

R. lateral ventricle

Anterior (frontal) horn
Body
Inferior (temporal) horn
Posterior (occipital) horn
} L. lateral ventricle

Cerebral aqueduct (of Sylvius)

4th ventricle

L. lateral aperture (foramen of Luschka)

L. lateral recess

Median aperture (foramen of Magendie)

L. interventricular foramen (of Monro)
3rd ventricle
Optic recess
Interthalamic adhesion
Infundibular recess
Pineal recess
Suprapineal recess

Corpus callosum
R. lateral ventricle
Body of caudate nucleus
Choroid plexus of lateral ventricle
Stria terminalis
R. thalamostriate vein
Body of fornix
Tela choroidea of 3rd ventricle
Choroid plexus of 3rd ventricle
Thalamus
Putamen _ _ _ _ _ _ _ _ _ _ _ _
Globus pallidus (internal [i] and external [e] segments)
} Lentiform nucleus
Internal capsule
3rd ventricle
Hypothalamus
Tail of caudate nucleus
Optic tract
Choroid plexus of lateral ventricle
Inferior (temporal) horn of lateral ventricle
Fimbria of hippocampus
Hippocampus
Dentate gyrus
Subiculum
Parahippocampal cortex
Entorhinal cortex

e
i

Coronal section of brain (posterior view; arrow in left interventricular foramen)

■ Ependyma ■ Pia mater

FIGURE I.42: VENTRICULAR ANATOMY

The lateral ventricles are C-shaped, reflecting their association with the developing telencephalon as it sweeps upward, back, and then down and forward as the temporal lobe. The position of the lateral ventricles in relation to the head and body of the caudate nucleus is an important radiological landmark in a variety of conditions (hydrocephalus, caudate atrophy in Huntington's disease, and shifting of the midline with a tumor). CSF flows through the foramen of Monro into the narrow third ventricle,

then into the cerebral aqueduct and the fourth ventricle. Blockage of flow in the aqueduct can precipitate internal hydrocephalus, with swelling of the ventricles above. The escape sites for CSF to flow into the subarachnoid (SA) space cisterns are the medial foramen of Magendie and the lateral foramina of Luschka, where blockage of CSF flow can occur. The choroid plexus, extending into the ventricles, produces the CSF.

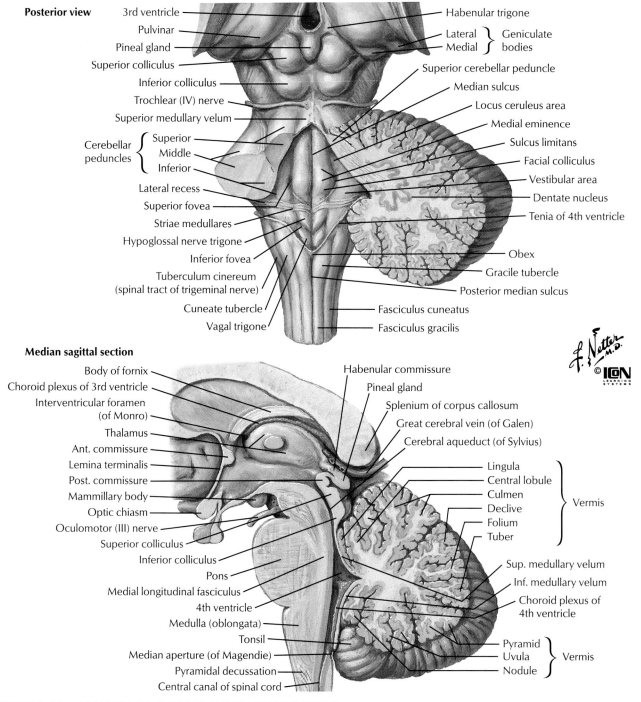

FIGURE I.43: ANATOMY OF THE FOURTH VENTRICLE

The rhombus-shaped fourth ventricle extends through the pons and the medulla. The foramina of Magendie and Luschka must remain patent for proper flow of CSF into the cisterns. Bilaterally symmetrical protrusions, depressions, and sulci on the floor of the ventricle define the underlying anatomy of brain stem regions. Vital brain stem centers for cardiovascular, respiratory, and metabolic functions just below the floor of the ventricle can be damaged from tumors in the region. The lateral margins of the ventricle are embraced by the huge cerebellar peduncles interconnecting the cerebellum with the brain stem and the diencephalon. These relationships are important for interpreting imaging studies in the compact brain stem regions, where diagnosis of tumors and vascular lesions is challenging.

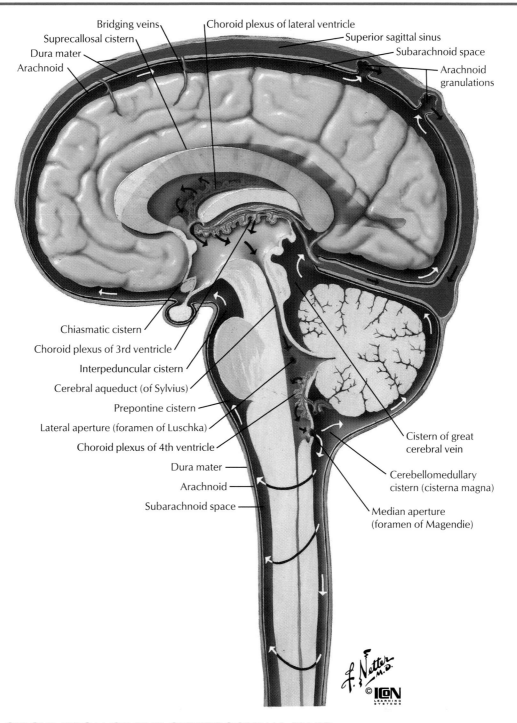

Bridging veins
Suprecallosal cistern
Dura mater
Arachnoid
Choroid plexus of lateral ventricle
Superior sagittal sinus
Subarachnoid space
Arachnoid granulations

Chiasmatic cistern
Choroid plexus of 3rd ventricle
Interpeduncular cistern
Cerebral aqueduct (of Sylvius)
Prepontine cistern
Lateral aperture (foramen of Luschka)
Choroid plexus of 4th ventricle
Dura mater
Arachnoid
Subarachnoid space

Cistern of great cerebral vein
Cerebellomedullary cistern (cisterna magna)
Median aperture (foramen of Magendie)

FIGURE I.44: CIRCULATION OF THE CEREBROSPINAL FLUID

Cerebrospinal fluid flowing through the ventricles (lateral to third to cerebral aqueduct to fourth) passes through several points where obstruction could precipitate internal hydrocephalus and increased intracranial pressure. CSF flow from the fourth ventricle into the cisterns of the SA space provides external cushioning to prevent injury to underlying CNS tissue from minor trauma. Some cisterns (e.g., the lumbar cistern) provide sites for withdrawal of CSF (lumbar puncture). The absorption of CSF from the SA space into the venous drainage through the arachnoid granulations is driven by flow through these one-way valves. Production, flow, and absorption of CSF must be in precise balance; disruption of this process results in external hydrocephalus. Flow of the CSF in the ventricles also can act as a fluid-delivery system for downstream influences of specific mediators (e.g., prostaglandins, interleukins) and is an internal paracrine communication channel for some structures close to the ventricles.

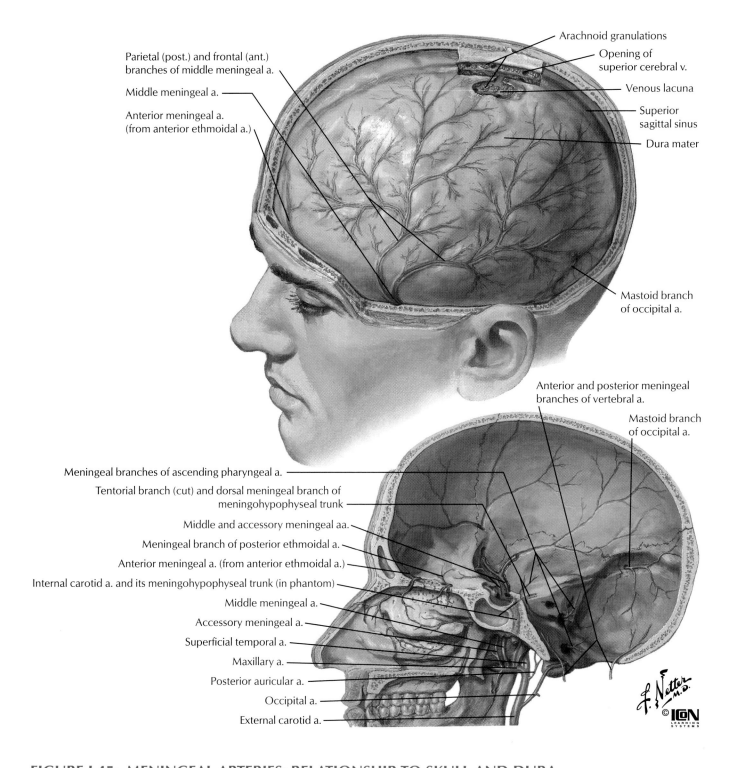

Arachnoid granulations

Opening of superior cerebral v.

Venous lacuna

Superior sagittal sinus

Dura mater

Parietal (post.) and frontal (ant.) branches of middle meningeal a.

Middle meningeal a.

Anterior meningeal a. (from anterior ethmoidal a.)

Mastoid branch of occipital a.

Anterior and posterior meningeal branches of vertebral a.

Mastoid branch of occipital a.

Meningeal branches of ascending pharyngeal a.

Tentorial branch (cut) and dorsal meningeal branch of meningohypophyseal trunk

Middle and accessory meningeal aa.

Meningeal branch of posterior ethmoidal a.

Anterior meningeal a. (from anterior ethmoidal a.)

Internal carotid a. and its meningohypophyseal trunk (in phantom)

Middle meningeal a.

Accessory meningeal a.

Superficial temporal a.

Maxillary a.

Posterior auricular a.

Occipital a.

External carotid a.

FIGURE I.45: MENINGEAL ARTERIES: RELATIONSHIP TO SKULL AND DURA

Meningeal arteries are found in the outer portion of the dura and supply it with blood. They also help supply adjacent skull and have some anastomoses with cerebral arteries. The skull has grooves or sulci for the meningeal vessels. This relationship reflects an important functional consequence of skull fractures. Fractures can rip a meningeal artery (usually the middle meningeal artery) and allow arterial blood to accumulate above the dura. Such an epidural hematoma is a space-occupying mass, and it can produce increased intracranial pressure and risk of herniation of the brain, particularly across the tentorium cerebelli. Even very fine fractures can have this dangerous consequence.

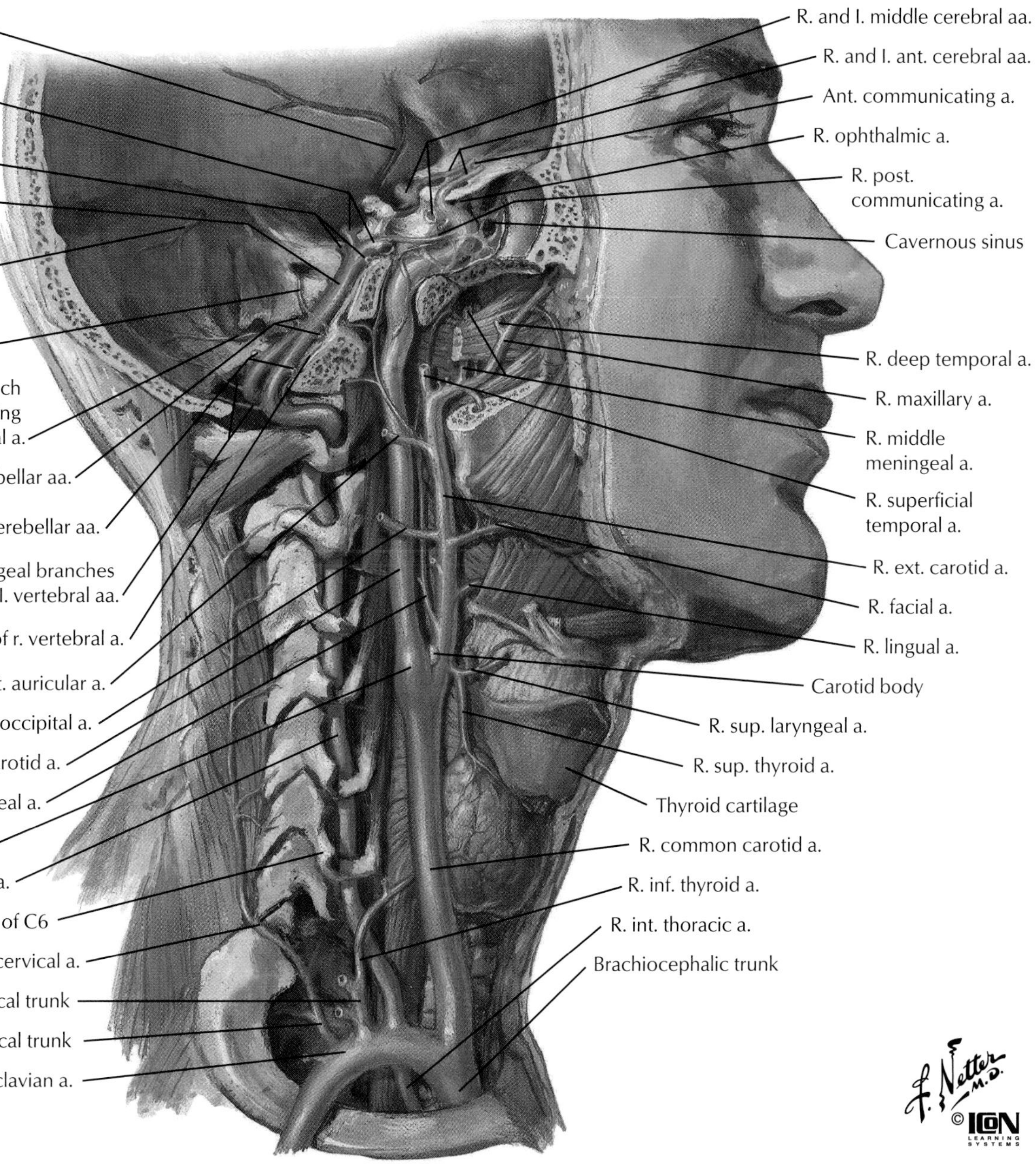

L. middle meningeal a.
R. and l. post. cerebral aa.
R. and l. sup. cerebellar aa.
Basilar a.
Mastoid branch of l. occipital a.
L. Int. auditory (labyrinthine) a.
Post. meningeal branch of l. ascending pharyngeal a.
R. and l. ant. inf. cerebellar aa.
R. and l. post. inf. cerebellar aa.
Post. meningeal branches of r. and l. vertebral aa.
Ant. meningeal branch of r. vertebral a.
R. post. auricular a.
R. occipital a.
R. int. carotid a.
R. ascending pharyngeal a.
R. carotid sinus
R. vertebral a.
Transverse process of C6
R. deep cervical a.
R. thyrocervical trunk
R. costocervical trunk
R. subclavian a.
R. and l. middle cerebral aa.
R. and l. ant. cerebral aa.
Ant. communicating a.
R. ophthalmic a.
R. post. communicating a.
Cavernous sinus
R. deep temporal a.
R. maxillary a.
R. middle meningeal a.
R. superficial temporal a.
R. ext. carotid a.
R. facial a.
R. lingual a.
Carotid body
R. sup. laryngeal a.
R. sup. thyroid a.
Thyroid cartilage
R. common carotid a.
R. inf. thyroid a.
R. int. thoracic a.
Brachiocephalic trunk

FIGURE I.46: ARTERIAL SUPPLY TO THE BRAIN AND THE MENINGES

The internal carotid and vertebral arteries ascend through the neck and enter the skull to supply the brain with blood. The tortuous bends and sites of branching of these arteries (such as the bifurcation of the common carotid artery into the internal and the external carotids) produce turbulent blood flow, and atherosclerosis can occur at these locations. The bifurcation of the common carotid is particularly vulnerable to plaque formation and occlusion, threatening the major anterior part of the brain with ischemia, which would result in a "stroke." Studies of blood flow through these arteries are important diagnostic tools. Magnetic resonance arteriography (MRA) and Doppler flow studies have replaced the older dye studies for cerebral angiography, for most purposes.

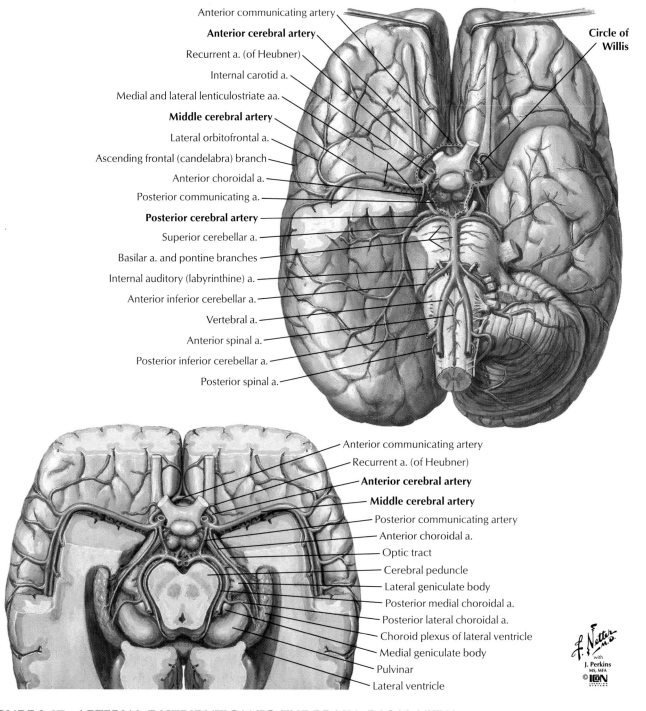

FIGURE I.47: ARTERIAL DISTRIBUTION TO THE BRAIN: BASAL VIEW

(Top) The anterior circulation (middle and anterior cerebral arteries [MCA, ACA]) and the posterior circulation (the vertebrobasilar system and its end branch, the posterior cerebral artery [PCA]) are shown. The right temporal pole is removed to show the course of the MCA through the lateral fissure. The circle of Willis (the paired ACAs, MCAs, and PCAs and the anterior and the 2 posterior communicating arteries) appears to allow free flow of blood around the anterior and posterior circula-

tion of both sides, but it is usually not sufficiently patent to allow bypass of an occluded zone. (Bottom) The circle of Willis and the course of the choroidal arteries are shown. The arteries supplying the brain are end arteries and do not have sufficient anastomotic channels with other arteries to sustain blood flow. The occlusion of an artery supplying a specific territory of the brain results in functional damage that affects the performance of the structures deprived of adequate blood flow.

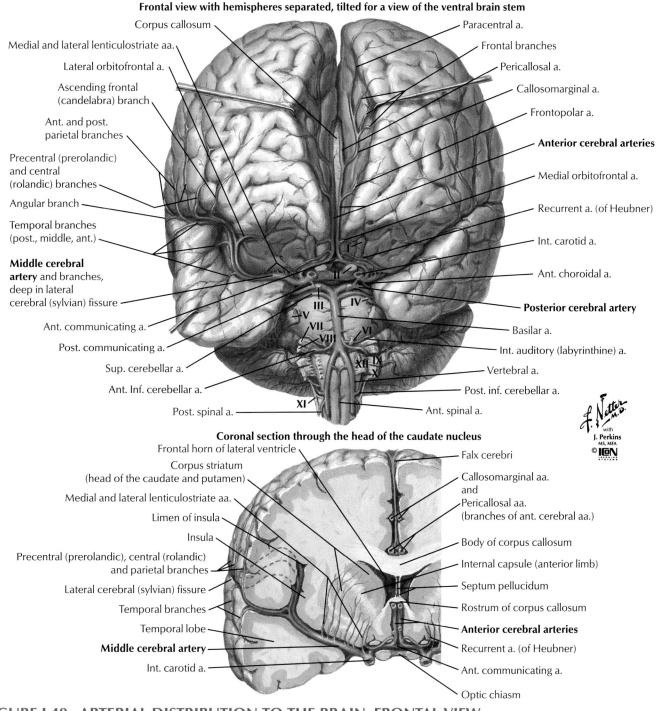

Frontal view with hemispheres separated, tilted for a view of the ventral brain stem

Corpus callosum
Medial and lateral lenticulostriate aa.
Lateral orbitofrontal a.
Ascending frontal (candelabra) branch
Ant. and post. parietal branches
Precentral (prerolandic) and central (rolandic) branches
Angular branch
Temporal branches (post., middle, ant.)
Middle cerebral artery and branches, deep in lateral cerebral (sylvian) fissure
Ant. communicating a.
Post. communicating a.
Sup. cerebellar a.
Ant. Inf. cerebellar a.
Post. spinal a.

Paracentral a.
Frontal branches
Pericallosal a.
Callosomarginal a.
Frontopolar a.
Anterior cerebral arteries
Medial orbitofrontal a.
Recurrent a. (of Heubner)
Int. carotid a.
Ant. choroidal a.
Posterior cerebral artery
Basilar a.
Int. auditory (labyrinthine) a.
Vertebral a.
Post. inf. cerebellar a.
Ant. spinal a.

Coronal section through the head of the caudate nucleus

Frontal horn of lateral ventricle
Corpus striatum (head of the caudate and putamen)
Medial and lateral lenticulostriate aa.
Limen of insula
Insula
Precentral (prerolandic), central (rolandic) and parietal branches
Lateral cerebral (sylvian) fissure
Temporal branches
Temporal lobe
Middle cerebral artery
Int. carotid a.

Falx cerebri
Callosomarginal aa. and
Pericallosal aa. (branches of ant. cerebral aa.)
Body of corpus callosum
Internal capsule (anterior limb)
Septum pellucidum
Rostrum of corpus callosum
Anterior cerebral arteries
Recurrent a. (of Heubner)
Ant. communicating a.
Optic chiasm

FIGURE I.48: ARTERIAL DISTRIBUTION TO THE BRAIN: FRONTAL VIEW AND CORONAL SECTION

The course of the ACA along the midline reflects its blood supply to the zone of the sensory and motor cortices, which are associated with the contralateral lower extremity; an ACA stroke thus affects the contralateral lower limb. The MCA courses laterally and gives branches to the entire convexity of the hemisphere. End branch infarcts of the MCA affect the contralateral upper extremity and, if on the left, language function. More proximal infarcts affecting the MCA distribution to the internal capsule cause full contralateral hemiplegia with drooping of the contralateral lower face; this results from damage to corticospinal and other corticomotor fibers in the posterior limb and to corticobulbar fibers in the genu. The lenticulostriate arteries ("arteries of stroke") are thin branches of the MCA that penetrate into the basal ganglia and the internal capsule regions in the forebrain. A stroke in this area produces the classic contralateral hemiplegia.

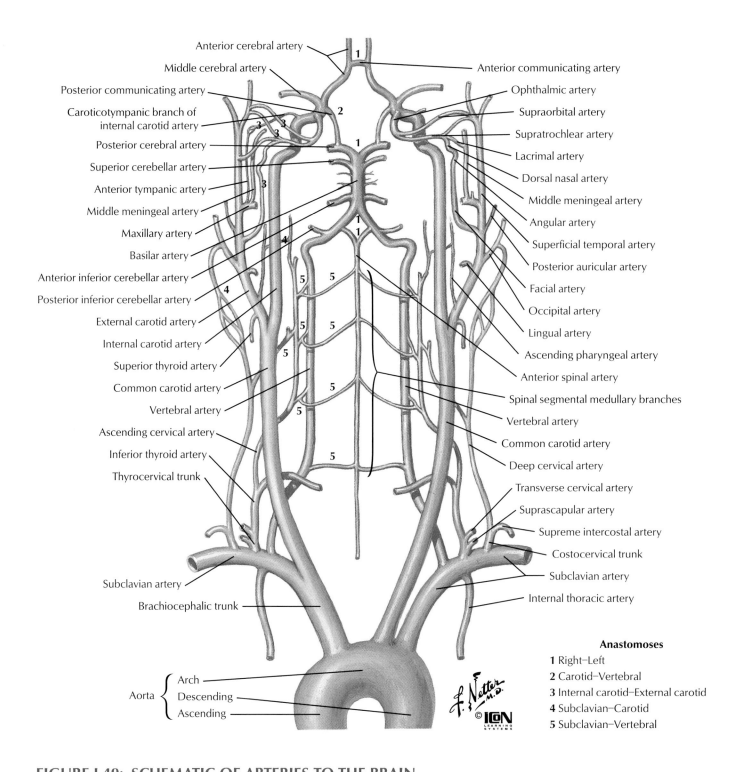

FIGURE I.49: SCHEMATIC OF ARTERIES TO THE BRAIN

This schematic diagram shows the entire layout of the arterial blood supply to the brain, including anastomoses. The circle of Willis is present in the upper central portion of this schematic. The relative separation of the anterior (MCA, ACA) and posterior (vertebro-basilar, PCA) circulation are evident in this diagram.

Vessels dissected out: inferior view

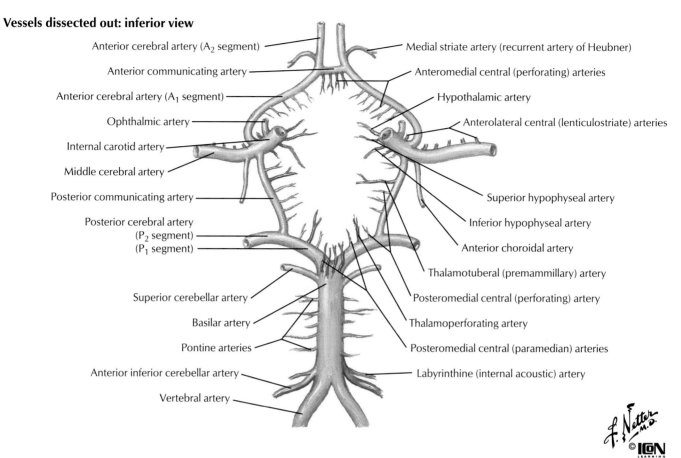

Anterior cerebral artery (A₂ segment)
Anterior communicating artery
Anterior cerebral artery (A₁ segment)
Ophthalmic artery
Internal carotid artery
Middle cerebral artery
Posterior communicating artery
Posterior cerebral artery
(P₂ segment)
(P₁ segment)
Superior cerebellar artery
Basilar artery
Pontine arteries
Anterior inferior cerebellar artery
Vertebral artery

Medial striate artery (recurrent artery of Heubner)
Anteromedial central (perforating) arteries
Hypothalamic artery
Anterolateral central (lenticulostriate) arteries
Superior hypophyseal artery
Inferior hypophyseal artery
Anterior choroidal artery
Thalamotuberal (premammillary) artery
Posteromedial central (perforating) artery
Thalamoperforating artery
Posteromedial central (paramedian) arteries
Labyrinthine (internal acoustic) artery

Vessels in situ: inferior view

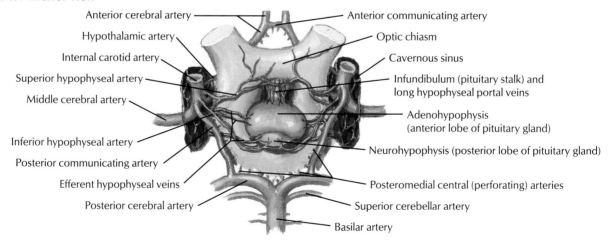

Anterior cerebral artery
Hypothalamic artery
Internal carotid artery
Superior hypophyseal artery
Middle cerebral artery
Inferior hypophyseal artery
Posterior communicating artery
Efferent hypophyseal veins
Posterior cerebral artery

Anterior communicating artery
Optic chiasm
Cavernous sinus
Infundibulum (pituitary stalk) and
long hypophyseal portal veins
Adenohypophysis
(anterior lobe of pituitary gland)
Neurohypophysis (posterior lobe of pituitary gland)
Posteromedial central (perforating) arteries
Superior cerebellar artery
Basilar artery

FIGURE I.50: SCHEMATIC OF THE CIRCLE OF WILLIS

The circle of Willis surrounds the optic tracts, the pituitary stalk, and the basal hypothalamus and is the most frequent site of cerebral aneurysms. It includes the 3 sets of paired cerebral arteries plus the anterior communicating artery interconnecting the ACAs and the posterior communicating arteries interconnecting the MCAs and the PCAs. The free flow of arterial blood through the communicating arteries is usually insufficient to perfuse the brain adequately in the face of an occlusion to a major cerebral artery. An aneurysm is a ballooning of an artery resulting from an inherent weakness in the arterial wall. A rupture can lead to a subarachnoid (SA) bleed, with loss of perfusion to vital CNS territories.

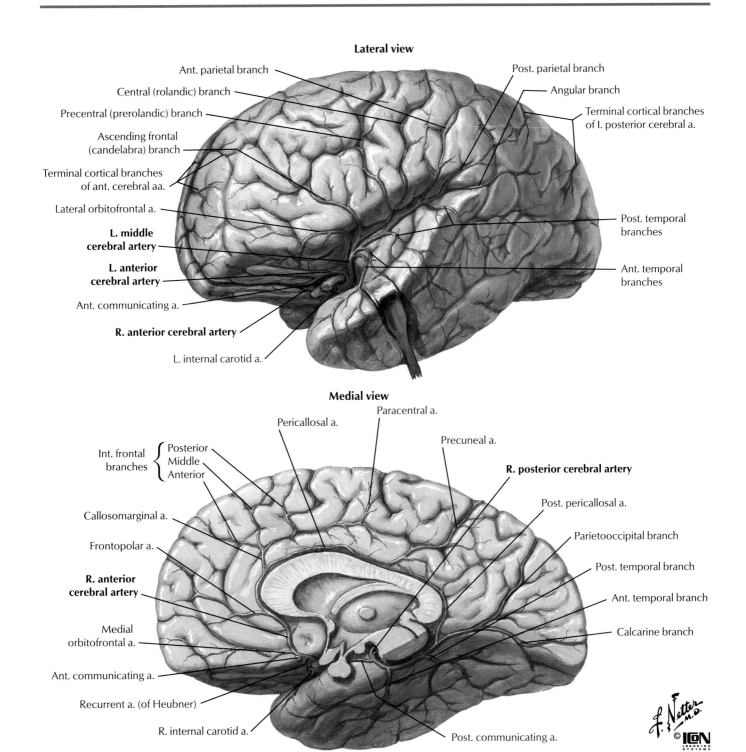

Lateral view

Ant. parietal branch

Central (rolandic) branch

Precentral (prerolandic) branch

Ascending frontal (candelabra) branch

Terminal cortical branches of ant. cerebral aa.

Lateral orbitofrontal a.

L. middle cerebral artery

L. anterior cerebral artery

Ant. communicating a.

R. anterior cerebral artery

L. internal carotid a.

Post. parietal branch

Angular branch

Terminal cortical branches of I. posterior cerebral a.

Post. temporal branches

Ant. temporal branches

Medial view

Paracentral a.

Pericallosal a.

Precuneal a.

Int. frontal branches { Posterior Middle Anterior }

R. posterior cerebral artery

Post. pericallosal a.

Callosomarginal a.

Parietooccipital branch

Frontopolar a.

Post. temporal branch

R. anterior cerebral artery

Ant. temporal branch

Medial orbitofrontal a.

Calcarine branch

Ant. communicating a.

Recurrent a. (of Heubner)

R. internal carotid a.

Post. communicating a.

FIGURE I.51: ARTERIAL DISTRIBUTION TO THE BRAIN: LATERAL AND MEDIAL VIEWS

(Top) The MCA sends the named branches along the surface of the hemispheric convexity into the frontal and parietal lobes and into the anterior and middle regions of the temporal lobes. Occlusion disrupts sensory and motor functions on the contralateral body, especially the upper extremity, or on the entire contralateral body if the internal capsule is affected. (Bottom) The ACA distributes to the midline region of the frontal and parietal lobes. Occlusion disrupts sensory and motor functions on the contralateral lower extremity. The PCA distributes to the occipital lobe and the inferior surface of the temporal lobe. Occlusion disrupts mainly visual functions from the contralateral visual field.

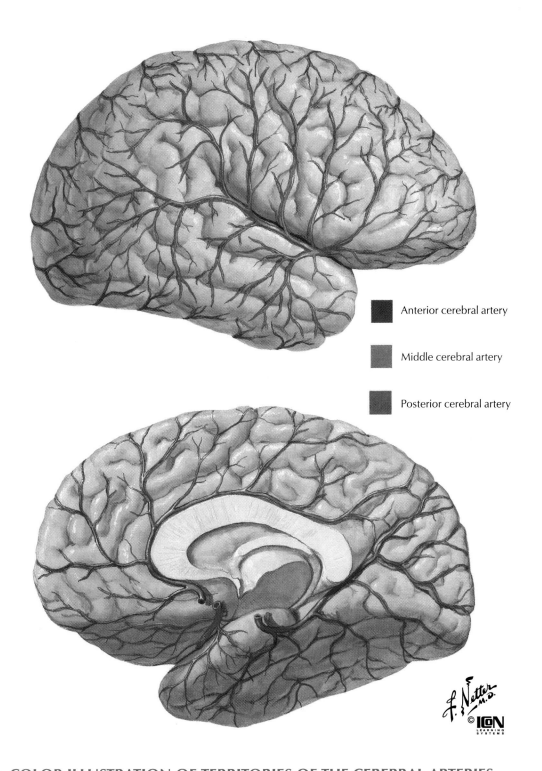

Anterior cerebral artery

Middle cerebral artery

Posterior cerebral artery

FIGURE I.52: COLOR ILLUSTRATION OF TERRITORIES OF THE CEREBRAL ARTERIES _____

The specific midline and lateral territories of distri-bution of the ACA, MCA, and PCA illustrate the exclusive zones supplied by these major arteries and make particularly clear the watershed zones at the junctions of the major cerebral arteries.

Femorocerebral Angiography

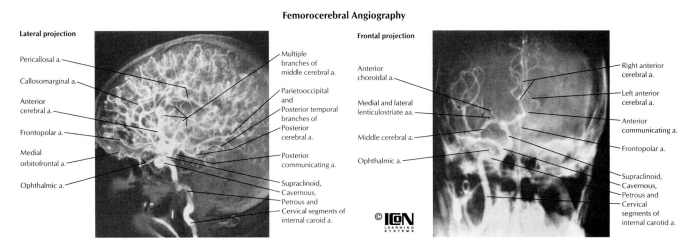

Lateral projection

- Pericallosal a.
- Callosomarginal a.
- Anterior cerebral a.
- Frontopolar a.
- Medial orbitofrontal a.
- Ophthalmic a.

- Multiple branches of middle cerebral a.
- Parietooccipital and Posterior temporal branches of Posterior cerebral a.
- Posterior communicating a.
- Supraclinoid, Cavernous, Petrous and Cervical segments of internal caroid a.

Frontal projection

- Anterior choroidal a.
- Medial and lateral lenticulostriate aa.
- Middle cerebral a.
- Ophthalmic a.

- Right anterior cerebral a.
- Left anterior cerebral a.
- Anterior communicating a.
- Frontopolar a.
- Supraclinoid, Cavernous, Petrous and Cervical segments of internal carotid a.

© ICON LEARNING SYSTEMS

FIGURE I.53: ANGIOGRAPHIC ANATOMY OF THE INTERNAL CAROTID CIRCULATION

The left plate is an angiogram lateral view of the internal carotid arterial circulation after injection of a radio-opaque contrast agent into the internal carotid artery. The major branches of the internal carotid artery, particularly the anterior cerebral and middle cerebral arteries, are delineated. The right plate is an angiogram frontal view of the internal carotid arterial circulation after injection of a radio-opaque contrast agent into the common carotid artery. The major branches of this arterial system are delineated. MR angiography is used commonly to investigate the status of the cerebral arteries, but does not provide the same level of detail for anatomical purposes that standard angiography provides.

Arteries of Posterior Cranial Fossa
Vertebral Angiograms: Arterial Phase

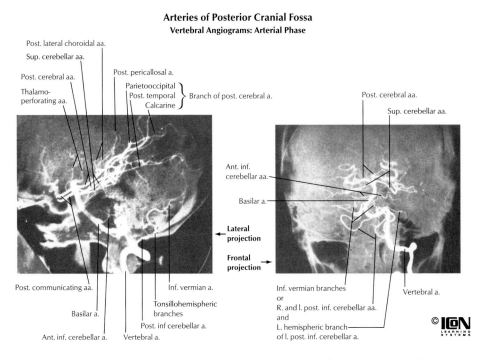

- Post. lateral choroidal aa.
- Sup. cerebellar aa.
- Post. cerebral aa.
- Thalamo-perforating aa.
- Post. pericallosal a.
- Parietooccipital
- Post. temporal } Branch of post. cerebral a.
- Calcarine
- Post. communicating aa.
- Basilar a.
- Ant. inf. cerebellar a.
- Vertebral a.
- Post. inf cerebellar a.
- Inf. vermian a.
- Tonsillohemispheric branches

- Ant. inf. cerebellar aa.
- Basilar a.
- Post. cerebral aa.
- Sup. cerebellar aa.
- Inf. vermian branches or R. and l. post. inf. cerebellar aa. and L. hemispheric branch of l. post. inf. cerebellar a.
- Vertebral a.

Lateral projection ←

Frontal projection

© ICON LEARNING SYSTEMS

FIGURE I.54: ANGIOGRAPHIC ANATOMY OF THE VERTEBROBASILAR SYSTEM

The upper figures show angiograms of both lateral and frontal views of the vertebro-basilar (posterior) circulation after injection of a radio-opaque contrast agent (dye) into the vertebral artery. The major arterial branches of this arterial system are delineated. The lower figure is an MR angiogram showing both the internal carotid and vertebro-basilar circulation. The major branches of these arteries are labeled. Angiograms with contrast agents provide more detailed anatomical information, but are more invasive than MR angiography. MR angiography is used with greater frequency, although use of contrast agents still occurs for specific diagnostic purposes.

Arteries of Posterior Cranial Fossa

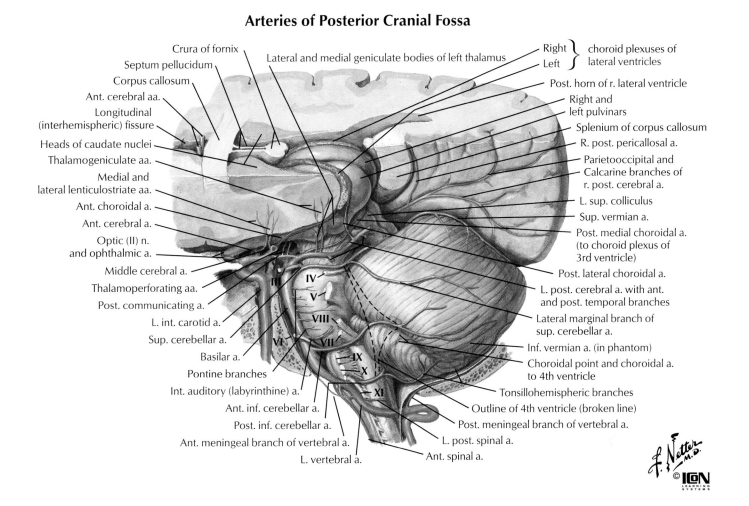

Crura of fornix
Septum pellucidum
Corpus callosum
Ant. cerebral aa.
Longitudinal (interhemispheric) fissure
Heads of caudate nuclei
Thalamogeniculate aa.
Medial and lateral lenticulostriate aa.
Ant. choroidal a.
Ant. cerebral a.
Optic (II) n. and ophthalmic a.
Middle cerebral a.
Thalamoperforating aa.
Post. communicating a.
L. int. carotid a.
Sup. cerebellar a.
Basilar a.
Pontine branches
Int. auditory (labyrinthine) a.
Ant. inf. cerebellar a.
Post. inf. cerebellar a.
Ant. meningeal branch of vertebral a.
L. vertebral a.

Lateral and medial geniculate bodies of left thalamus

III   IV   V   VIII   VI   VII   IX   X   XI

Right
Left
} choroid plexuses of lateral ventricles
Post. horn of r. lateral ventricle
Right and left pulvinars
Splenium of corpus callosum
R. post. pericallosal a.
Parietooccipital and Calcarine branches of r. post. cerebral a.
L. sup. colliculus
Sup. vermian a.
Post. medial choroidal a. (to choroid plexus of 3rd ventricle)
Post. lateral choroidal a.
L. post. cerebral a. with ant. and post. temporal branches
Lateral marginal branch of sup. cerebellar a.
Inf. vermian a. (in phantom)
Choroidal point and choroidal a. to 4th ventricle
Tonsillohemispheric branches
Outline of 4th ventricle (broken line)
Post. meningeal branch of vertebral a.
L. post. spinal a.
Ant. spinal a.

FIGURE I.55: VERTEBROBASILAR ARTERIAL SYSTEM

The vertebral arteries unite at the midline to form the basilar artery. Medial penetrating branches extend into medial zones of the brain stem, supplying wedge-like territories. Infarcts in these branches can produce "alternating hemiplegias," with contralateral motor deficits (corticospinal system damage above the decussation of the pyramids) and ipsilateral brain stem/cranial nerve signs and symptoms. The vertebral and basilar arteries give rise to the larger short and long circumferential branches, such as the posterior inferior cerebellar artery (PICA), the anterior inferior cerebellar artery (AICA), and the superior cerebellar artery (SCA). Strokes in these arterial territories produce a constellation of ipsilateral brain stem sensory, motor, and autonomic symptoms and contralateral somatosensory symptoms. For example, a PICA infarct results in loss of pain and temperature sensation on the contralateral body and the ipsilateral face. The end branch of the basilar artery is the PCA, distributing to the visual cortex and the inferior temporal lobe. Occlusion results in contralateral hemianopia.

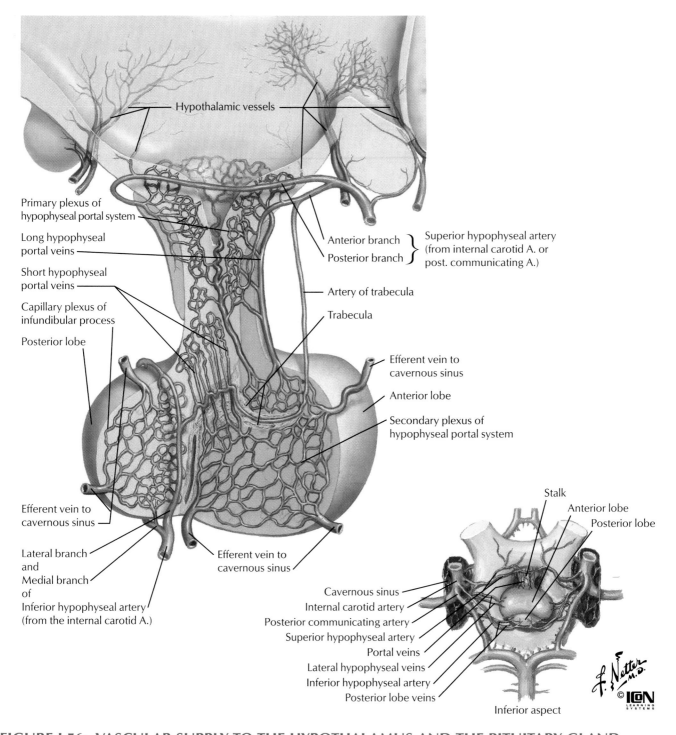

Hypothalamic vessels

Primary plexus of
hypophyseal portal system

Long hypophyseal
portal veins

Short hypophyseal
portal veins

Capillary plexus of
infundibular process

Posterior lobe

Anterior branch
Posterior branch } Superior hypophyseal artery
(from internal carotid A. or
post. communicating A.)

Artery of trabecula

Trabecula

Efferent vein to
cavernous sinus

Anterior lobe

Secondary plexus of
hypophyseal portal system

Efferent vein to
cavernous sinus

Lateral branch
and
Medial branch
of
Inferior hypophyseal artery
(from the internal carotid A.)

Efferent vein to
cavernous sinus

Stalk
Anterior lobe
Posterior lobe

Cavernous sinus
Internal carotid artery
Posterior communicating artery
Superior hypophyseal artery
Portal veins
Lateral hypophyseal veins
Inferior hypophyseal artery
Posterior lobe veins

Inferior aspect

FIGURE I.56: VASCULAR SUPPLY TO THE HYPOTHALAMUS AND THE PITUITARY GLAND

The superior hypophyseal arteries (from the ICA or the posterior communicating artery) supply the hypothalamus and the infundibular stalk and anastomose with branches of the inferior hypophyseal artery (from the ICA). A unique aspect of this arterial distribution is the hypophyseal portal system, whose primary plexus derives from small arterioles and capillaries that then send branches into the anterior pituitary gland. This plexus allows neurons that produce hypothalamic releasing and inhibitory factors to secrete these factors into the hypophyseal portal system, which delivers a very high concentration directly into the secondary plexus in the anterior pituitary. Thus, anterior pituitary cells are bathed in releasing and inhibitory factors in very high concentration. This private vascular communication channel allows the hypothalamus to exert fine control, both directly and through feedback, over the secretion of anterior pituitary hormones.

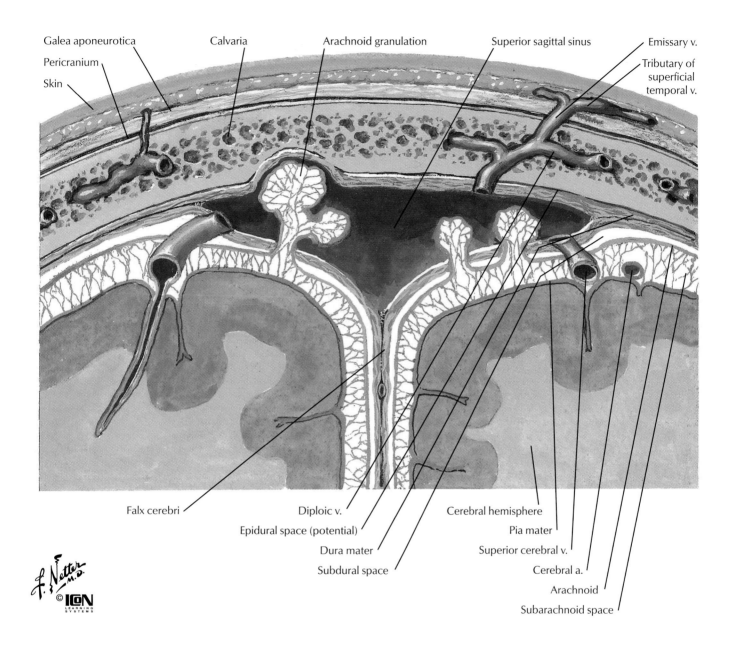

Galea aponeurotica   Calvaria   Arachnoid granulation   Superior sagittal sinus   Emissary v.

Pericranium

Skin

Tributary of superficial temporal v.

Falx cerebri   Diploic v.   Cerebral hemisphere

Epidural space (potential)   Pia mater

Dura mater   Superior cerebral v.

Subdural space   Cerebral a.

Arachnoid

Subarachnoid space

FIGURE I.57: MENINGES AND SUPERFICIAL CEREBRAL VEINS

The superior sagittal sinus and other dural sinuses receive venous blood from a variety of veins, including superficial cerebral veins draining blood from the cortical surface, meningeal veins draining blood from the meninges, diploic veins draining blood from channels located between the inner and outer tables of the calvaria, and emissary veins, which link the venous sinuses and diploic veins with veins on the surface of the skull. These channels do not have valves and permit free communication between these venous systems and the venous sinuses. This is a significant factor in the possible spread of infections from foci outside the cranium to the venous sinuses.

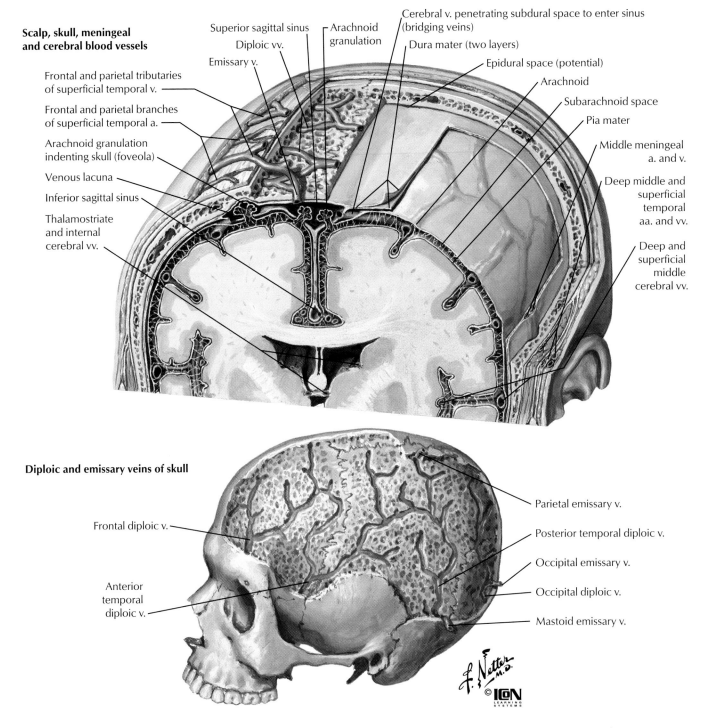

Scalp, skull, meningeal and cerebral blood vessels

Superior sagittal sinus

Diploic vv.

Emissary v.

Arachnoid granulation

Cerebral v. penetrating subdural space to enter sinus (bridging veins)

Dura mater (two layers)

Epidural space (potential)

Arachnoid

Subarachnoid space

Pia mater

Middle meningeal a. and v.

Deep middle and superficial temporal aa. and vv.

Deep and superficial middle cerebral vv.

Frontal and parietal tributaries of superficial temporal v.

Frontal and parietal branches of superficial temporal a.

Arachnoid granulation indenting skull (foveola)

Venous lacuna

Inferior sagittal sinus

Thalamostriate and internal cerebral vv.

Diploic and emissary veins of skull

Frontal diploic v.

Anterior temporal diploic v.

Parietal emissary v.

Posterior temporal diploic v.

Occipital emissary v.

Occipital diploic v.

Mastoid emissary v.

FIGURE I.58: SUPERFICIAL CEREBRAL, MENINGEAL, DIPLOIC, AND EMISSARY VEINS

Venous blood drains from the skull, the meninges, and the cerebral cortex into the superior sagittal sinus and other dural sinuses. This area is vulnerable to infections and contamination from drainage from superficial venous networks into the central venous sinus channels.

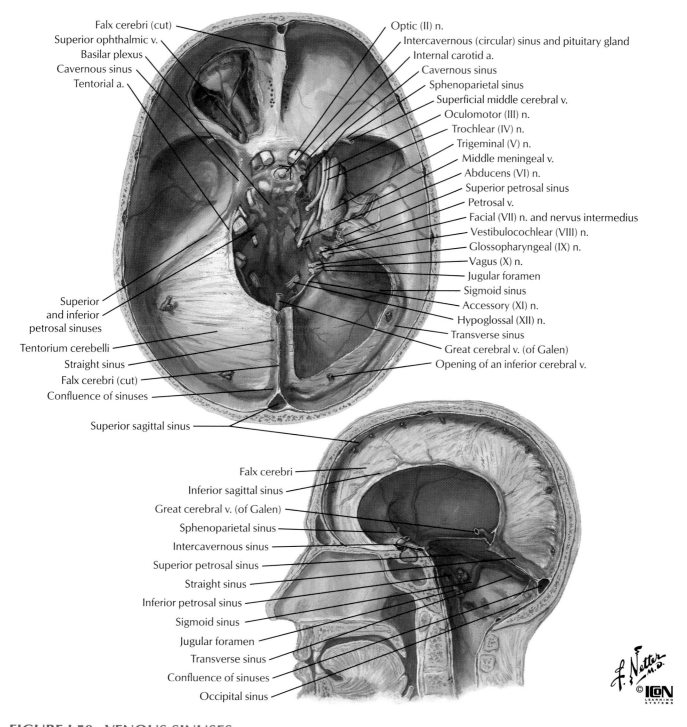

Falx cerebri (cut)
Superior ophthalmic v.
Basilar plexus
Cavernous sinus
Tentorial a.

Optic (II) n.
Intercavernous (circular) sinus and pituitary gland
Internal carotid a.
Cavernous sinus
Sphenoparietal sinus
Superficial middle cerebral v.
Oculomotor (III) n.
Trochlear (IV) n.
Trigeminal (V) n.
Middle meningeal v.
Abducens (VI) n.
Superior petrosal sinus
Petrosal v.
Facial (VII) n. and nervus intermedius
Vestibulocochlear (VIII) n.
Glossopharyngeal (IX) n.
Vagus (X) n.
Jugular foramen
Sigmoid sinus
Accessory (XI) n.
Hypoglossal (XII) n.
Transverse sinus
Great cerebral v. (of Galen)
Opening of an inferior cerebral v.

Superior and inferior petrosal sinuses
Tentorium cerebelli
Straight sinus
Falx cerebri (cut)
Confluence of sinuses

Superior sagittal sinus

Falx cerebri
Inferior sagittal sinus
Great cerebral v. (of Galen)
Sphenoparietal sinus
Intercavernous sinus
Superior petrosal sinus
Straight sinus
Inferior petrosal sinus
Sigmoid sinus
Jugular foramen
Transverse sinus
Confluence of sinuses
Occipital sinus

FIGURE I.59: VENOUS SINUSES

The falx cerebri and the tentorium cerebelli, protrusions of fused inner and outer dural membranes, confine the anterior, middle, and posterior fossae of the skull. Outer (superior sagittal) and inner (inferior sagittal) venous channels found in split layers of the dura drain blood from the superficial and the deep regions of the CNS, respectively, into the jugular veins. The great cerebral vein of Galen and the straight sinus merge with the transverse sinus into the confluence of sinuses to drain the deep,

posterior regions of the CNS. Infection can be introduced into the cerebral circulation through these sinuses. Venous sinus thrombosis can cause stasis (a backup of the venous pressure), which causes inadequate perfusion of the regions where drainage should occur. The protrusions of dura are tough, rigid membranes through which portions of the brain can herniate when intracranial pressure increases.

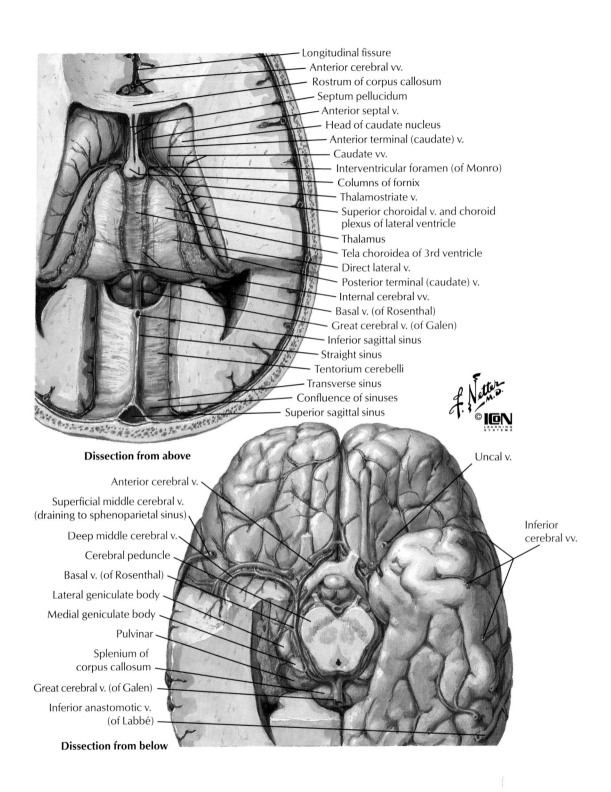

Longitudinal fissure
Anterior cerebral vv.
Rostrum of corpus callosum
Septum pellucidum
Anterior septal v.
Head of caudate nucleus
Anterior terminal (caudate) v.
Caudate vv.
Interventricular foramen (of Monro)
Columns of fornix
Thalamostriate v.
Superior choroidal v. and choroid plexus of lateral ventricle
Thalamus
Tela choroidea of 3rd ventricle
Direct lateral v.
Posterior terminal (caudate) v.
Internal cerebral vv.
Basal v. (of Rosenthal)
Great cerebral v. (of Galen)
Inferior sagittal sinus
Straight sinus
Tentorium cerebelli
Transverse sinus
Confluence of sinuses
Superior sagittal sinus

Dissection from above

Uncal v.

Anterior cerebral v.
Superficial middle cerebral v. (draining to sphenoparietal sinus)
Deep middle cerebral v.
Cerebral peduncle
Basal v. (of Rosenthal)
Lateral geniculate body
Medial geniculate body
Pulvinar
Splenium of corpus callosum
Great cerebral v. (of Galen)
Inferior anastomotic v. (of Labbé)

Inferior cerebral vv.

Dissection from below

FIGURE I.60: DEEP VENOUS DRAINAGE OF THE BRAIN

(Top) This superior view of the thalamus and the basal ganglia reveals the venous drainage of deeper forebrain regions into the posterior venous sinuses. (Bottom) This basal view of the brain with the brain stem removed illustrates the drainage of forebrain and mesencephalic venous blood into the great cerebral vein of Galen, heading toward the straight sinus.

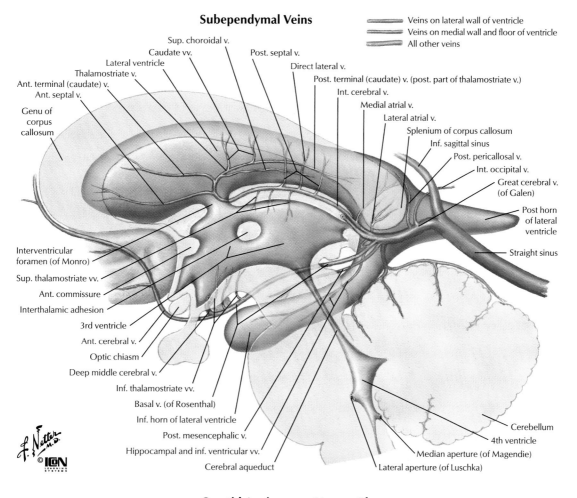

Subependymal Veins

Veins on lateral wall of ventricle
Veins on medial wall and floor of ventricle
All other veins

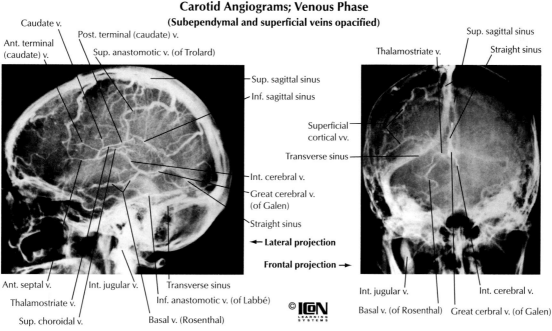

Carotid Angiograms; Venous Phase
(Subependymal and superficial veins opacified)

← **Lateral projection**

Frontal projection →

FIGURE I.61: DEEP VENOUS DRAINAGE OF THE BRAIN: RELATIONSHIP TO VENTRICLES

Subependymal regions of the CNS drain venous blood into the inferior sagittal sinus (left) or the great cerebral vein of Galen (right), both of which drain into the straight sinus. Occlusion of a vein in this region causes a blockage of drainage and a backup of perfusion, with resultant ischemia of the tissue in the regions of drainage.

Veins of Posterior Cranial Fossa

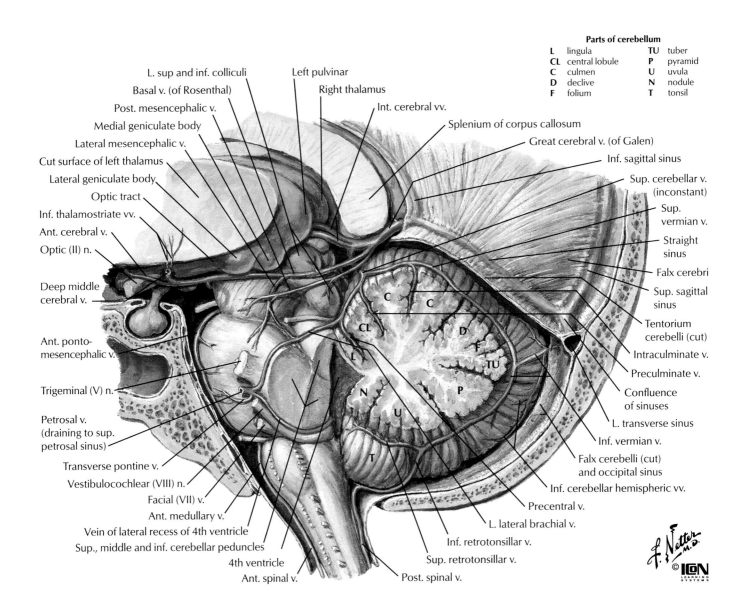

Parts of cerebellum

L	lingula	TU	tuber
CL	central lobule	P	pyramid
C	culmen	U	uvula
D	declive	N	nodule
F	folium	T	tonsil

L. sup and inf. colliculi
Basal v. (of Rosenthal)
Post. mesencephalic v.
Medial geniculate body
Lateral mesencephalic v.
Cut surface of left thalamus
Lateral geniculate body
Optic tract
Inf. thalamostriate vv.
Ant. cerebral v.
Optic (II) n.
Deep middle cerebral v.
Ant. ponto-mesencephalic v.
Trigeminal (V) n.
Petrosal v. (draining to sup. petrosal sinus)
Transverse pontine v.
Vestibulocochlear (VIII) n.
Facial (VII) v.
Ant. medullary v.
Vein of lateral recess of 4th ventricle
Sup., middle and inf. cerebellar peduncles
4th ventricle
Ant. spinal v.

Left pulvinar
Right thalamus
Int. cerebral vv.
Splenium of corpus callosum
Great cerebral v. (of Galen)
Inf. sagittal sinus
Sup. cerebellar v. (inconstant)
Sup. vermian v.
Straight sinus
Falx cerebri
Sup. sagittal sinus
Tentorium cerebelli (cut)
Intraculminate v.
Preculminate v.
Confluence of sinuses
L. transverse sinus
Inf. vermian v.
Falx cerebelli (cut) and occipital sinus
Inf. cerebellar hemispheric vv.
Precentral v.
L. lateral brachial v.
Inf. retrotonsillar v.
Sup. retrotonsillar v.
Post. spinal v.

FIGURE I.62: VENOUS DRAINAGE OF THE BRAIN STEM AND THE CEREBELLUM

The venous drainage of the cerebellum and the brain stem is anatomically diverse. The veins of the posterior fossa drain the cerebellum and the brain stem. The superior group drains the superior cerebellum and the upper brain stem posteriorly into the great cerebral vein of Galen and the straight sinus or laterally into the transverse and superior petrosal sinuses. The anterior, or petrosal, group drains the anterior brain stem, the superior and inferior surfaces of the cerebellar hemispheres, and the lateral regions associated with the fourth ventricle into the superior petrosal sinus. The posterior, or tentorial, group drains the inferior portion of the cerebellar vermis and the medial portion of the superior and inferior cerebellar hemispheres into the transverse sinus or the straight sinus.

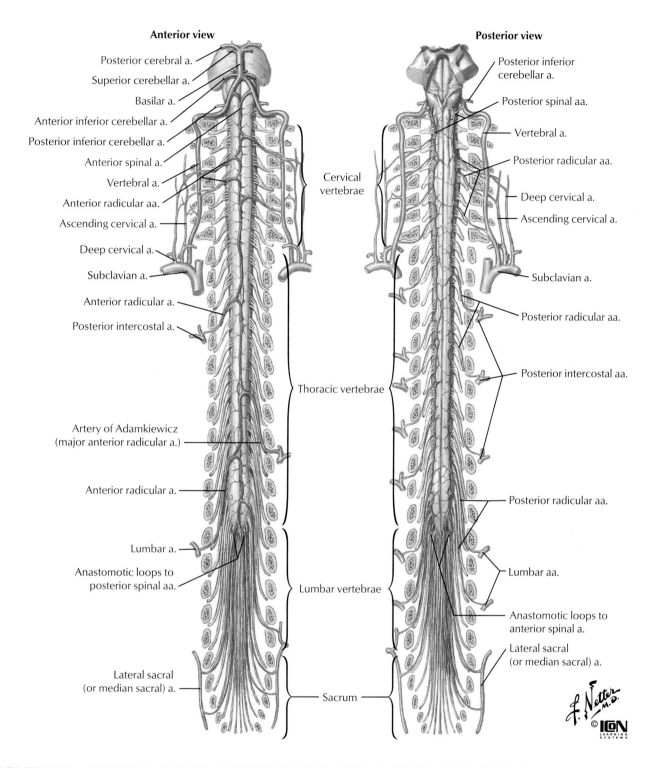

Anterior view

- Posterior cerebral a.
- Superior cerebellar a.
- Basilar a.
- Anterior inferior cerebellar a.
- Posterior inferior cerebellar a.
- Anterior spinal a.
- Vertebral a.
- Anterior radicular aa.
- Ascending cervical a.
- Deep cervical a.
- Subclavian a.
- Anterior radicular a.
- Posterior intercostal a.
- Artery of Adamkiewicz (major anterior radicular a.)
- Anterior radicular a.
- Lumbar a.
- Anastomotic loops to posterior spinal aa.
- Lateral sacral (or median sacral) a.

Cervical vertebrae

Thoracic vertebrae

Lumbar vertebrae

Sacrum

Posterior view

- Posterior inferior cerebellar a.
- Posterior spinal aa.
- Vertebral a.
- Posterior radicular aa.
- Deep cervical a.
- Ascending cervical a.
- Subclavian a.
- Posterior radicular aa.
- Posterior intercostal aa.
- Posterior radicular aa.
- Lumbar aa.
- Anastomotic loops to anterior spinal a.
- Lateral sacral (or median sacral) a.

FIGURE I.63: ARTERIAL BLOOD SUPPLY TO THE SPINAL CORD: LONGITUDINAL VIEW

The major arterial blood supply to the spinal cord derives from the anterior spinal artery (ASA) and the paired posterior spinal arteries (PSAs), both branches of the vertebral artery. The actual blood flow through these arteries, derived from the posterior circulation, is inadequate to maintain the spinal cord beyond the cervical segments. Radicular arteries, deriving from the aorta, provide major anastomoses with the ASA and the PSAs and supplement the blood flow to the spinal cord. Impaired flow through these critical radicular arteries, especially during surgical procedures with abrupt disruption of blood flow through the aorta, can result in spinal cord infarct.

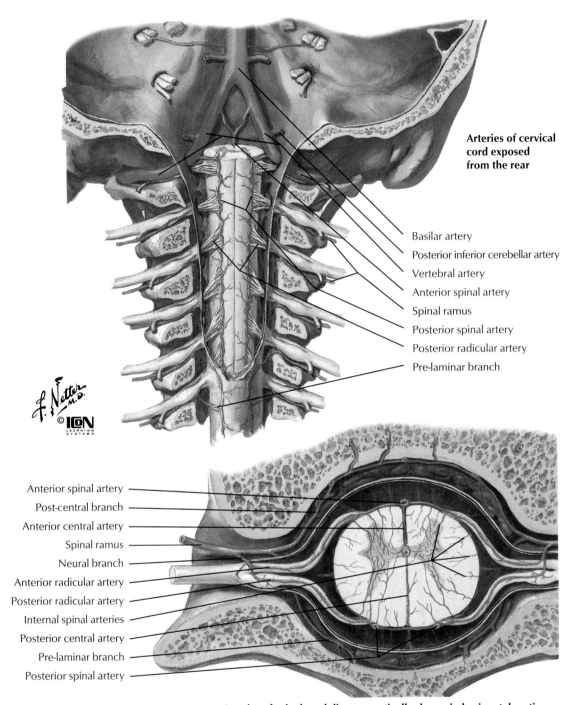

Arteries of cervical
cord exposed
from the rear

Basilar artery
Posterior inferior cerebellar artery
Vertebral artery
Anterior spinal artery
Spinal ramus
Posterior spinal artery
Posterior radicular artery
Pre-laminar branch

Anterior spinal artery
Post-central branch
Anterior central artery
Spinal ramus
Neural branch
Anterior radicular artery
Posterior radicular artery
Internal spinal arteries
Posterior central artery
Pre-laminar branch
Posterior spinal artery

Arteries of spinal cord diagrammatically shown in horizontal section

FIGURE I.64: ANTERIOR AND POSTERIOR SPINAL ARTERIES AND THEIR DISTRIBUTION ——

The ASA and PSAs travel in the SA space and send branches into the spinal cord. The ASA sends alternating branches into the anterior median fissure to supply the anterior two-thirds of the spinal cord. Occlusion results in ipsilateral flaccid paralysis in muscles supplied by the affected segments, ipsilateral spastic paralysis below the affected level (upper motor neuron axonal damage), and contralateral loss of pain and temperature sensation below the affected level (damage to the anterolateral spinothalamic/spinoreticular system). The PSA branches supply the dorsal third of the spinal cord. Occlusion affects the ipsilateral perception of fine discriminative touch, vibratory sensation, and joint position sense below the level of the lesion (from damage to fasciculi gracilis and cuneatus, the dorsal columns).

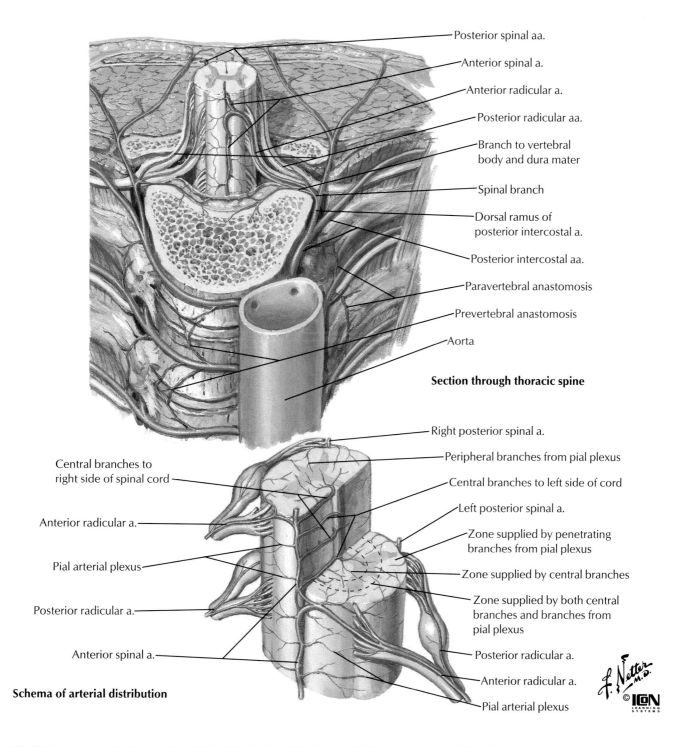

Posterior spinal aa.

Anterior spinal a.

Anterior radicular a.

Posterior radicular aa.

Branch to vertebral body and dura mater

Spinal branch

Dorsal ramus of posterior intercostal a.

Posterior intercostal aa.

Paravertebral anastomosis

Prevertebral anastomosis

Aorta

Section through thoracic spine

Central branches to right side of spinal cord

Anterior radicular a.

Pial arterial plexus

Posterior radicular a.

Anterior spinal a.

Schema of arterial distribution

Right posterior spinal a.

Peripheral branches from pial plexus

Central branches to left side of cord

Left posterior spinal a.

Zone supplied by penetrating branches from pial plexus

Zone supplied by central branches

Zone supplied by both central branches and branches from pial plexus

Posterior radicular a.

Anterior radicular a.

Pial arterial plexus

FIGURE I.65: ARTERIAL SUPPLY TO THE SPINAL CORD: CROSS-SECTIONAL VIEW

The major contribution to the arterial blood supply of the spinal cord derives from the aorta via the radicular arteries (top). This intercostal blood supply also distributes to adjacent bony and muscular structures. The penetrating vessels supplying the spinal cord derive from central branches of the ASA and from a pial plexus of vessels that surrounds the exterior of the spinal cord.

Veins of Spinal Cord and Vertebrae

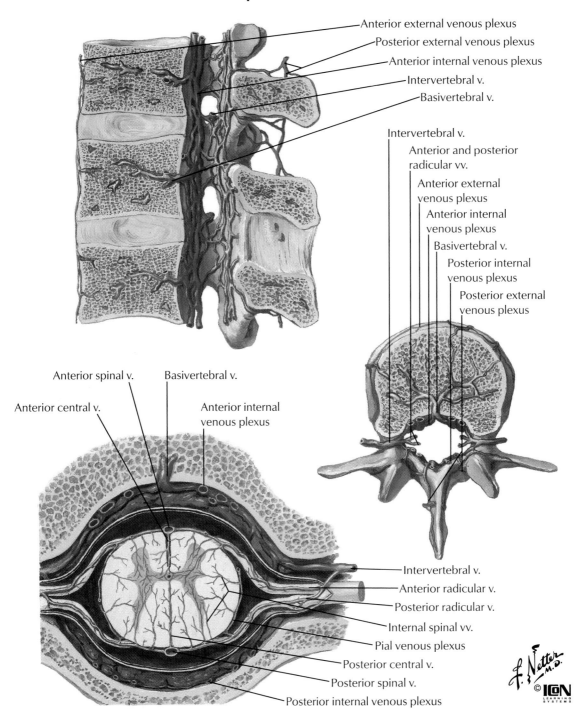

Anterior external venous plexus
Posterior external venous plexus
Anterior internal venous plexus
Intervertebral v.
Basivertebral v.

Intervertebral v.
Anterior and posterior radicular vv.
Anterior external venous plexus
Anterior internal venous plexus
Basivertebral v.
Posterior internal venous plexus
Posterior external venous plexus

Anterior spinal v.   Basivertebral v.
Anterior central v.   Anterior internal venous plexus

Intervertebral v.
Anterior radicular v.
Posterior radicular v.
Internal spinal vv.
Pial venous plexus
Posterior central v.
Posterior spinal v.
Posterior internal venous plexus

FIGURE I.66: VENOUS DRAINAGE OF THE SPINAL CORD

An external and an internal plexus of veins extends along the length of the vertebral column, forming a series of venous "rings" with extensive anastomoses around each vertebra. Blood from the spinal cord, the vertebrae, and the ligaments drains into these plexuses. Changes in intrathoracic pressure and CSF pressure can be conveyed through these venous plexuses, affecting the venous volume. Ultimately, these venous plexuses drain through the intervertebral veins into vertebral, posterior intercostal, subcostal, and lumbar and lateral sacral veins.

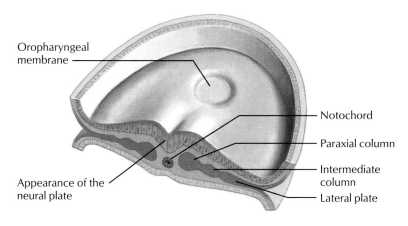

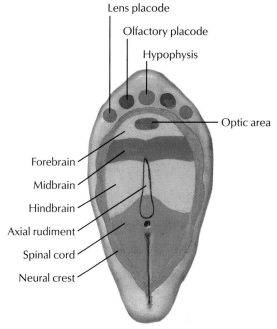

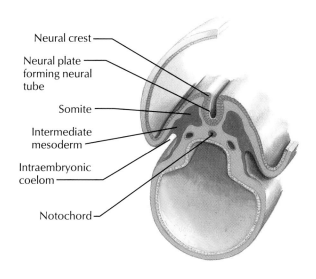

**Developmental fates of
local regions of ectoderm
of embryonic disc at 18 days**

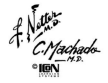

FIGURE I.67: FORMATION OF THE NEURAL PLATE, NEURAL TUBE, AND NEURAL CREST

The neural plate, neural tube, and neural crest form at the 18-day stage of embryonic development. The underlying notochord induces the neural plate, and a midline neural groove forms. The elevated lateral margins become the neural folds, tissue destined to become the neural crest with a future contribution to many components of the PNS. At this very early stage of embryonic development, these neural precursors are vulnerable to toxic or other forms of insult.

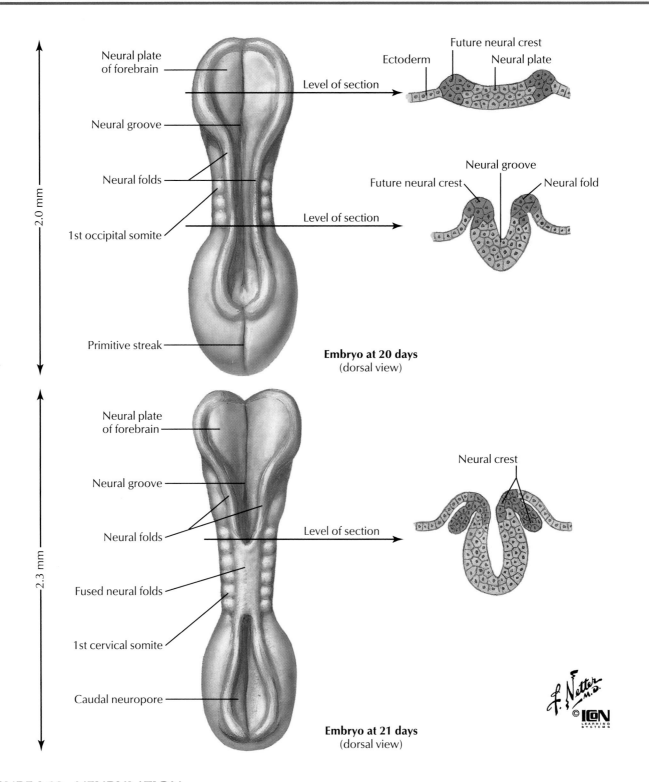

Embryo at 20 days
(dorsal view)

Embryo at 21 days
(dorsal view)

FIGURE I.68: NEURULATION

In the 21- to 22-day-old embryo, the neural plate, with its midline neural groove, thickens and begins to fold and elevate along either side, allowing the 2 lateral edges to fuse at the dorsal midline to form the completed neural tube. The central canal, the site of the future development of the ventricular system, is in the center of the neural tube. This process of neurulation continues both caudally and rostrally. Disruption can occur because of failure of full neural tube formation caudally (spina bifida) or rostrally (anencephaly).

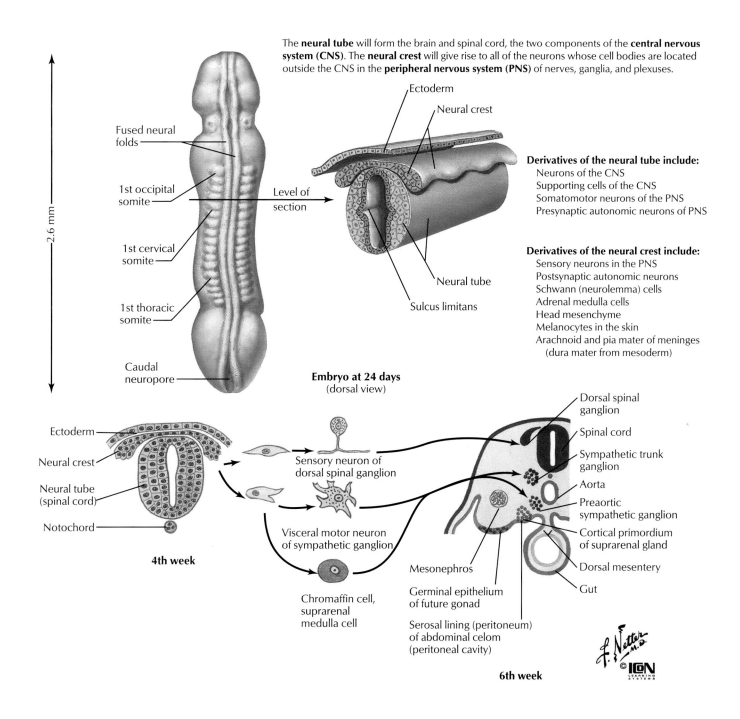

The **neural tube** will form the brain and spinal cord, the two components of the **central nervous system (CNS)**. The **neural crest** will give rise to all of the neurons whose cell bodies are located outside the CNS in the **peripheral nervous system (PNS)** of nerves, ganglia, and plexuses.

Derivatives of the neural tube include:
Neurons of the CNS
Supporting cells of the CNS
Somatomotor neurons of the PNS
Presynaptic autonomic neurons of PNS

Derivatives of the neural crest include:
Sensory neurons in the PNS
Postsynaptic autonomic neurons
Schwann (neurolemma) cells
Adrenal medulla cells
Head mesenchyme
Melanocytes in the skin
Arachnoid and pia mater of meninges
(dura mater from mesoderm)

Embryo at 24 days
(dorsal view)

4th week

6th week

FIGURE I.69: NEURAL TUBE DEVELOPMENT AND NEURAL CREST FORMATION

The dorsal and ventral halves of the neural tube are separated by the sulcus limitans, an external protrusion from the central canal that demarcates the alar plate from the basal plate. This important landmark persists at some sites in the adult ventricular system. The alar plate is the source of generation of many neurons with sensory function. The basal plate is the source of generation of many neurons with motor or autonomic function in the spinal cord and the brain stem. The neural crest cells at the edge of the neural folds unite to become a dorsal crest, the neural crest above the neural tube. The neural tube and the neural crest separate from the originating ectoderm. The neural crest gives rise to many cell types in the periphery.

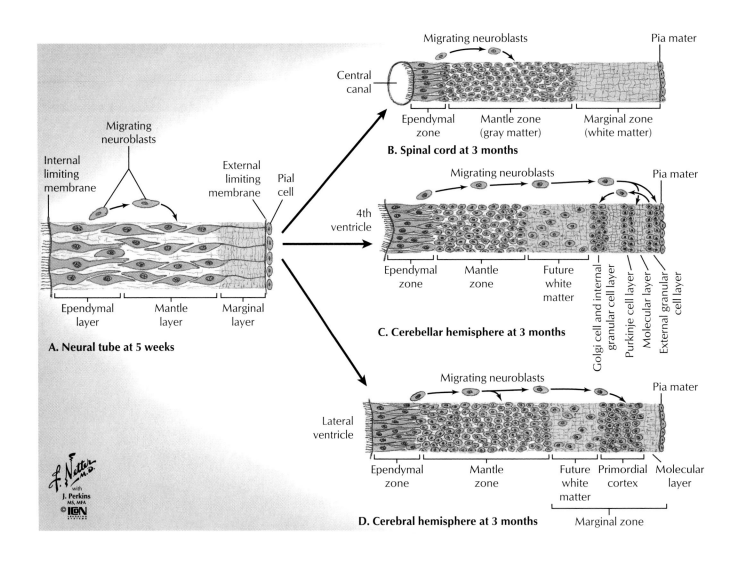

B. Spinal cord at 3 months

C. Cerebellar hemisphere at 3 months

A. Neural tube at 5 weeks

D. Cerebral hemisphere at 3 months

FIGURE I.70: NEURAL PROLIFERATION AND DIFFERENTIATION:
WALLS OF THE NEURAL TUBE

Early in development (5 weeks), neuroblasts in the ependymal layer lining the central canal move back and forth from the ependymal surface to the pial surface, replicating as they go. Neural migration follows distinctive patterns in different regions of the neural tube. In the spinal cord, neurons migrate into the inner mantle zone, leaving the outer marginal zone as a site for axonal pathways. In the cerebellar cortex, some neurons migrate to a location on the outer pial surface as an external granular layer, from which granule cells then migrate inward to synapse with other neurons present in the deeper layers of the cerebellar cortex. In the cerebral cortex, neurons migrate to the outer zone, where the gray matter remains on the surface, external to the white matter. These developmental patterns reflect the anatomical organization of the mature structures, their blood supply, and their vulnerability to a variety of insults.

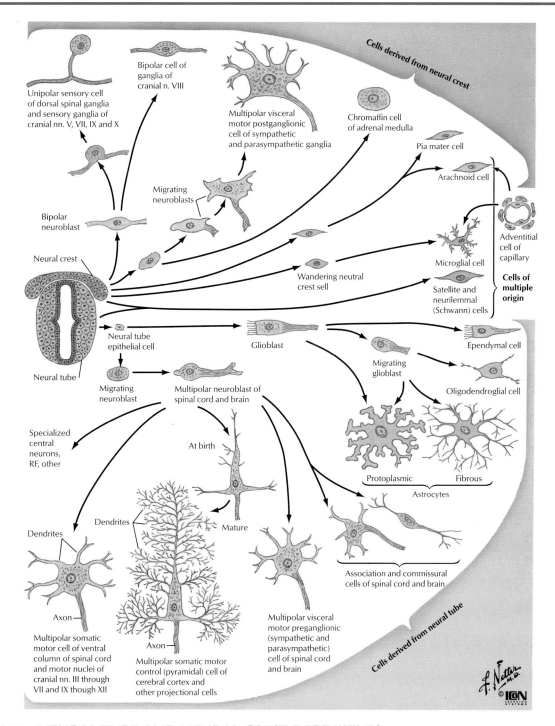

FIGURE I.71: NEURAL TUBE AND NEURAL CREST DERIVATIVES

Neural tube ependymal cells give rise to neuroblasts from which the neurons of the CNS are derived. They also give rise to the glioblasts from which the mature ependymal cells, astrocytes, and oligodendroglia are derived. Microglia, the "scavenger" cells of the CNS, are derived mainly from mesodermal precursors. Cells of glial origin are the predominant cells that give rise to CNS tumors. The neural crest cells give rise to many peripheral neural structures, including primary sensory neurons, postganglionic autonomic neurons (sympathetic and parasympathetic), adrenal medullary chromaffin cells, pial and arachnoid cells, Schwann cells (the supporting cells of the PNS), and other specialized cell types. Neural crest cells can be damaged selectively in some disorders (e.g., familial dysautonomia) and also can give rise to specific tumor cell types, such as pheochromocytomas.

Central nervous system at 28 days

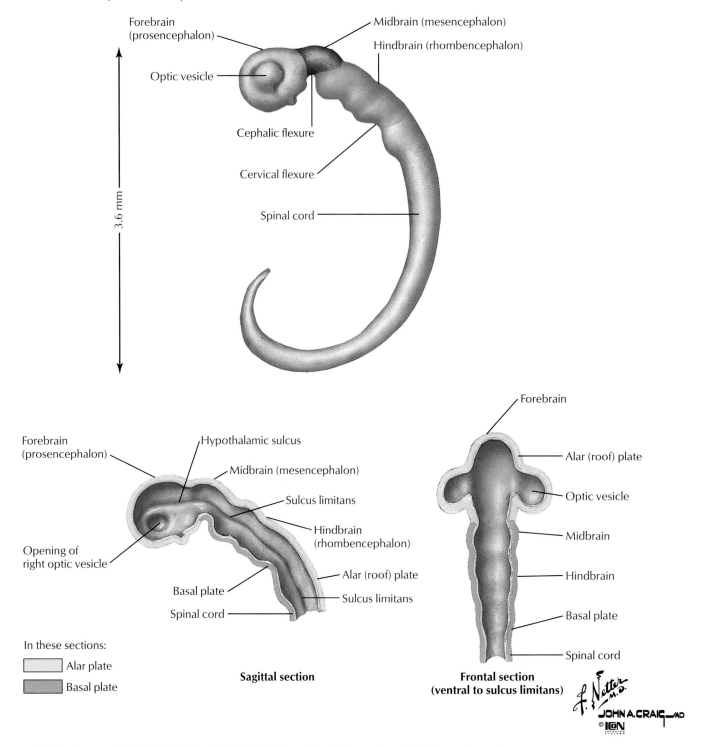

FIGURE I.72: EARLY BRAIN DEVELOPMENT: THE 28-DAY-OLD EMBRYO

Some components of the neural tube expand differentially, resulting in bends or flexures that separate the neural tube into caudal to rostral components. The cervical flexure, caudally, and the cephalic flexure, rostrally, result from the differential expansion. Three regions of rapid cellular proliferation develop—the forebrain (prosencephalon) rostrally, the mesencephalon (midbrain) in the middle, and the hindbrain (rhombencephalon) caudally. The ventricular system bends and expands to accommodate increasing neural growth. An outgrowth of the caudal part of the prosencephalon extends from the future diencephalon to become the optic vesicle, giving rise to the future retina and its central connections.

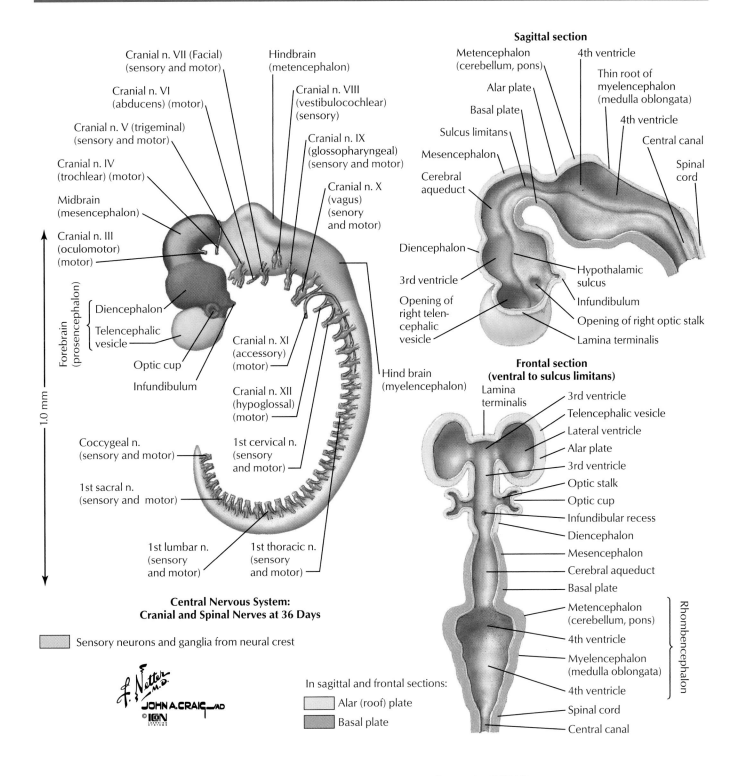

Cranial n. VII (Facial) (sensory and motor)
Cranial n. VI (abducens) (motor)
Cranial n. V (trigeminal) (sensory and motor)
Cranial n. IV (trochlear) (motor)
Midbrain (mesencephalon)
Cranial n. III (oculomotor) (motor)

Forebrain (prosencephalon)
Diencephalon
Telencephalic vesicle
Optic cup
Infundibulum

Hindbrain (metencephalon)
Cranial n. VIII (vestibulocochlear) (sensory)
Cranial n. IX (glossopharyngeal) (sensory and motor)
Cranial n. X (vagus) (senory and motor)

Cranial n. XI (accessory) (motor)
Cranial n. XII (hypoglossal) (motor)
1st cervical n. (sensory and motor)
Hind brain (myelencephalon)

Coccygeal n. (sensory and motor)
1st sacral n. (sensory and motor)
1st lumbar n. (sensory and motor)
1st thoracic n. (sensory and motor)

1.0 mm

Central Nervous System: Cranial and Spinal Nerves at 36 Days

Sensory neurons and ganglia from neural crest

Sagittal section
Metencephalon (cerebellum, pons)
Alar plate
Basal plate
Sulcus limitans
Mesencephalon
Cerebral aqueduct
Diencephalon
3rd ventricle
Opening of right telencephalic vesicle

4th ventricle
Thin root of myelencephalon (medulla oblongata)
4th ventricle
Central canal
Spinal cord
Hypothalamic sulcus
Infundibulum
Opening of right optic stalk
Lamina terminalis

Frontal section (ventral to sulcus limitans)
Lamina terminalis
3rd ventricle
Telencephalic vesicle
Lateral ventricle
Alar plate
3rd ventricle
Optic stalk
Optic cup
Infundibular recess
Diencephalon
Mesencephalon
Cerebral aqueduct
Basal plate
Metencephalon (cerebellum, pons)
4th ventricle
Myelencephalon (medulla oblongata)
4th ventricle
Spinal cord
Central canal
Rhombencephalon

In sagittal and frontal sections:
Alar (roof) plate
Basal plate

JOHN A. CRAIG ᴍᴅ
©ICN

FIGURE I.73: EARLY BRAIN DEVELOPMENT: THE 36-DAY-OLD EMBRYO

By day 36, the prosencephalon begins to expand rapidly as the future diencephalon (thalamus and hypothalamus) and telencephalon (basal ganglia, limbic forebrain, olfactory system, and cerebral cortex). This rapid growth is accompanied by the formation of the thin, third ventricle for the diencephalon and the C-shaped lateral ventricles from the rostral end of the original central canal for the telencephalon. The rhombencephalon further develops into 2 distinct regions, the metencephalon (future pons and cerebellum) and the myelencephalon (future medulla). Distinct spinal nerves and cranial nerves begin to form as sensory and motor neurons differentiate and begin to connect with their targets in the periphery.

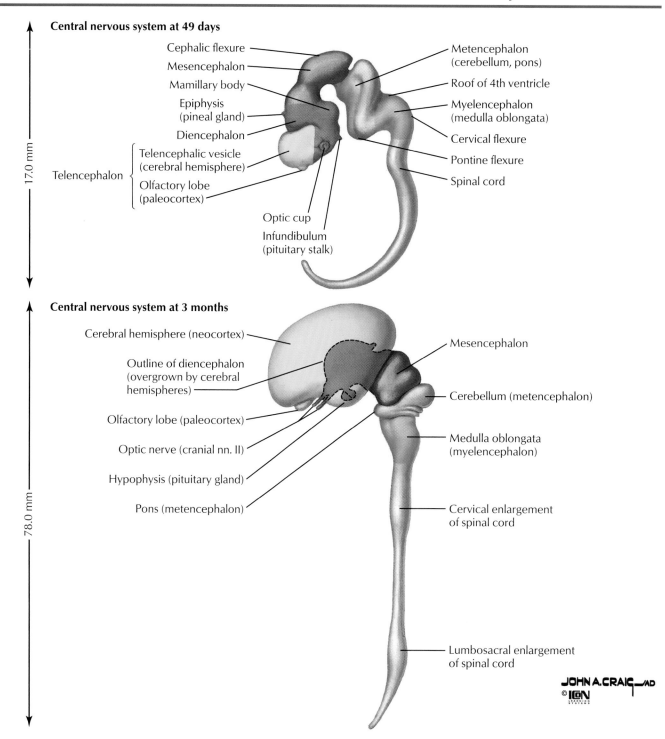

Central nervous system at 49 days

Cephalic flexure
Mesencephalon
Mamillary body
Epiphysis (pineal gland)
Diencephalon
Telencephalon
Telencephalic vesicle (cerebral hemisphere)
Olfactory lobe (paleocortex)
Optic cup
Infundibulum (pituitary stalk)

Metencephalon (cerebellum, pons)
Roof of 4th ventricle
Myelencephalon (medulla oblongata)
Cervical flexure
Pontine flexure
Spinal cord

17.0 mm

Central nervous system at 3 months

Cerebral hemisphere (neocortex)
Outline of diencephalon (overgrown by cerebral hemispheres)
Olfactory lobe (paleocortex)
Optic nerve (cranial nn. II)
Hypophysis (pituitary gland)
Pons (metencephalon)

Mesencephalon
Cerebellum (metencephalon)
Medulla oblongata (myelencephalon)
Cervical enlargement of spinal cord
Lumbosacral enlargement of spinal cord

78.0 mm

JOHN A. CRAIG—AD
© ICN

FIGURE I.74: EARLY BRAIN DEVELOPMENT: THE 49-DAY-OLD AND THE 3-MONTH-OLD EMBRYOS

By 49 days of age, the diencephalon and the telencephalon differentiate into distinct components: the dorsal thalamus and the ventral hypothalamus, and the olfactory lobe and the future cerebral hemispheres, respectively. The metencephalon (pons) and the myelencephalon (medulla) develop further and fold, separated by the pontine flexure dorsally. Between 49 days and 3 months, massive development of the telencephalon overrides and

covers the diencephalon. The cerebellum forms from the rhombic lips of the metencephalon, as neurons travel dorsally to overlie the future pons and eventually most of the brain stem. The mesencephalon expands dorsally, forming the superior and inferior colliculi (quadrigeminal bodies). The continuing growth of the spinal cord as it connects with peripheral tissues in the developing limbs forms the cervical and lumbosacral enlargements.

Forebrain at 7 Weeks (transverse section)

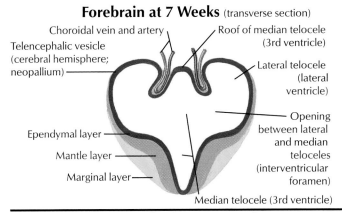

Choroidal vein and artery

Roof of median telocele (3rd ventricle)

Telencephalic vesicle (cerebral hemisphere; neopallium)

Lateral telocele (lateral ventricle)

Opening between lateral and median teloceles (interventricular foramen)

Ependymal layer

Mantle layer

Marginal layer

Median telocele (3rd ventricle)

Telencephalon at 7½ Weeks (transverse section)

Choroidal vein and artery

Roof of 3rd ventricle

Telencephalic vesicle (cerebral hemisphere; neopallium)

Hippocampus (archipallium)

Lateral ventricle

Choroid plexus

Ependymal layer

Interventricular foramen

Mantle layer

Corpus striatum (basal ganglion)

Marginal layer

3rd ventricle

Anterior lobe of hypophysis (pituitary gland)

Infundibulum (pituitary stalk)

Forebrain at 2 Months (coronal section; anterior view)

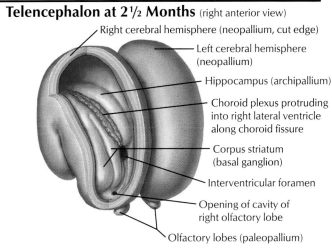

Epiphysis (pineal gland)

Diencephalon

Cerebral hemisphere (neopallium, cut edge)

Roof of 3rd ventricle

Hippocampus (archipallium)

Choroid plexus

Choroid fissure

Thalamus

Lateral ventricle

Corpus striatum (basal ganglion)

Interventricular foramen

3rd ventricle

Optic (nerve) stalk

Lamina terminalis

Telencephalon at 2½ Months (right anterior view)

Right cerebral hemisphere (neopallium, cut edge)

Left cerebral hemisphere (neopallium)

Hippocampus (archipallium)

Choroid plexus protruding into right lateral ventricle along choroid fissure

Corpus striatum (basal ganglion)

Interventricular foramen

Opening of cavity of right olfactory lobe

Olfactory lobes (paleopallium)

Right Cerebral Hemisphere at 3 Months (medial aspect)

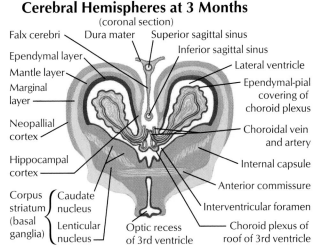

Corpus callosum

Medial surface of right cerebral hemisphere (neopallium)

Commissure of fornix (hippocampal commissure)

Choroidal vessels passing to choroid plexus, which protrudes into right lateral ventricle along choroid fissure

Fornix

Anterior commissure

Lamina terminalis

Hippocampus (archipallium)

Olfactory lobe (paleopallium)

Stria terminalis

3rd ventricle

Thalamus (cut surface)

Line of division between diencephalon and telencephalon

Cerebral Hemispheres at 3 Months (coronal section)

Falx cerebri

Dura mater

Superior sagittal sinus

Inferior sagittal sinus

Ependymal layer

Lateral ventricle

Mantle layer

Ependymal-pial covering of choroid plexus

Marginal layer

Neopallial cortex

Choroidal vein and artery

Hippocampal cortex

Internal capsule

Corpus striatum (basal ganglia) { Caudate nucleus, Lenticular nucleus }

Anterior commissure

Interventricular foramen

Optic recess of 3rd ventricle

Choroid plexus of roof of 3rd ventricle

FIGURE I.75: FOREBRAIN DEVELOPMENT: 7 WEEKS THROUGH 3 MONTHS

Neurons of the developing telencephalon move rostrally, dorsally, and then around the diencephalon in a C-shaped course toward the anterior pole of the temporal lobe. The hippocampus forms in a dorsal and anterior position and migrates in a C-shaped course into the anterior temporal lobe, leaving the fornix in its wake. The amygdala develops in a similar manner, giving rise to the stria terminalis in a C-shape. The lateral ventricles follow the same C-shaped developmental process anatomically. The caudate nucleus also extends around the telencephalon in a C-shaped pattern, with the head of the caudate remaining anterior and the much smaller body and tail following as a thinner C-shaped structure that ends ventrally in the temporal horn of the lateral ventricle. The corpus callosum and the anterior commissure connect the 2 hemispheres. The internal capsule funnels centrally in the core of the forebrain on either side and continues caudally as the cerebral peduncle.

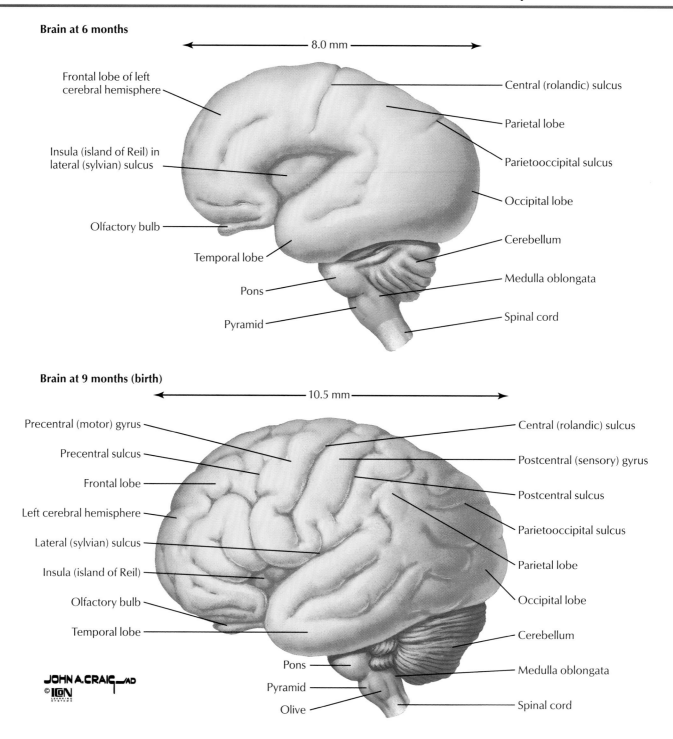

Brain at 6 months

8.0 mm

Frontal lobe of left cerebral hemisphere

Insula (island of Reil) in lateral (sylvian) sulcus

Olfactory bulb

Temporal lobe

Pons

Pyramid

Central (rolandic) sulcus

Parietal lobe

Parietooccipital sulcus

Occipital lobe

Cerebellum

Medulla oblongata

Spinal cord

Brain at 9 months (birth)

10.5 mm

Precentral (motor) gyrus

Precentral sulcus

Frontal lobe

Left cerebral hemisphere

Lateral (sylvian) sulcus

Insula (island of Reil)

Olfactory bulb

Temporal lobe

Pons

Pyramid

Olive

Central (rolandic) sulcus

Postcentral (sensory) gyrus

Postcentral sulcus

Parietooccipital sulcus

Parietal lobe

Occipital lobe

Cerebellum

Medulla oblongata

Spinal cord

JOHN A. CRAIG AD
© ICON

FIGURE I.76: THE 6-MONTH AND THE 9-MONTH CENTRAL NERVOUS SYSTEM

At 6 months, the brain stem has differentiated into the medulla, the pons, and the midbrain, with the cerebellum overlying them dorsally. Even though the diencephalon is rapidly developing, the overlying telencephalon shows massive growth rostrally, then caudally, downward and forward into the temporal lobe. From 6 to 9 months, the cerebral cortex forms its characteristic convolutions with gyri and sulci, and the cerebellar cortex forms its distinctive folds, the folia. Within the forebrain, the major components of the basal ganglia, the limbic structures (e.g., amygdala and hippocampal formation), the olfactory system, and the cerebral cortex develop rapidly. Most neurons are present at birth, except for some populations of granular cells in the cerebellum, the hippocampal dentate gyrus, and the cerebral cortex, which form postnatally in response to environmental stimuli. The in utero and postnatal environments provide major influences on neuronal development and function.

Frontal section (ventral to sulcus limitans) at 36 days

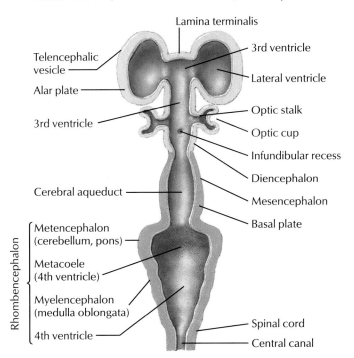

Lamina terminalis
Telencephalic vesicle
3rd ventricle
Lateral ventricle
Alar plate
Optic stalk
3rd ventricle
Optic cup
Infundibular recess
Diencephalon
Mesencephalon
Cerebral aqueduct
Basal plate
Rhombencephalon
Metencephalon (cerebellum, pons)
Metacoele (4th ventricle)
Myelencephalon (medulla oblongata)
Spinal cord
4th ventricle
Central canal

Ependymal lining of cavities of brain at 3 months

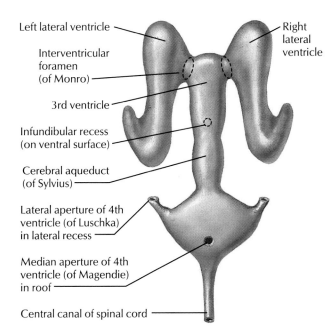

Left lateral ventricle
Right lateral ventricle
Interventricular foramen (of Monro)
3rd ventricle
Infundibular recess (on ventral surface)
Cerebral aqueduct (of Sylvius)
Lateral aperture of 4th ventricle (of Luschka) in lateral recess
Median aperture of 4th ventricle (of Magendie) in roof
Central canal of spinal cord

Ependymal lining of cavities of brain at 9 months (birth)

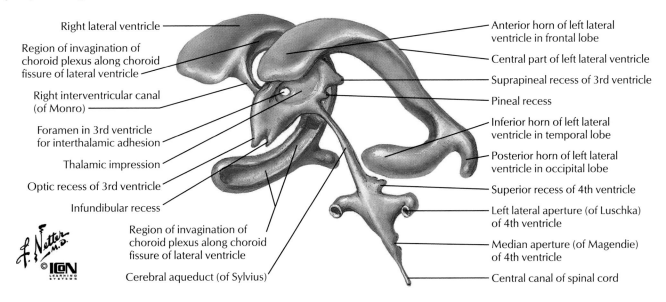

Right lateral ventricle
Region of invagination of choroid plexus along choroid fissure of lateral ventricle
Right interventricular canal (of Monro)
Foramen in 3rd ventricle for interthalamic adhesion
Thalamic impression
Optic recess of 3rd ventricle
Infundibular recess
Region of invagination of choroid plexus along choroid fissure of lateral ventricle
Cerebral aqueduct (of Sylvius)
Anterior horn of left lateral ventricle in frontal lobe
Central part of left lateral ventricle
Suprapineal recess of 3rd ventricle
Pineal recess
Inferior horn of left lateral ventricle in temporal lobe
Posterior horn of left lateral ventricle in occipital lobe
Superior recess of 4th ventricle
Left lateral aperture (of Luschka) of 4th ventricle
Median aperture (of Magendie) of 4th ventricle
Central canal of spinal cord

FIGURE I.77: DEVELOPMENT OF THE VENTRICLES

The rapid growth of the brain stem and the forebrain alters the uniform appearance of the ventricles. The C-shaped lateral ventricles follow the growth of the telencephalon, with limited access into the third ventricle through the interventricular foramen of Monro. The narrow cerebral aqueduct remains very small in the upper mesencephalon and opens into the rhombus-shaped and expanding fourth ventricle. The foramina of Magendie (medial) and Luschka (lateral) open the ventricular system into the developing cisterns of the subarachnoid (SA) space at the medial and lateral margins of the fourth ventricle, respectively. CSF reenters the venous system through the arachnoid granulations, one-way valves allowing drainage from the SA space into the dural (venous) sinuses, especially the superior sagittal sinus.

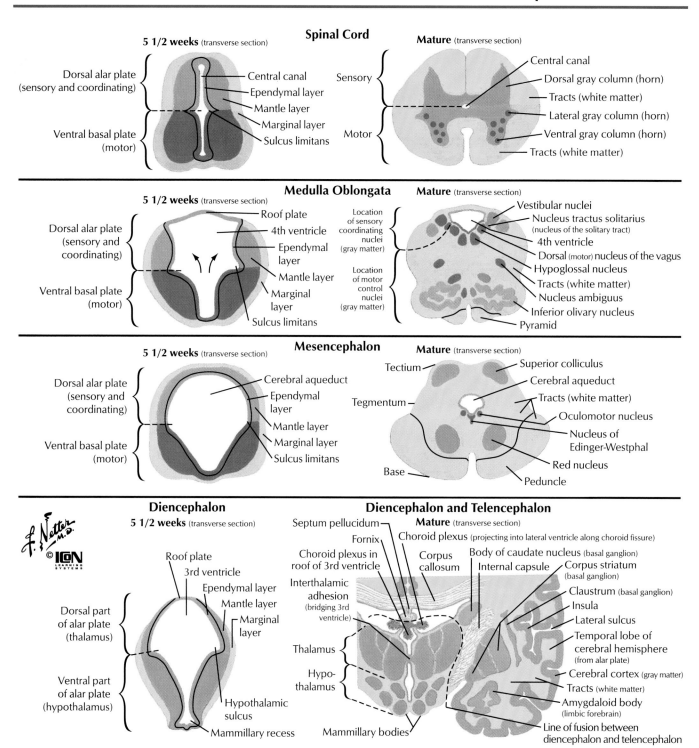

FIGURE I.78: COMPARISON OF 5½-WEEK AND ADULT CENTRAL NERVOUS SYSTEM REGIONS

At 5½ weeks, the ventricular system becomes comparatively smaller as neuronal growth occurs. In adults, the central canal of the spinal cord is virtually obliterated. The fourth ventricle opens up laterally; the sulcus limitans demarcates motor nuclei (medially) and sensory nuclei (laterally). The cerebral aqueduct remains very small. The third ventricle narrows to a slit. The lateral ventricles expand massively into a C-shaped form. The basal plate forms motor and autonomic structures whose axons leave the CNS. The alar plate forms sensory derivatives in the spinal cord and the brain stem, and structures that migrate ventrally (inferior olive, pontine nuclei, and red nucleus). The rhombic lips, an alar derivative of the metencephalon, give rise to the cerebellum. The diencephalon and the telencephalon are also alar plate derivatives.

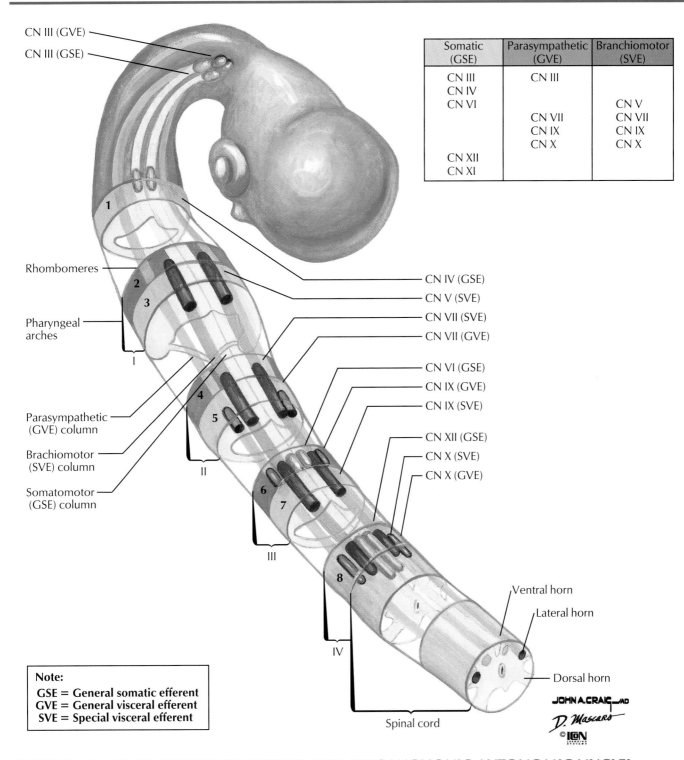

Somatic (GSE)	Parasympathetic (GVE)	Branchiomotor (SVE)
CN III	CN III	
CN IV		CN V
CN VI	CN VII	CN VII
	CN IX	CN IX
	CN X	CN X
CN XII		
CN XI		

Note:
GSE = General somatic efferent
GVE = General visceral efferent
SVE = Special visceral efferent

FIGURE I.79: DEVELOPMENT OF MOTOR AND PREGANGLIONIC AUTONOMIC NUCLEI IN THE BRAIN STEM AND THE SPINAL CORD

Gray matter columns develop in the spinal cord for somatic lower motor neurons (ventral horn) and preganglionic autonomic neurons (lateral horn). These columns extend rostrally into the brain stem, maintaining the same general positional relationship to each other but organized into a series of separate but aligned nuclei. A third group of nuclei develop in the rhombencephalon as branchiomotor neurons supplying pharyngeal arch muscles. Both the somatic motor and the branchiomotor neurons are classified as lower motor neurons and have axons exiting the CNS to synapse on skeletal muscle fibers.

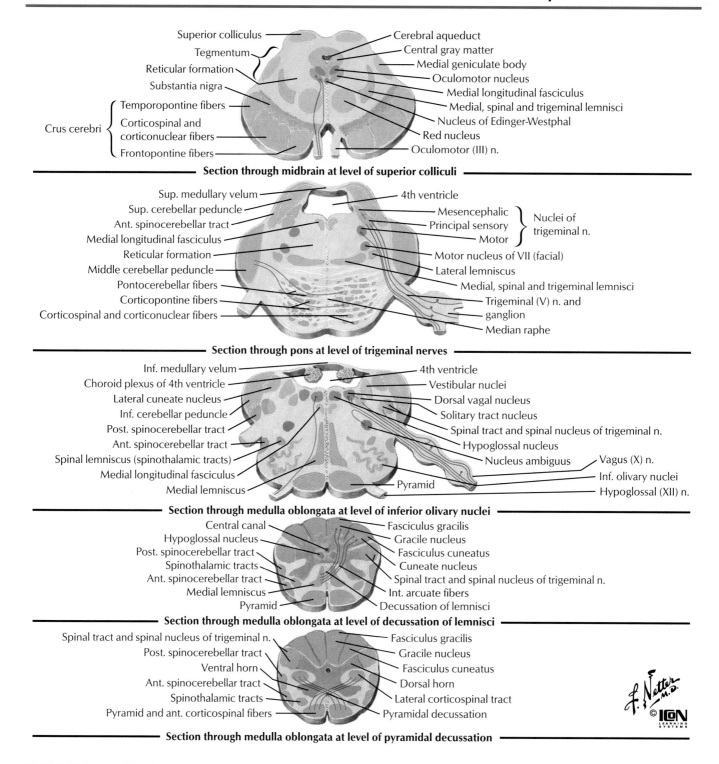

Superior colliculus — Cerebral aqueduct
Tegmentum — Central gray matter
Reticular formation — Medial geniculate body
Substantia nigra — Oculomotor nucleus
Crus cerebri {
Temporopontine fibers — Medial longitudinal fasciculus
Corticospinal and corticonuclear fibers — Medial, spinal and trigeminal lemnisci
Nucleus of Edinger-Westphal
Frontopontine fibers — Red nucleus
Oculomotor (III) n.

Section through midbrain at level of superior colliculi

Sup. medullary velum — 4th ventricle
Sup. cerebellar peduncle — Mesencephalic
Ant. spinocerebellar tract — Principal sensory } Nuclei of trigeminal n.
Medial longitudinal fasciculus — Motor
Reticular formation — Motor nucleus of VII (facial)
Middle cerebellar peduncle — Lateral lemniscus
Pontocerebellar fibers — Medial, spinal and trigeminal lemnisci
Corticopontine fibers — Trigeminal (V) n. and ganglion
Corticospinal and corticonuclear fibers — Median raphe

Section through pons at level of trigeminal nerves

Inf. medullary velum — 4th ventricle
Choroid plexus of 4th ventricle — Vestibular nuclei
Lateral cuneate nucleus — Dorsal vagal nucleus
Inf. cerebellar peduncle — Solitary tract nucleus
Post. spinocerebellar tract — Spinal tract and spinal nucleus of trigeminal n.
Ant. spinocerebellar tract — Hypoglossal nucleus
Spinal lemniscus (spinothalamic tracts) — Nucleus ambiguus — Vagus (X) n.
Medial longitudinal fasciculus — Pyramid — Inf. olivary nuclei
Medial lemniscus — Hypoglossal (XII) n.

Section through medulla oblongata at level of inferior olivary nuclei

Central canal — Fasciculus gracilis
Hypoglossal nucleus — Gracile nucleus
Post. spinocerebellar tract — Fasciculus cuneatus
Spinothalamic tracts — Cuneate nucleus
Ant. spinocerebellar tract — Spinal tract and spinal nucleus of trigeminal n.
Medial lemniscus — Int. arcuate fibers
Pyramid — Decussation of lemnisci

Section through medulla oblongata at level of decussation of lemnisci

Spinal tract and spinal nucleus of trigeminal n. — Fasciculus gracilis
Post. spinocerebellar tract — Gracile nucleus
Ventral horn — Fasciculus cuneatus
Ant. spinocerebellar tract — Dorsal horn
Spinothalamic tracts — Lateral corticospinal tract
Pyramid and ant. corticospinal fibers — Pyramidal decussation

Section through medulla oblongata at level of pyramidal decussation

FIGURE I.80: ALAR AND BASAL PLATE DERIVATIVES IN THE BRAIN STEM

"The general pattern of alar and basal plate derivatives seen in the spinal cord continues into the brain stem. The alar plate derivatives are the sensory nuclei, the rhombic lip from which the cerebellum is derived, and nuclei which migrate ventrally to form structures such as the inferior olivary nuclei, the pontine nuclei, the red nucleus, and others. The basal plate derivatives are the motor and preganglionic autonomic nuclei."

5¹/₂ weeks

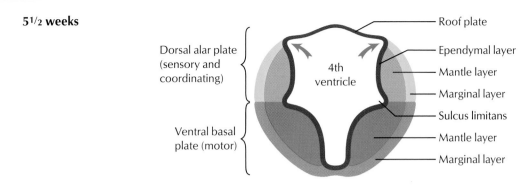

- Roof plate
- Ependymal layer
- Mantle layer
- Marginal layer
- Sulcus limitans
- Mantle layer
- Marginal layer

Dorsal alar plate (sensory and coordinating)

Ventral basal plate (motor)

4th ventricle

3¹/₂ months

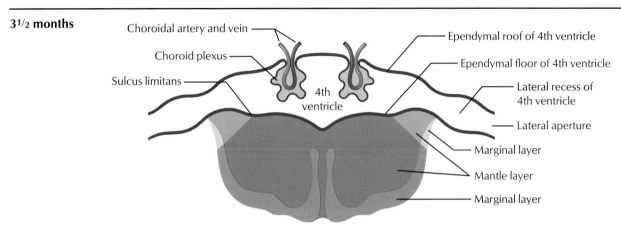

- Choroidal artery and vein
- Choroid plexus
- Sulcus limitans
- 4th ventricle
- Ependymal roof of 4th ventricle
- Ependymal floor of 4th ventricle
- Lateral recess of 4th ventricle
- Lateral aperture
- Marginal layer
- Mantle layer
- Marginal layer

Mature

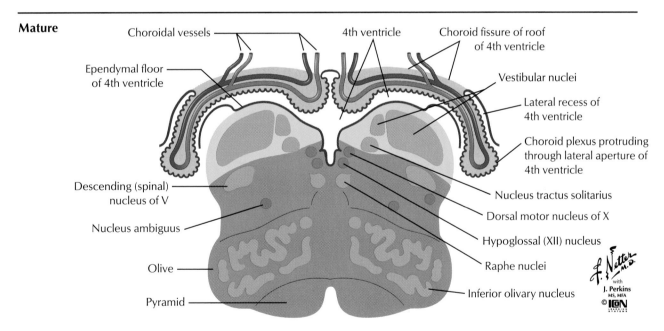

- Choroidal vessels
- 4th ventricle
- Choroid fissure of roof of 4th ventricle
- Ependymal floor of 4th ventricle
- Vestibular nuclei
- Lateral recess of 4th ventricle
- Choroid plexus protruding through lateral aperture of 4th ventricle
- Descending (spinal) nucleus of V
- Nucleus ambiguus
- Olive
- Pyramid
- Nucleus tractus solitarius
- Dorsal motor nucleus of X
- Hypoglossal (XII) nucleus
- Raphe nuclei
- Inferior olivary nucleus

FIGURE I.81: DEVELOPMENT OF THE FOURTH VENTRICLE

The expansion of the fourth ventricle from the original central canal of the rhombencephalon into its mature form is a complex process. The sulcus limitans is conspicuous early in development (5¹/₂ weeks), and the original lateral walls expand outward and lay down horizontally (3¹/₂ months) as the roof plate expands to either side; as a result, the sulcus limitans becomes a landmark at the dorsal boundary of the medulla on the floor of the fourth ventricle, separating the motor structures medially from the sensory structures laterally. The lateral aperture of the fourth ventricle opens into the SA space. In their mature form (lower illustration), these paired lateral apertures, the foramina of Luschka, are major channels between the internal and the external circulation of the CSF and must remain open to prevent internal hydrocephalus.

Differentiation and Growth of Neurons at 26 Days

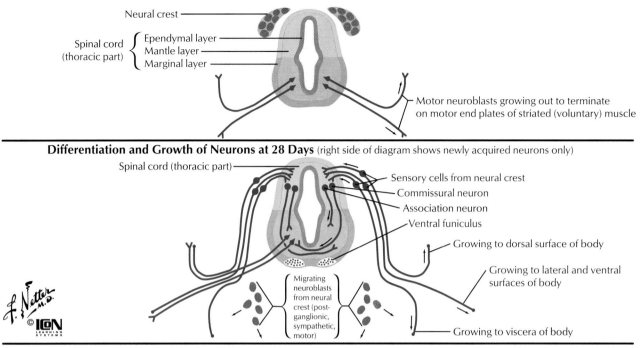

Neural crest

Spinal cord (thoracic part)
- Ependymal layer
- Mantle layer
- Marginal layer

Motor neuroblasts growing out to terminate on motor end plates of striated (voluntary) muscle

Differentiation and Growth of Neurons at 28 Days (right side of diagram shows newly acquired neurons only)

Spinal cord (thoracic part)

Sensory cells from neural crest
Commissural neuron
Association neuron
Ventral funiculus

Growing to dorsal surface of body

Growing to lateral and ventral surfaces of body

Migrating neuroblasts from neural crest (post-ganglionic, sympathetic, motor)

Growing to viscera of body

Differentiation and Growth of Neurons at 5 to 7 Weeks (right side of diagram shows neurons acquired since 28th day only)

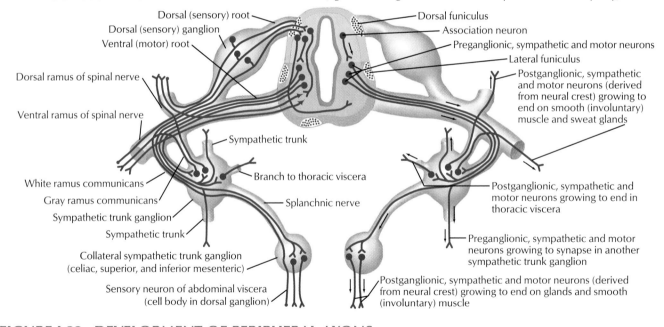

Dorsal (sensory) root
Dorsal (sensory) ganglion
Ventral (motor) root

Dorsal ramus of spinal nerve

Ventral ramus of spinal nerve

Dorsal funiculus
Association neuron
Preganglionic, sympathetic and motor neurons
Lateral funiculus
Postganglionic, sympathetic and motor neurons (derived from neural crest) growing to end on smooth (involuntary) muscle and sweat glands

Sympathetic trunk

Branch to thoracic viscera

White ramus communicans
Gray ramus communicans
Sympathetic trunk ganglion
Sympathetic trunk

Splanchnic nerve

Postganglionic, sympathetic and motor neurons growing to end in thoracic viscera

Collateral sympathetic trunk ganglion (celiac, superior, and inferior mesenteric)

Sensory neuron of abdominal viscera (cell body in dorsal ganglion)

Preganglionic, sympathetic and motor neurons growing to synapse in another sympathetic trunk ganglion

Postganglionic, sympathetic and motor neurons (derived from neural crest) growing to end on glands and smooth (involuntary) muscle

FIGURE I.82: DEVELOPMENT OF PERIPHERAL AXONS

Peripheral axon development is a complex process of neurite extension, trophic and chemotactic factors, axonal guidance, and maintenance by innervated target tissues. Dorsal root ganglion cells are bipolar; a peripheral axonal process associates with simple or complex sensory receptor cells, and a central axonal process extends into the CNS. The lower motor neurons send axons to the developing skeletal muscles through the ventral roots or the motor cranial nerves, forming neuromuscular junctions. Central preganglionic axons exit in the ventral roots and terminate on sympathetic ganglion cells in the sympathetic chain or collateral ganglia or parasympathetic intramural ganglia. Postganglionic axons form connections with target tissues, including smooth muscle, cardiac muscle, secretory glands, some metabolic cells (hepatocytes), and immune cells in lymphoid organs. Sensory, motor, and autonomic symptoms can occur in peripheral neuropathies based on disruption of these connections.

II. REGIONAL NEUROSCIENCE

A. PERIPHERAL NERVOUS SYSTEM (PNS)

A.1. INTRODUCTION AND BASIC ORGANIZATION

A.2. SOMATIC NERVOUS SYSTEM

A.3. AUTONOMIC NERVOUS SYSTEM (ANS)

D. DIENCEPHALON

E. TELENCEPHALON

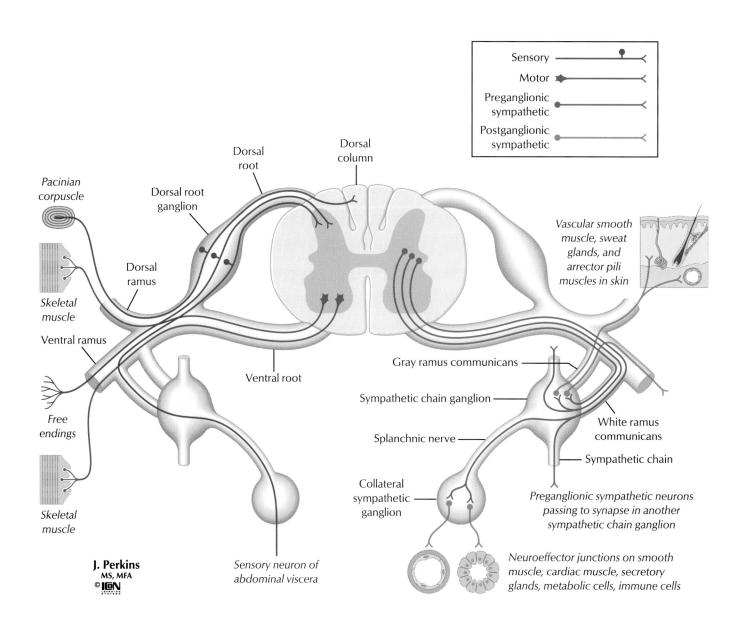

Sensory

Motor

Preganglionic
sympathetic

Postganglionic
sympathetic

Dorsal
root

Dorsal
column

Pacinian
corpuscle

Dorsal root
ganglion

Vascular smooth
muscle, sweat
glands, and
arrector pili
muscles in skin

Dorsal
ramus

Skeletal
muscle

Ventral ramus

Gray ramus communicans

Free
endings

Ventral root

Sympathetic chain ganglion

White ramus
communicans

Splanchnic nerve

Sympathetic chain

Skeletal
muscle

Collateral
sympathetic
ganglion

Preganglionic sympathetic neurons
passing to synapse in another
sympathetic chain ganglion

J. Perkins
MS, MFA
©ICN

Sensory neuron of
abdominal viscera

Neuroeffector junctions on smooth
muscle, cardiac muscle, secretory
glands, metabolic cells, immune cells

FIGURE II.1: SCHEMATIC OF THE SPINAL CORD WITH SENSORY, MOTOR, AND AUTONOMIC COMPONENTS OF PERIPHERAL NERVES

Peripheral nerves consist of axons from primary sensory neurons, lower motor neurons (LMNs), and preganglionic and postganglionic autonomic neurons. The primary sensory axons have sensory receptors (transducing elements) at their peripheral ends contiguous with their initial segments. The proximal portion of the axon enters the CNS and terminates in secondary sensory nuclei associated with reflex, cerebellar, and lemniscal channels. LMNs in the anterior horn of the spinal cord send axons, via the ventral (anterior) roots, to travel in peripheral nerves to skeletal muscles, with which they form neuromuscular junctions. Autonomic preganglionic neurons send axons via the ventral roots to terminate in autonomic ganglia. Postganglionic neurons send axons into splanchnic or peripheral nerves and form neuroeffector junctions with smooth muscle, cardiac muscle, secretory glands, metabolic cells, and cells of the immune system.

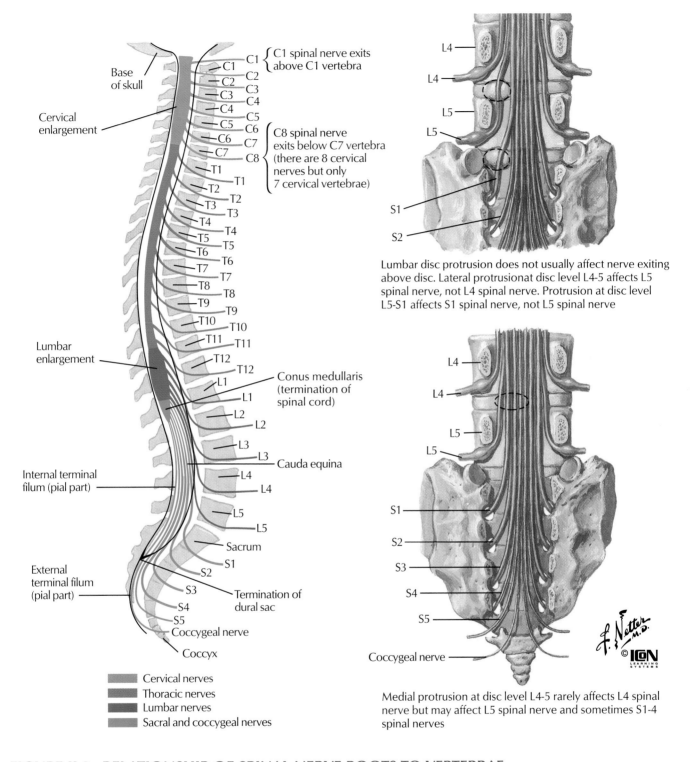

Lumbar disc protrusion does not usually affect nerve exiting above disc. Lateral protrusion at disc level L4-5 affects L5 spinal nerve, not L4 spinal nerve. Protrusion at disc level L5-S1 affects S1 spinal nerve, not L5 spinal nerve

Medial protrusion at disc level L4-5 rarely affects L4 spinal nerve but may affect L5 spinal nerve and sometimes S1-4 spinal nerves

FIGURE II.2: RELATIONSHIP OF SPINAL NERVE ROOTS TO VERTEBRAE

The dorsal (posterior) and ventral (anterior) roots of the spinal cord segments extend from the spinal cord as groups of peripheral axons invested initially with meninges. As the axons enter the PNS, they associate with Schwann cells for myelination and support. The roots exit through the intervertebral foramina, compact openings between the vertebrae where herniated disks (nucleus pulposus) can impinge on the nerve roots, producing sensory and/or motor symptoms. Sensory and motor axons enter the dorsal and ventral rami of peripheral nerves. Autonomic axons course from the ventral roots into the white (preganglionic) rami communicantes, and postganglionic axons course through the gray rami communicantes.

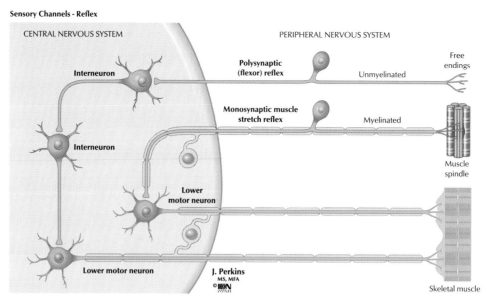

FIGURE II.3: SENSORY CHANNELS: REFLEX

Primary sensory axons communicate with secondary sensory neurons in reflex, cerebellar, and lemniscal channels carrying transduced information from the periphery into the CNS. The reflex channels interconnect primary sensory axons with anterior horn cells (LMNs), through one or more synapses, to achieve an unconscious reflex motor response to sensory input. These responses can be elicited in an isolated spinal cord devoid of connections from the brain. The monosynaptic reflex channels connect primary sensory axons from muscle spindles directly with LMNs involved in muscle stretch reflex contraction; this is the only monosynaptic reflex seen in the human CNS. Polysynaptic reflex channels are directed particularly toward flexor (withdrawal) responses through one or more interneurons to produce coordinated patterns of muscle activity able to remove a portion of the body from a potentially damaging or offending stimulus. This polysynaptic channel can spread ipsilaterally and contralaterally through many segments.

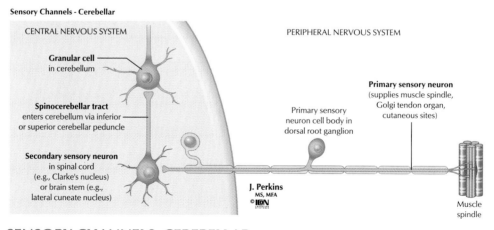

FIGURE II.4: SENSORY CHANNELS: CEREBELLAR

Primary somatosensory axons carrying unconsciously processed information from muscles, joints, tendons, ligaments, and cutaneous sources enter the CNS via dorsal roots and synapse with secondary sensory neurons in the spinal cord or the caudal brain stem. These neurons convey information from the periphery to the ipsilateral cerebellum by sending secondary sensory axonal projections through spinocerebellar pathways. The dorsal and ventral spinocerebellar tracts carry information from the lower body (T6 and below). The rostral spinocerebellar tract and the cuneocerebellar tract carry information from the upper body (above T6). Polysynaptic indirect spinocerebellar pathways (spino-olivo-cerebellar and spino-reticulo-cerebellar) also are present.

Sensory Channels - Lemniscal

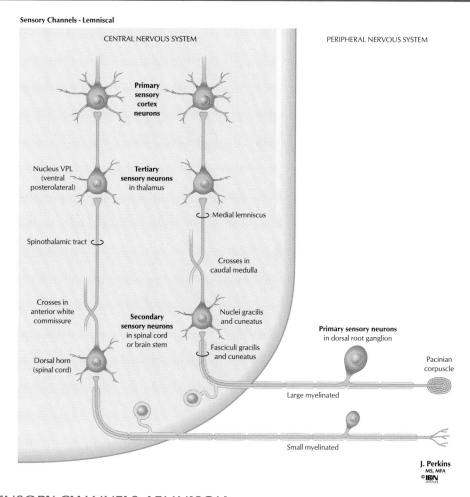

FIGURE II.5: SENSORY CHANNELS: LEMNISCAL

Primary sensory axons carrying information destined for conscious perception arise from receptors in superficial and deep tissue. These axons enter the CNS via the dorsal roots and terminate on secondary sensory nuclei in the spinal cord or the brain stem. Secondary sensory axons from these nuclei cross the midline (decussate), ascend as lemniscal pathways, and terminate in the contralateral thalamus. These thalamic nuclei then project to specific regions of the primary sensory cortex, where fine-grained analysis of incoming consciously perceived information takes place. Somatosensory information is directed into either protopathic or epicritic channels. Epicritic information (fine discriminative sensation, vibratory sensation, joint position sense) is transduced by primary sensory neurons that send myelinated axons to neurons in the medulla, nuclei gracilis (lower body, T6 and below), and nuclei cuneatus (upper body, above T6). Nuclei gracilis and cuneatus give rise to the medial lemniscus, a crossed secondary sensory pathway that terminates in the ventral postero-lateral (VPL) nucleus of the thalamus. This thalamic nucleus has reciprocal connections with cortical neurons in the postcentral gyrus (Brodmann areas 3, 1, and 2). Protopathic information (pain, temperature sensation, light moving touch) is transduced by primary sensory ganglion cells that project to neurons in the dorsal horn of the spinal cord via small myelinated and unmyelinated axons. These spinal cord neurons give rise to the spinothalamic tract (spinal lemniscus), a secondary sensory pathway that terminates in separate neuronal sites in the VPL nucleus of the thalamus. This portion of the VPL nucleus communicates with the primary sensory cortex and a secondary area of the somatosensory cortex posterior to the lateral postcentral gyrus. Some unmyelinated nociceptive protopathic axons that terminate in the dorsal horn of the spinal cord interconnect with a cascade of spinal cord interneurons that project mainly into the reticular formation of the brain stem (spinoreticular pathway). This more diffuse pain system is processed through nonspecific thalamic nuclei, leading to perception of excruciating, long-lasting pain.

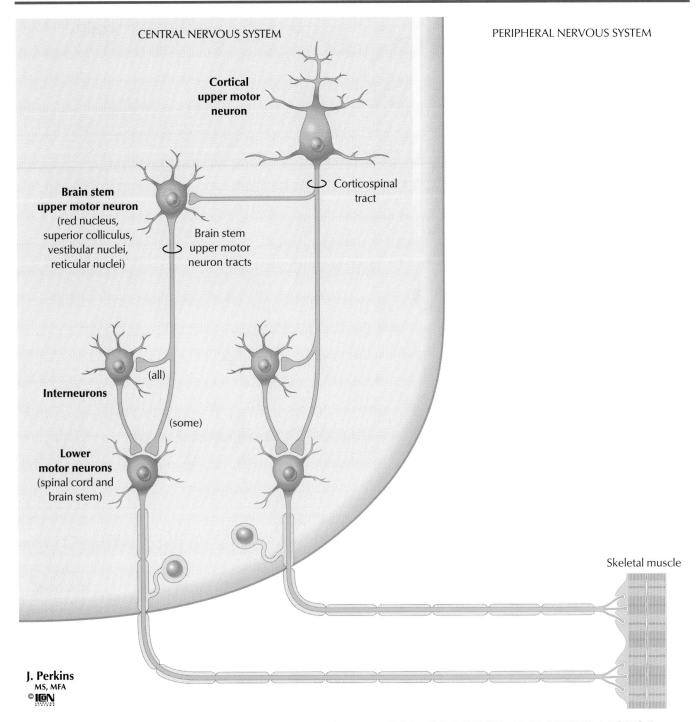

CENTRAL NERVOUS SYSTEM

PERIPHERAL NERVOUS SYSTEM

Cortical upper motor neuron

Corticospinal tract

Brain stem upper motor neuron (red nucleus, superior colliculus, vestibular nuclei, reticular nuclei)

Brain stem upper motor neuron tracts

Interneurons

(all)

(some)

Lower motor neurons (spinal cord and brain stem)

Skeletal muscle

J. Perkins
MS, MFA
©ICN

FIGURE II.6: MOTOR CHANNELS: BASIC ORGANIZATION OF LOWER AND UPPER MOTOR NEURONS

Lower motor neurons are found in the anterior horn of the spinal cord or in motor cranial nerve nuclei in the brain stem. Their axons exit via the ventral roots or the cranial nerves to supply skeletal muscles. LMN synapses with muscle fibers form neuromuscular junctions and release the neuro-transmitter acetylcholine (ACh), which acts on nicotinic receptors on the skeletal muscle fibers. A motor unit consists of an LMN, its axon, and the muscle fibers the axon innervates. LMNs are regulated and coordinated by groups of upper motor neurons (UMNs) found in the brain. Brain stem UMNs regulate basic tone and posture. Cortical UMNs (from corticospinal and cortico-bulbar tracts) regulate consciously directed, or volitional, movements. The cerebellum and the basal ganglia aid in pattern selection and coordi-nation of movement via connections with these UMNs; they do not connect with LMNs directly.

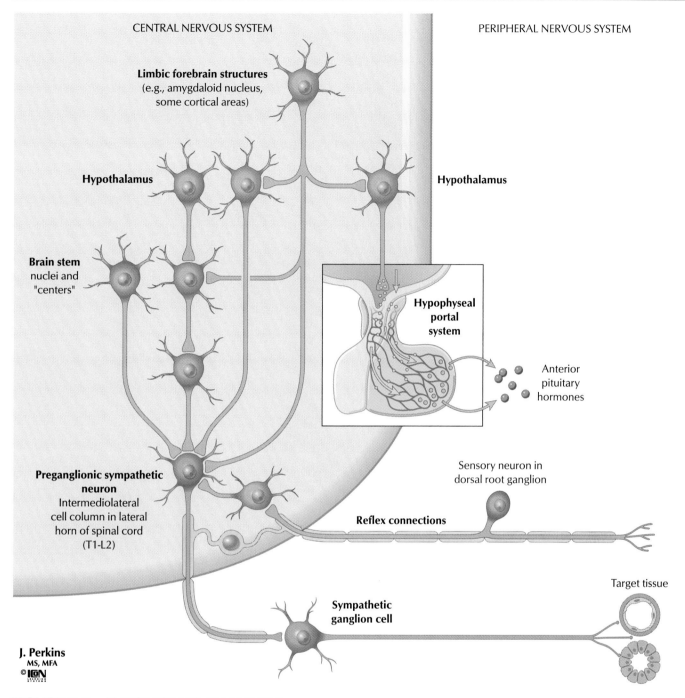

CENTRAL NERVOUS SYSTEM

PERIPHERAL NERVOUS SYSTEM

Limbic forebrain structures
(e.g., amygdaloid nucleus,
some cortical areas)

Hypothalamus

Hypothalamus

Brain stem
nuclei and
"centers"

**Hypophyseal
portal
system**

Anterior
pituitary
hormones

Sensory neuron in
dorsal root ganglion

**Preganglionic sympathetic
neuron**
Intermediolateral
cell column in lateral
horn of spinal cord
(T1-L2)

Reflex connections

Target tissue

**Sympathetic
ganglion cell**

J. Perkins
MS, MFA
©IGN

FIGURE II.7: AUTONOMIC CHANNELS

Preganglionic neurons for the sympathetic nervous system (SNS) are found in the lateral horn (intermediolateral cell column) of the thoracolumbar (T1-L2) spinal cord. For the parasympathetic nervous system (PsNS), these neurons are found in nuclei of cranial nerves (CNs) III, VII, IX, and X and in S2-S4 intermediate gray matter of the spinal cord (a craniosacral system). Preganglionic axons exit the CNS via cranial nerves or ventral roots and terminate in chain ganglia or collateral ganglia (SNS) or in intramural ganglia in or near the organ innervated (PsNS). Postganglionic axons innervate smooth muscle, cardiac muscle, secretory glands, metabolic cells, and cells of the immune system. The SNS is a fight-or-flight system that responds to emergency demands. The PsNS is a homeostatic, reparative system active in the more quiescent digestive and eliminative functions. Preganglionic responses are coordinated by autonomic "UMN" equivalents from the brain stem (autonomic centers), the hypothalamus, and limbic forebrain structures. These central regulatory systems coordinate autonomic responses that affect both visceral functions and neuroendocrine outflow from the pituitary gland.

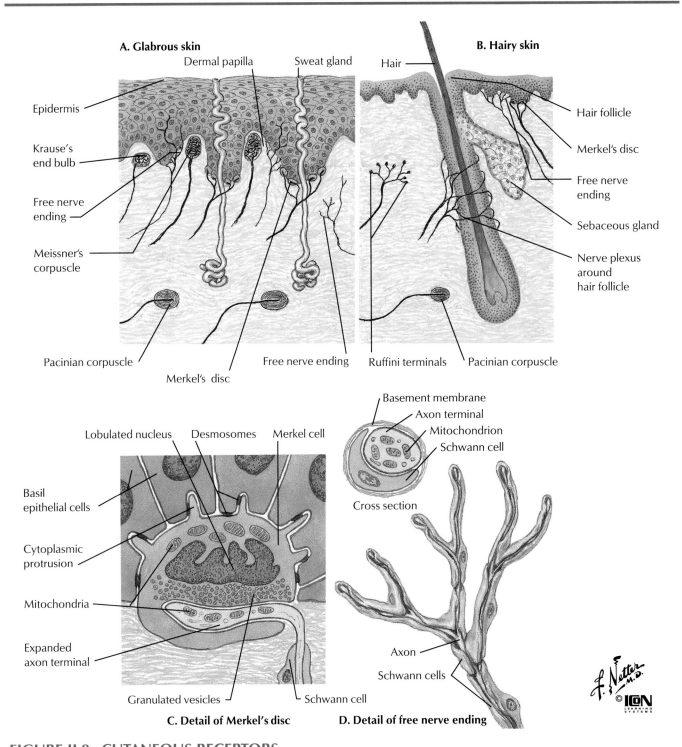

A. Glabrous skin

Dermal papilla — Sweat gland

Epidermis

Krause's
end bulb

Free nerve
ending

Meissner's
corpuscle

Pacinian corpuscle

Merkel's disc

Free nerve ending

B. Hairy skin

Hair

Hair follicle

Merkel's disc

Free nerve
ending

Sebaceous gland

Nerve plexus
around
hair follicle

Ruffini terminals   Pacinian corpuscle

C. Detail of Merkel's disc

Lobulated nucleus   Desmosomes   Merkel cell

Basil
epithelial cells

Cytoplasmic
protrusion

Mitochondria

Expanded
axon terminal

Granulated vesicles — Schwann cell

D. Detail of free nerve ending

Basement membrane
Axon terminal
Mitochondrion
Schwann cell

Cross section

Axon

Schwann cells

FIGURE II.8: CUTANEOUS RECEPTORS

Glabrous skin and hairy skin contain a variety of sensory receptors for detecting mechanical, thermal, or nociceptive (consciously perceived as painful) stimuli applied at the body surface. These receptors include bare nerve endings (nociception, thermal sensation) and encapsulated endings. The latter include pacinian corpuscles (fast-adapting mechanoreceptors for detecting vibration or brief touch), Merkel's disks (slowly adapting mechanoreceptors for detecting maintained deformation or sustained touch at the skin), Meissner's corpuscles (fast-adapting mechanoreceptors for detecting moving touch), Ruffini endings (slowly adapting mechanoreceptors for detecting steady pressure applied to hairy skin), hair follicle receptors (rapidly adapting), and end bulbs of Krause (possibly thermoreceptors). The initial segment of the primary sensory axon is immediately adjacent to the sensory receptor.

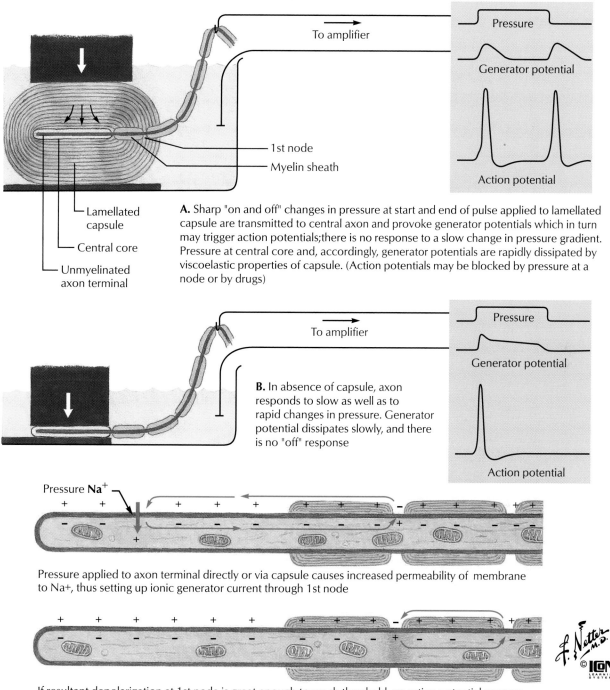

A. Sharp "on and off" changes in pressure at start and end of pulse applied to lamellated capsule are transmitted to central axon and provoke generator potentials which in turn may trigger action potentials; there is no response to a slow change in pressure gradient. Pressure at central core and, accordingly, generator potentials are rapidly dissipated by viscoelastic properties of capsule. (Action potentials may be blocked by pressure at a node or by drugs)

B. In absence of capsule, axon responds to slow as well as to rapid changes in pressure. Generator potential dissipates slowly, and there is no "off" response

Pressure applied to axon terminal directly or via capsule causes increased permeability of membrane to Na+, thus setting up ionic generator current through 1st node

If resultant depolarization at 1st node is great enough to reach threshold, an action potential appears which is propagated along nerve fiber

FIGURE II.9: PACINIAN CORPUSCLES

Pacinian corpuscles are mechanoreceptors that transform mechanical force or displacement in large-diameter primary sensory axons into action potentials. The mechanical stimulus is modified by the viscoelastic properties of the contributing lamellae of the pacinian corpuscle and the associated accessory cells. An action potential results when a generator potential of sufficient magnitude to bring the initial segment of the axon to threshold is elicited. The onset and cessation of mechanical deformation enhance ionic permeability in the axon, optimizing the physiological response of the pacinian corpuscle to vibratory stimuli.

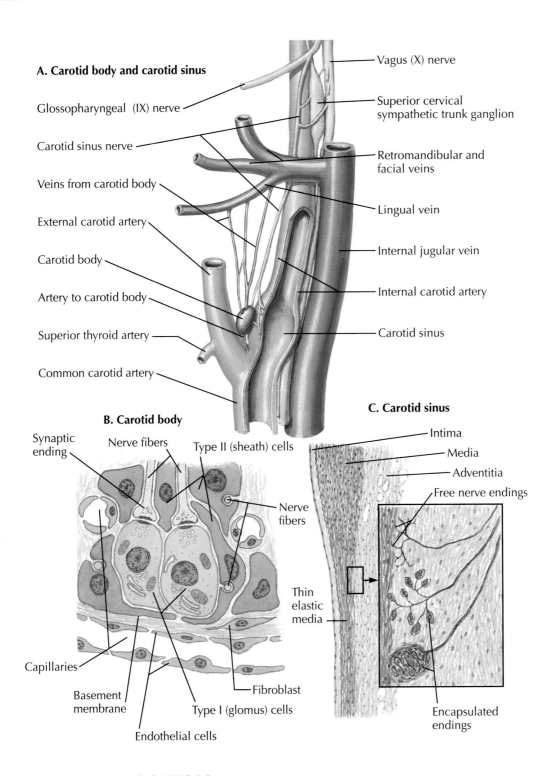

A. Carotid body and carotid sinus

Vagus (X) nerve

Glossopharyngeal (IX) nerve

Superior cervical sympathetic trunk ganglion

Carotid sinus nerve

Veins from carotid body

Retromandibular and facial veins

External carotid artery

Lingual vein

Carotid body

Internal jugular vein

Artery to carotid body

Internal carotid artery

Superior thyroid artery

Carotid sinus

Common carotid artery

C. Carotid sinus

B. Carotid body

Intima

Synaptic ending

Nerve fibers

Type II (sheath) cells

Media

Adventitia

Free nerve endings

Nerve fibers

Thin elastic media

Capillaries

Basement membrane

Type I (glomus) cells

Fibroblast

Endothelial cells

Encapsulated endings

FIGURE II.10: INTEROCEPTORS

Interoceptors, including internal nociceptors, chemoreceptors, and stretch receptors, inform the CNS about the internal state of the body. The carotid body, a specialized chemoreceptor for detecting carbon dioxide (in a hypoxic state) or, to a lesser extent, low blood pH resulting in increased respiration, is associated with afferents of CN IX projecting to caudal nucleus solitarius in the medulla. The carotid sinus, a thin-walled region of the carotid artery, contains encapsulated and bare nerve endings that act as stretch receptors. These stretch receptors respond to increased arterial pressure as baroreceptors, eliciting a reflex brady-cardia and a decrease in blood pressure via primary afferents of CN IX projecting to caudal nucleus solitarius.

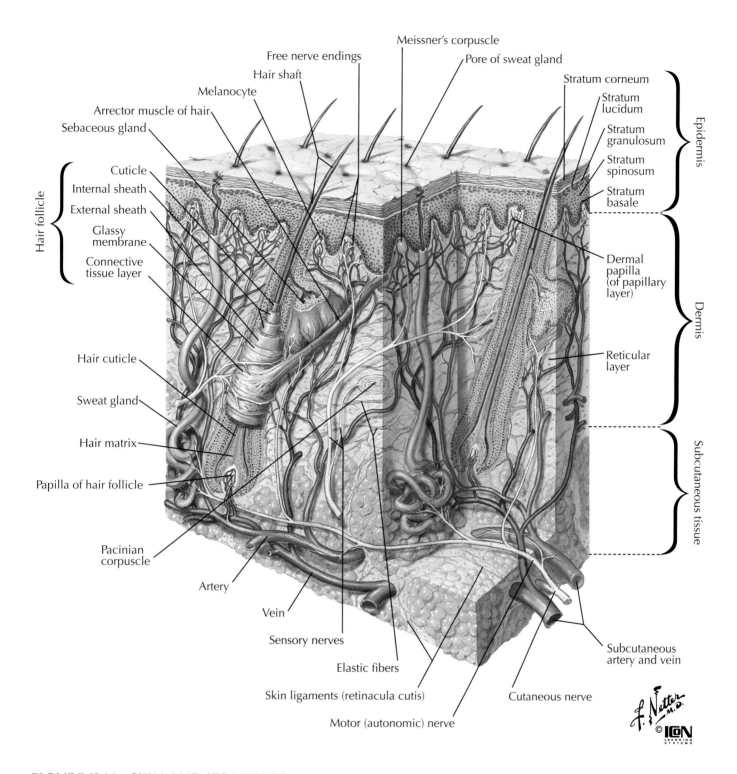

Meissner's corpuscle
Free nerve endings
Pore of sweat gland
Hair shaft
Stratum corneum
Melanocyte
Stratum lucidum
Arrector muscle of hair
Stratum granulosum
Sebaceous gland
Stratum spinosum
Stratum basale
Epidermis

Cuticle
Internal sheath
External sheath
Glassy membrane
Connective tissue layer
Hair follicle

Dermal papilla (of papillary layer)
Dermis

Hair cuticle
Reticular layer

Sweat gland

Hair matrix

Papilla of hair follicle
Subcutaneous tissue

Pacinian corpuscle
Artery
Vein
Sensory nerves
Elastic fibers
Skin ligaments (retinacula cutis)
Motor (autonomic) nerve
Cutaneous nerve
Subcutaneous artery and vein

FIGURE II.11: SKIN AND ITS NERVES

The skin is supplied with a variety of receptor types (see Figure II.8) that transduce slowly and rapidly adapting mechanical stimuli and deformation into electrical impulses in primary afferent fibers. The bare nerve endings are associated mainly with nociceptors, peripheral arborizations of unmyelinated axons. Some nociceptors and thermoreceptors are associated with small myelinated axons. These axons contribute somatosensory information collectively to the spinothalamic/spinoreticular lemniscal system for protopathic sensation. The more complex encapsulated receptors contribute somatosensory information to the dorsal column/medial lemniscal system for epicritic sensation and are associated with larger myelinated axons.

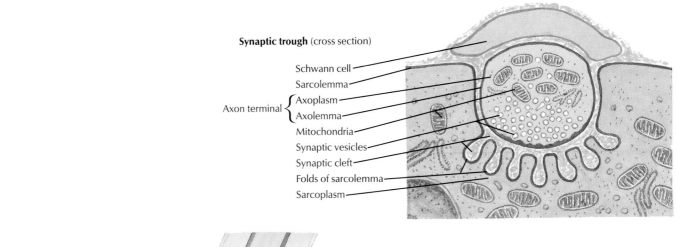

Synaptic trough (cross section)

Schwann cell
Sarcolemma
Axon terminal { Axoplasm
                Axolemma
Mitochondria
Synaptic vesicles
Synaptic cleft
Folds of sarcolemma
Sarcoplasm

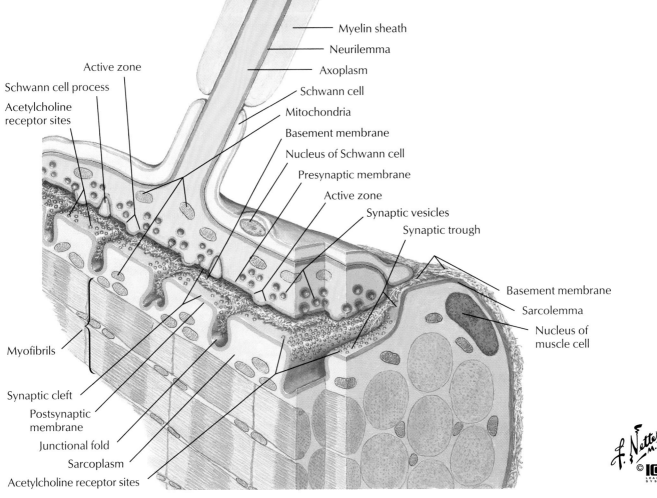

Active zone
Schwann cell process
Acetylcholine receptor sites

Myelin sheath
Neurilemma
Axoplasm
Schwann cell
Mitochondria
Basement membrane
Nucleus of Schwann cell
Presynaptic membrane
Active zone
Synaptic vesicles
Synaptic trough

Basement membrane
Sarcolemma
Nucleus of muscle cell

Myofibrils
Synaptic cleft
Postsynaptic membrane
Junctional fold
Sarcoplasm
Acetylcholine receptor sites

FIGURE II.12: NEUROMUSCULAR NEUROTRANSMISSION

Axons of LMNs that synapse on skeletal muscle fibers form expanded terminals called neuromuscular junctions (motor endplates). The motor axon loses its myelin sheath and expands into an extended terminal that resides in a trough in the muscle fiber and is covered with a layer of Schwann cell cytoplasm. The postsynaptic membrane is thrown into secondary folds. When an action potential invades the motor terminal, hundreds of synaptic vesicles release their packets of ACh simultaneously into the synaptic cleft. The ACh binds to nicotinic receptors on the muscle sarcolemma, initiating a motor endplate potential (EPP), which is normally of sufficient magnitude to result in the firing of a muscle action potential, leading to contraction of the muscle fiber. A single muscle fiber has only one neuromuscular junction, but a motor axon may innervate multiple muscle fibers.

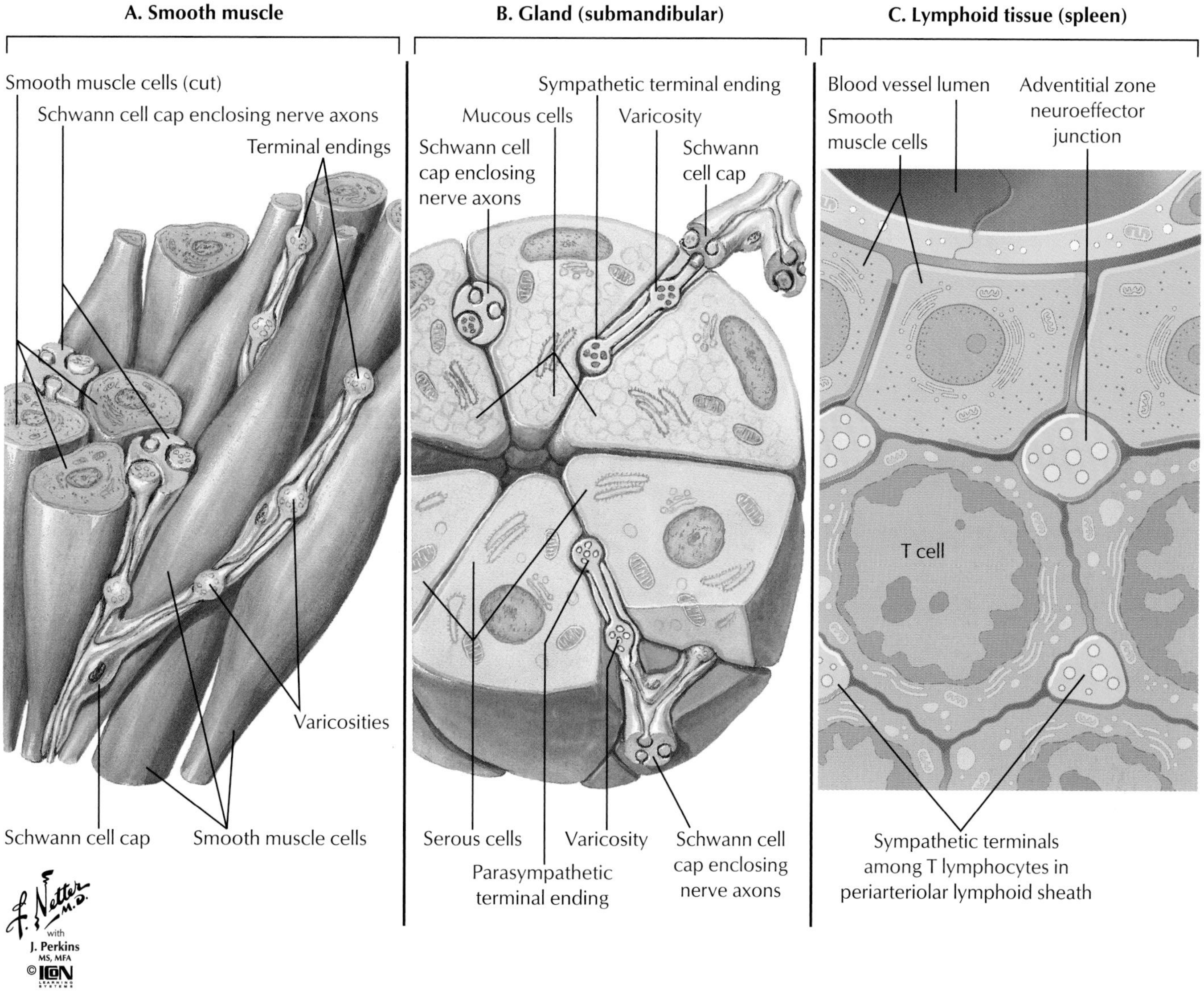

A. Smooth muscle

Smooth muscle cells (cut)
Schwann cell cap enclosing nerve axons
Terminal endings

Varicosities

Schwann cell cap   Smooth muscle cells

B. Gland (submandibular)

Sympathetic terminal ending
Mucous cells   Varicosity
Schwann cell cap enclosing nerve axons   Schwann cell cap

Serous cells   Varicosity   Schwann cell cap enclosing nerve axons
Parasympathetic terminal ending

C. Lymphoid tissue (spleen)

Blood vessel lumen   Adventitial zone neuroeffector junction
Smooth muscle cells

T cell

Sympathetic terminals among T lymphocytes in periarteriolar lymphoid sheath

J. Netter M.D.
with
J. Perkins
MS, MFA
© ICN

FIGURE II.13: NEUROEFFECTOR JUNCTIONS

Autonomic postganglionic axons form neuroeffector junctions with cardiac muscle, smooth muscle (A), secretory glands (B), metabolic cells such as hepatocytes, and cells of the immune system (C). These nerve endings use mainly norepinephrine for the SNS and ACh for the PsNS. These endings do not form classic CNS or motor endplate synapses but terminate as neuroeffector junctions, releasing neurotransmitter into interstitial spaces. This permits widespread diffusion of the neurotransmitter as a paracrine secretion, initiating postsynaptic responses on cells with appropriate receptors (including many types of immune cells). Some close appositions also are found, such as SNS endings on lymphocytes. Smooth muscle cells that are not innervated are coupled by gap junctions and can contract together when the innervated smooth muscle cell contracts.

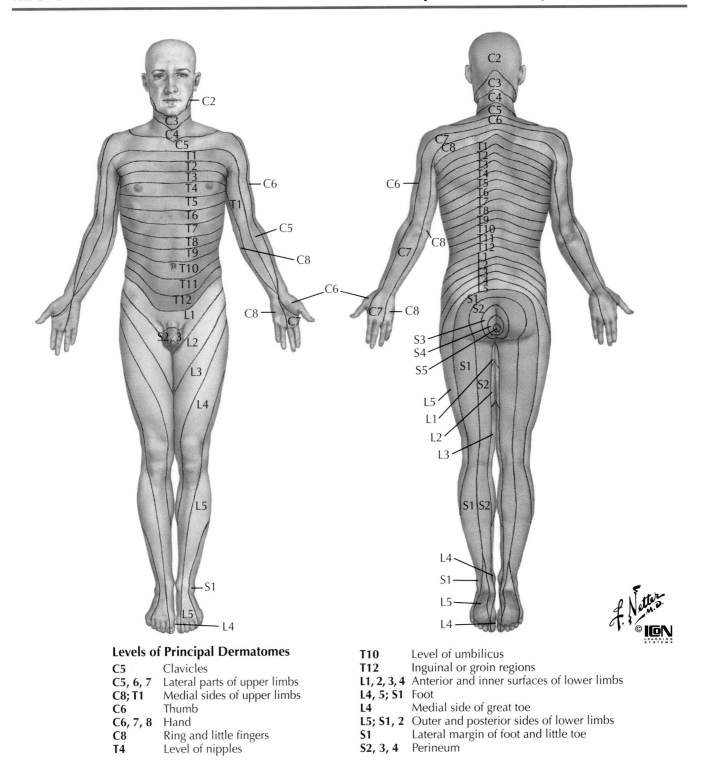

Levels of Principal Dermatomes

C5	Clavicles
C5, 6, 7	Lateral parts of upper limbs
C8; T1	Medial sides of upper limbs
C6	Thumb
C6, 7, 8	Hand
C8	Ring and little fingers
T4	Level of nipples

T10	Level of umbilicus
T12	Inguinal or groin regions
L1, 2, 3, 4	Anterior and inner surfaces of lower limbs
L4, 5; S1	Foot
L4	Medial side of great toe
L5; S1, 2	Outer and posterior sides of lower limbs
S1	Lateral margin of foot and little toe
S2, 3, 4	Perineum

FIGURE II.14: DERMATOMAL DISTRIBUTION

A dermatome is the cutaneous area supplied by a single spinal nerve root; the cell bodies are located in dorsal root ganglia. The spinal nerve roots are distributed to structures according to their association with spinal cord segments. The nerve roots supplying neighboring dermatomes overlap. Thus, sectioning or dysfunction of a single dorsal root produces hypoesthesia (diminished sensation), not anesthesia (total loss of sensation), in the region predominantly supplied by that dermatome. Dermatomal anesthesia requires damage to at least 3 dorsal roots: the central dorsal root and the roots above and below it. Knowledge of dermatomes is important for identifying the location of peripheral nerve root lesions and distinguishing them from peripheral nerve lesions.

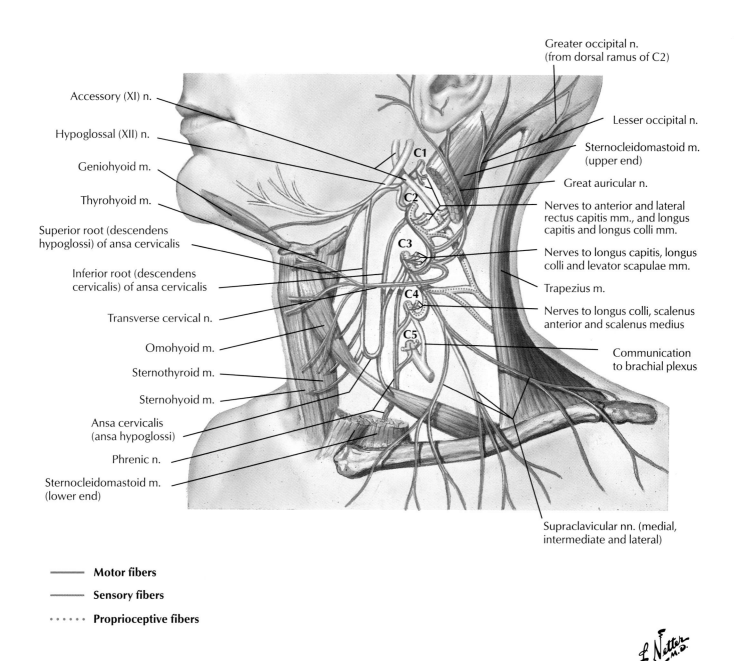

Greater occipital n.
(from dorsal ramus of C2)

Accessory (XI) n.

Hypoglossal (XII) n.

Geniohyoid m.

Thyrohyoid m.

Superior root (descendens
hypoglossi) of ansa cervicalis

Inferior root (descendens
cervicalis) of ansa cervicalis

Transverse cervical n.

Omohyoid m.

Sternothyroid m.

Sternohyoid m.

Ansa cervicalis
(ansa hypoglossi)

Phrenic n.

Sternocleidomastoid m.
(lower end)

Lesser occipital n.

Sternocleidomastoid m.
(upper end)

Great auricular n.

Nerves to anterior and lateral
rectus capitis mm., and longus
capitis and longus colli mm.

Nerves to longus capitis, longus
colli and levator scapulae mm.

Trapezius m.

Nerves to longus colli, scalenus
anterior and scalenus medius

Communication
to brachial plexus

Supraclavicular nn. (medial,
intermediate and lateral)

C1
C2
C3
C4
C5

———— Motor fibers

———— Sensory fibers

· · · · · Proprioceptive fibers

FIGURE II.15: CERVICAL PLEXUS

The cervical plexus lies deep to the sternocleido-mastoid muscle. Its branches convey motor fibers to many cervical muscles and to the diaphragm. Its sensory fibers convey exteroceptive information from parts of the scalp, neck, and chest, as well as proprioceptive information from muscles, tendons, and joints. Sympathetic sudomotor and vasomotor fibers travel with this plexus to blood vessels and glands. The superficial branches perforate the cervical fascia to supply cutaneous structures; the deep branches supply mainly muscles and joints.

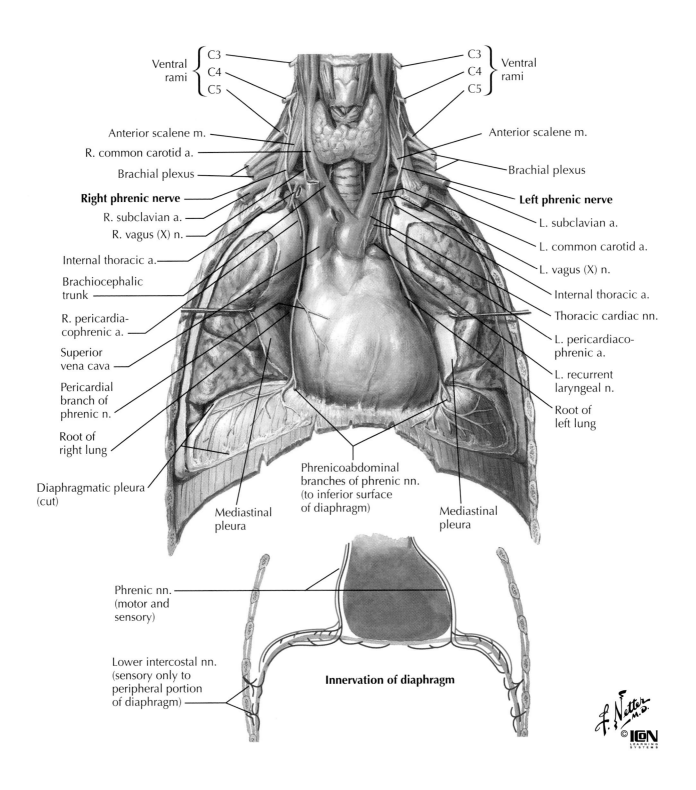

Ventral rami { C3 C4 C5 }

Ventral rami { C3 C4 C5 }

Anterior scalene m.
R. common carotid a.
Brachial plexus
Right phrenic nerve
R. subclavian a.
R. vagus (X) n.
Internal thoracic a.
Brachiocephalic trunk
R. pericardia-cophrenic a.
Superior vena cava
Pericardial branch of phrenic n.
Root of right lung
Diaphragmatic pleura (cut)

Anterior scalene m.
Brachial plexus
Left phrenic nerve
L. subclavian a.
L. common carotid a.
L. vagus (X) n.
Internal thoracic a.
Thoracic cardiac nn.
L. pericardiaco-phrenic a.
L. recurrent laryngeal n.
Root of left lung

Mediastinal pleura

Phrenicoabdominal branches of phrenic nn. (to inferior surface of diaphragm)

Mediastinal pleura

Phrenic nn. (motor and sensory)

Innervation of diaphragm

Lower intercostal nn. (sensory only to peripheral portion of diaphragm)

FIGURE II.16: PHRENIC NERVE

The left and right phrenic nerves are the motor nerves that supply both sides of the diaphragm from the C3, C4, and C5 ventral roots. The phrenic nerve also contains many sensory nerve fibers, which supply the fibrous pericardium, the media- stinal pleura, and central areas of the diaphrag- matic pleura. Sympathetic postganglionic nerve fibers also travel with this nerve. Damage to the phrenic nerves abolishes inspiration, which results in respiratory failure.

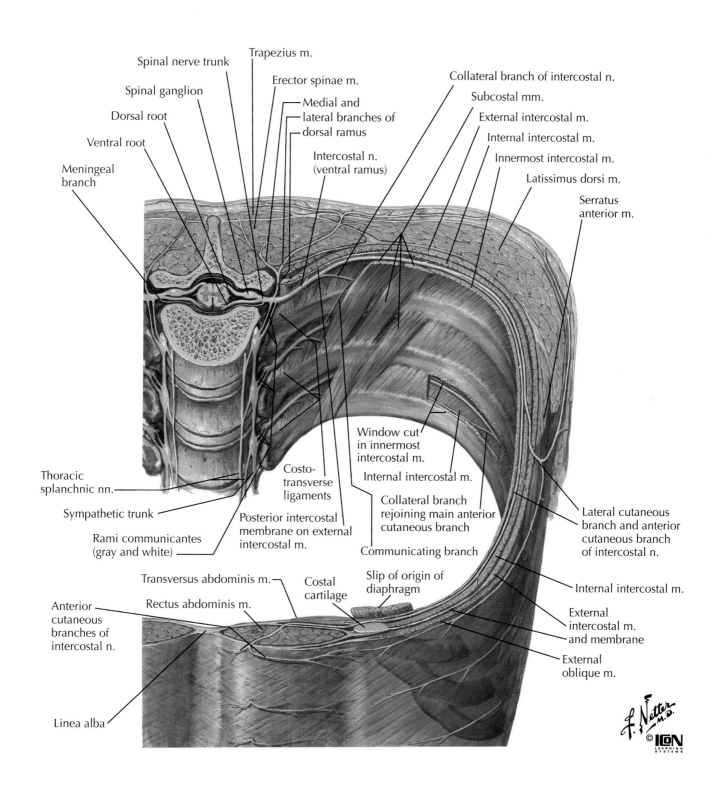

Spinal nerve trunk
Trapezius m.
Spinal ganglion
Dorsal root
Erector spinae m.
Medial and lateral branches of dorsal ramus
Ventral root
Intercostal n. (ventral ramus)
Meningeal branch
Collateral branch of intercostal n.
Subcostal mm.
External intercostal m.
Internal intercostal m.
Innermost intercostal m.
Latissimus dorsi m.
Serratus anterior m.

Thoracic splanchnic nn.
Costo-transverse ligaments
Sympathetic trunk
Posterior intercostal membrane on external intercostal m.
Rami communicantes (gray and white)

Window cut in innermost intercostal m.
Internal intercostal m.
Collateral branch rejoining main anterior cutaneous branch
Communicating branch
Lateral cutaneous branch and anterior cutaneous branch of intercostal n.

Transversus abdominis m.
Costal cartilage
Slip of origin of diaphragm
Anterior cutaneous branches of intercostal n.
Rectus abdominis m.
Internal intercostal m.
External intercostal m. and membrane
External oblique m.
Linea alba

FIGURE II.17: THORACIC NERVES

The 12 pairs of thoracic nerves are derived from the dorsal and ventral roots of their corresponding segments. These nerves do not form plexuses; they distribute cutaneous branches to the thoracic dermatomes and send other sensory fibers to deeper muscular structures, vessels, the periosteum, parietal pleura, the peritoneum, and breast tissue. The thoracic nerves also send motor fibers to muscles of the thoracic and the abdominal walls and carry preganglionic and postganglionic sympathetic nerve fibers into and out of the sympathetic chain.

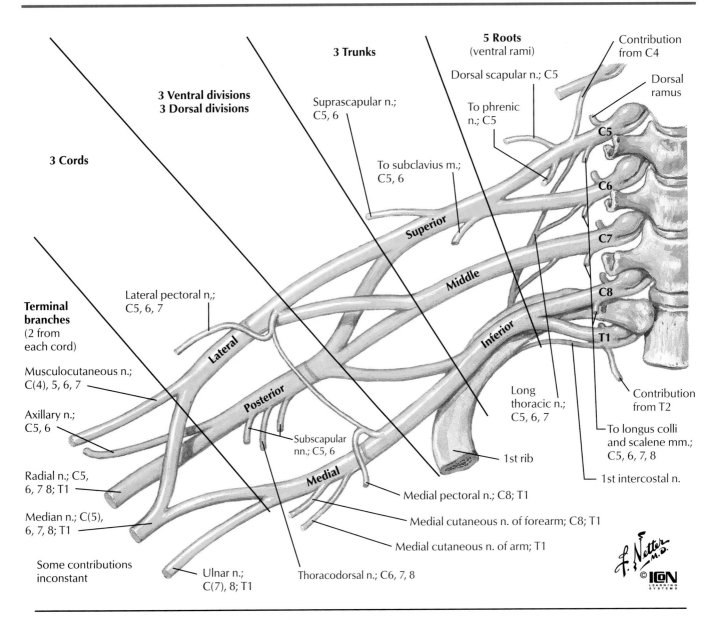

3 Trunks

5 Roots
(ventral rami)

Contribution
from C4

Dorsal scapular n.; C5

Dorsal
ramus

3 Ventral divisions
3 Dorsal divisions

Suprascapular n.;
C5, 6

To phrenic
n.; C5

C5

3 Cords

To subclavius m.;
C5, 6

Superior

C6

C7

Terminal
branches
(2 from
each cord)

Lateral pectoral n,;
C5, 6, 7

Middle

C8

Lateral

Inferior

T1

Musculocutaneous n.;
C(4), 5, 6, 7

Posterior

Long
thoracic n.;
C5, 6, 7

Contribution
from T2

Axillary n.;
C5, 6

Subscapular
nn.; C5, 6

To longus colli
and scalene mm.;
C5, 6, 7, 8

Radial n.; C5,
6, 7 8; T1

Medial

1st rib

1st intercostal n.

Medial pectoral n.; C8; T1

Median n.; C(5),
6, 7, 8; T1

Medial cutaneous n. of forearm; C8; T1

Medial cutaneous n. of arm; T1

Some contributions
inconstant

Ulnar n.;
C(7), 8; T1

Thoracodorsal n.; C6, 7, 8

Supraclavicular Branches		Infraclavicular Branches			
From plexus roots		*From lateral cord*		Ulnar	C(7), 8; T1
To longus colli and scalene mm	C 5, 6, 7, 8	Lateral pectoral	C5, 6, 7	Medial root of median	C8; T1
Dorsal scapular	C5	Musculocutaneous	C(4), 5, 6, 7	*From posterior cord*	
Branch to phrenic	C5	Lateral root of median	C(5), 6, 7	Upper subscapular	C5, 6, (7)
Long thoracic	C5, 6, 7	*From medial cord*		Lower subscapular	C5, 6
From superior trunk		Medial pectoral	C8; T1	Axillary (circumflex humeral)	C5, 6
Suprascapular	C5, 6	Medial cutaneous n. of arm	T1	Thoracodorsal	C6, 7, 8
To subclavius m.	C5, 6	Medial cutaneous n. of forearm	C8; T1	Radial	C5, 6, 7, 8

FIGURE II.18: BRACHIAL PLEXUS

The brachial plexus is formed by the union of the ventral roots of C5, C6, C7, C8, and T1, with a smaller contribution from C4. Sensory and sympathetic fibers also distribute with the brachial plexus. The roots give rise to 3 trunks, 3 ventral and 3 dorsal divisions, and 3 cords, as well as numerous terminal branches, the peripheral nerves. This plexus is vulnerable to birth injury (superior plexus para-lysis), with paralysis of the deltoid, biceps, brachial, and brachioradialis muscles, with sparing of the hands, and sensory loss over the deltoid area and the radial aspect of the forearm and the hand. Pressure of a cervical rib can cause inferior plexus injury (C8, T1 injury), which results in paralysis of small hand muscles and flexors of the hand, with ulnar sensory loss and possible Horner's syndrome.

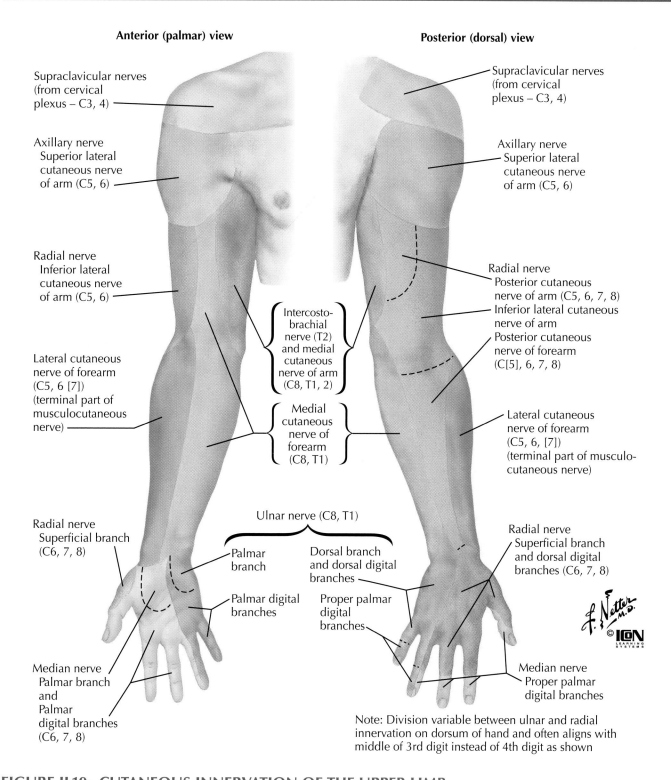

Anterior (palmar) view

Supraclavicular nerves
(from cervical
plexus – C3, 4)

Axillary nerve
Superior lateral
cutaneous nerve
of arm (C5, 6)

Radial nerve
Inferior lateral
cutaneous nerve
of arm (C5, 6)

Lateral cutaneous
nerve of forearm
(C5, 6 [7])
(terminal part of
musculocutaneous
nerve)

Radial nerve
Superficial branch
(C6, 7, 8)

Median nerve
Palmar branch
and
Palmar
digital branches
(C6, 7, 8)

Intercosto-
brachial
nerve (T2)
and medial
cutaneous
nerve of arm
(C8, T1, 2)

Medial
cutaneous
nerve of
forearm
(C8, T1)

Ulnar nerve (C8, T1)

Palmar
branch

Palmar digital
branches

Dorsal branch
and dorsal digital
branches

Proper palmar
digital
branches

Posterior (dorsal) view

Supraclavicular nerves
(from cervical
plexus – C3, 4)

Axillary nerve
Superior lateral
cutaneous nerve
of arm (C5, 6)

Radial nerve
Posterior cutaneous
nerve of arm (C5, 6, 7, 8)
Inferior lateral cutaneous
nerve of arm
Posterior cutaneous
nerve of forearm
(C[5], 6, 7, 8)

Lateral cutaneous
nerve of forearm
(C5, 6, [7])
(terminal part of musculocutaneous nerve)

Radial nerve
Superficial branch
and dorsal digital
branches (C6, 7, 8)

Median nerve
Proper palmar
digital branches

Note: Division variable between ulnar and radial
innervation on dorsum of hand and often aligns with
middle of 3rd digit instead of 4th digit as shown

FIGURE II.19: CUTANEOUS INNERVATION OF THE UPPER LIMB

The cutaneous innervation of the limb derives from the musculocutaneous, axillary, radial, median, and ulnar nerves. These nerves are the terminal branches of the brachial plexus. Unlike the dorsal nerve roots, the cutaneous sensory distribution of these peripheral nerves to the upper limb does not overlap. Thus, a peripheral nerve injury or compression results in a zone of anesthesia corresponding to its distribution.

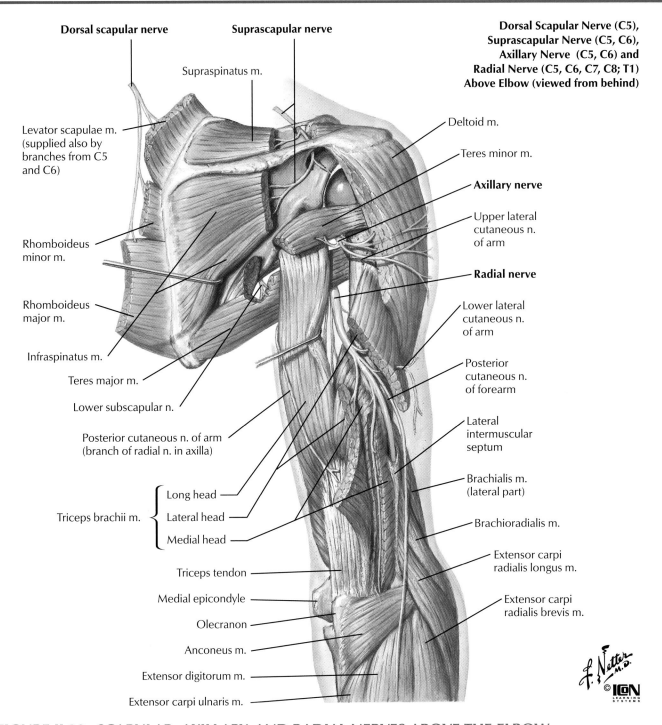

Dorsal scapular nerve

Suprascapular nerve

**Dorsal Scapular Nerve (C5),
Suprascapular Nerve (C5, C6),
Axillary Nerve (C5, C6) and
Radial Nerve (C5, C6, C7, C8; T1)
Above Elbow (viewed from behind)**

Supraspinatus m.

Levator scapulae m.
(supplied also by
branches from C5
and C6)

Rhomboideus
minor m.

Rhomboideus
major m.

Infraspinatus m.

Teres major m.

Lower subscapular n.

Posterior cutaneous n. of arm
(branch of radial n. in axilla)

Triceps brachii m.
{ Long head
Lateral head
Medial head }

Triceps tendon

Medial epicondyle

Olecranon

Anconeus m.

Extensor digitorum m.

Extensor carpi ulnaris m.

Deltoid m.

Teres minor m.

Axillary nerve

Upper lateral
cutaneous n.
of arm

Radial nerve

Lower lateral
cutaneous n.
of arm

Posterior
cutaneous n.
of forearm

Lateral
intermuscular
septum

Brachialis m.
(lateral part)

Brachioradialis m.

Extensor carpi
radialis longus m.

Extensor carpi
radialis brevis m.

FIGURE II.20: SCAPULAR, AXILLARY, AND RADIAL NERVES ABOVE THE ELBOW

The dorsal scapular nerve (C5) supplies the levator scapulae and rhomboid muscles; it aids in elevation and adduction of the scapula toward the spinal column. A nerve lesion leads to lateral displacement of the vertebral border of the scapula and rhomboid atrophy. The suprascapular nerve (C5, C6) supplies the supraspinatus and the infraspinatus muscles; it aids in lifting and in outward rotation of the arm. A lesion results in weakness in the first 15° of abduction and in external rotation of the arm. The axillary nerve (C5, C6) supplies the

deltoid and teres minor muscles; it aids in abduction of the arm to the horizontal and in outward rotation of the arm. A lesion results in deltoid atrophy and weakness in abduction from 15° to 90°. The radial nerve (C5, C6, C7, C8) supplies the triceps, anconeus, brachioradialis, extensor carpi radialis, extensor digitorum, and supinator muscles; and it aids in extension and flexion of the elbow. A lesion leads to paralysis of extension and flexion of the elbow and paralysis of supination of the forearm.

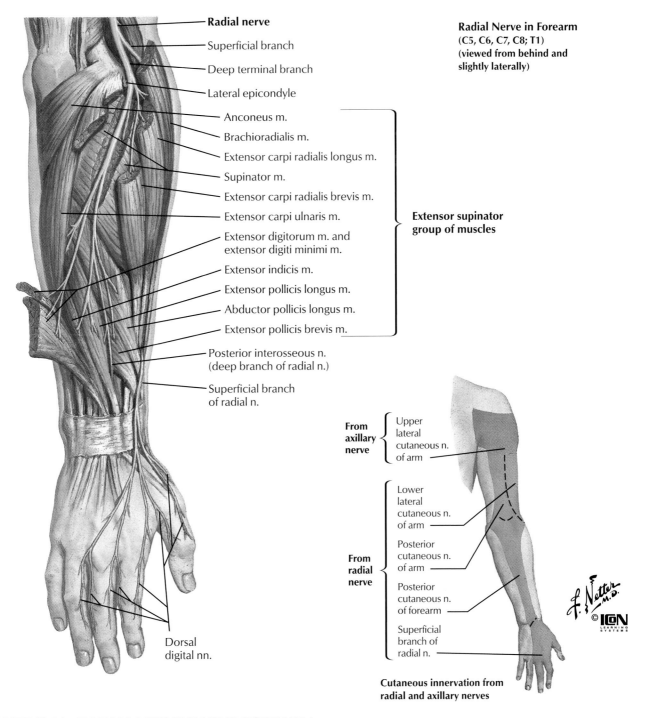

Radial nerve
Superficial branch
Deep terminal branch
Lateral epicondyle
Anconeus m.
Brachioradialis m.
Extensor carpi radialis longus m.
Supinator m.
Extensor carpi radialis brevis m.
Extensor carpi ulnaris m.
Extensor digitorum m. and extensor digiti minimi m.
Extensor indicis m.
Extensor pollicis longus m.
Abductor pollicis longus m.
Extensor pollicis brevis m.
Posterior interosseous n. (deep branch of radial n.)
Superficial branch of radial n.
Dorsal digital nn.

Radial Nerve in Forearm (C5, C6, C7, C8; T1) (viewed from behind and slightly laterally)

Extensor supinator group of muscles

From axillary nerve — Upper lateral cutaneous n. of arm

From radial nerve — Lower lateral cutaneous n. of arm; Posterior cutaneous n. of arm; Posterior cutaneous n. of forearm; Superficial branch of radial n.

Cutaneous innervation from radial and axillary nerves

FIGURE II.21: RADIAL NERVE IN THE FOREARM

In the forearm, the radial nerve (C6, C7, C8) supplies motor fibers to the (1) extensor carpi radialis, (2) extensor digitorum, (3) extensor digiti V, (4) extensor carpi ulnaris, (5) supinator, (6) abductor pollicis longus, (7) extensor pollicis brevis and longus, and (8) extensor indicis proprius muscles. It supplies the posterior upper arm, an elongated zone of the posterior forearm, and the posterior hand, thumb, and lateral 2½ fingers. A lesion results in paralysis of extension and flexion of the elbow, paralysis of supination of the forearm, paralysis of extension of the wrist and fingers, paralysis of abduction of the thumb, and loss of sensation over the radial aspect of the posterior forearm and the dorsum of the hand.

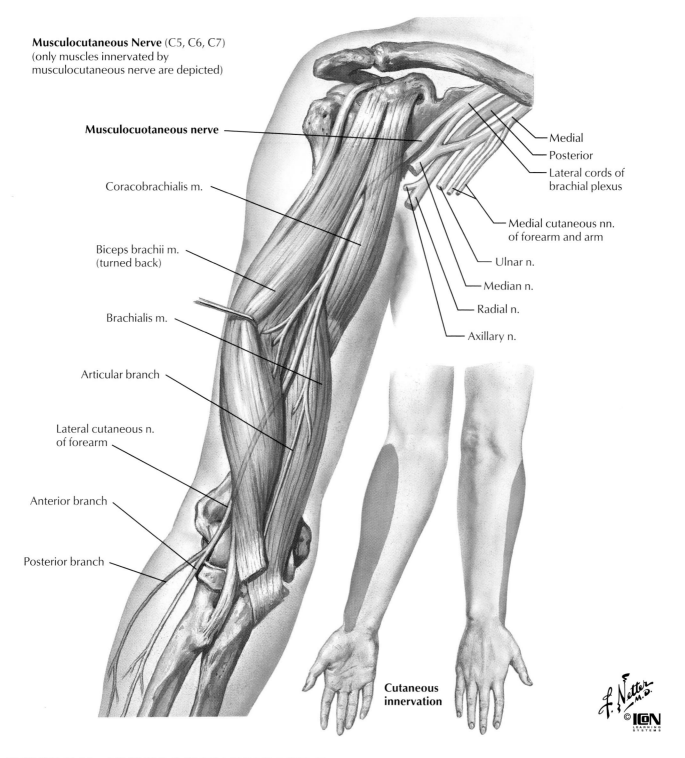

Musculocutaneous Nerve (C5, C6, C7)
(only muscles innervated by
musculocutaneous nerve are depicted)

Musculocuotaneous nerve

Coracobrachialis m.

Biceps brachii m.
(turned back)

Brachialis m.

Articular branch

Lateral cutaneous n.
of forearm

Anterior branch

Posterior branch

Medial
Posterior
Lateral cords of
brachial plexus

Medial cutaneous nn.
of forearm and arm

Ulnar n.

Median n.

Radial n.

Axillary n.

Cutaneous
innervation

FIGURE II.22: MUSCULOCUTANEOUS NERVE

The musculocutaneous nerve (C5, C6) supplies motor fibers to the biceps brachii, coracobrachialis, and brachialis muscles; it aids in flexion of the upper and lower arm, supination of the lower arm, and elevation and adduction of the arm. This nerve supplies sensory innervation to the lateral forearm. A lesion results in wasting of the muscles supplied, weakness of flexion of the supinated arm, and loss of sensation on the lateral forearm.

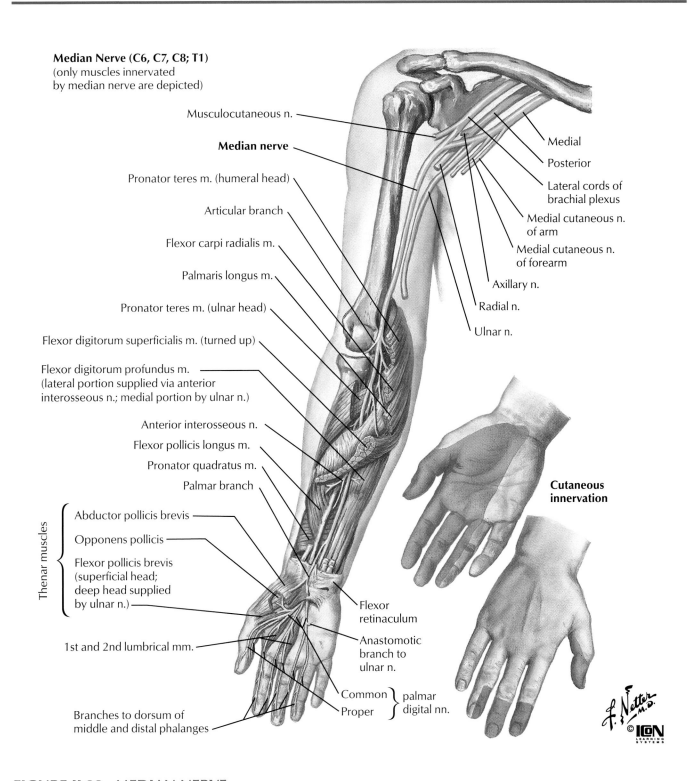

Median Nerve (C6, C7, C8; T1)
(only muscles innervated
by median nerve are depicted)

Musculocutaneous n.

Median nerve

Pronator teres m. (humeral head)

Articular branch

Flexor carpi radialis m.

Palmaris longus m.

Pronator teres m. (ulnar head)

Flexor digitorum superficialis m. (turned up)

Flexor digitorum profundus m.
(lateral portion supplied via anterior
interosseous n.; medial portion by ulnar n.)

Anterior interosseous n.
Flexor pollicis longus m.
Pronator quadratus m.
Palmar branch

Thenar muscles {
Abductor pollicis brevis
Opponens pollicis
Flexor pollicis brevis
(superficial head;
deep head supplied
by ulnar n.)

1st and 2nd lumbrical mm.

Branches to dorsum of
middle and distal phalanges

Medial
Posterior
Lateral cords of
brachial plexus
Medial cutaneous n.
of arm
Medial cutaneous n.
of forearm
Axillary n.
Radial n.
Ulnar n.

Cutaneous
innervation

Flexor
retinaculum

Anastomotic
branch to
ulnar n.

Common } palmar
Proper } digital nn.

FIGURE II.23: MEDIAN NERVE

The median nerve (C5-T1) supplies motor fibers to the (1) flexor carpi radialis, (2) pronator teres, (3) palmaris longus, (4) flexor digitorum superficialis and profundus, (5) flexor pollicis longus, (6) abductor pollicis brevis, (7) flexor pollicis brevis, (8) opponens pollicis brevis, and (9) lumbrical muscles of the index and middle fingers. It supplies sensory innervation to the palm and the adjacent thumb, the index and middle fingers, and the lateral half of the fourth finger. A lesion (from carpal tunnel syndrome) results in weakness in flexion of the fingers, and abduction and opposition of the thumb and loss of sensation, or painful sensation in the radial distribution in the hand. A higher lesion also produces weakness in pronation of the forearm.

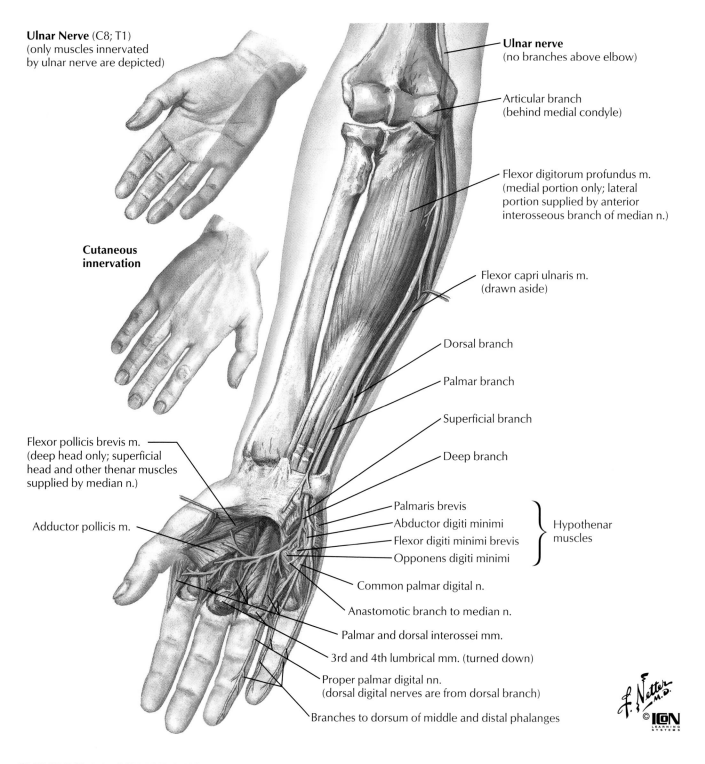

Ulnar Nerve (C8; T1)
(only muscles innervated
by ulnar nerve are depicted)

Cutaneous
innervation

Flexor pollicis brevis m.
(deep head only; superficial
head and other thenar muscles
supplied by median n.)

Adductor pollicis m.

Ulnar nerve
(no branches above elbow)

Articular branch
(behind medial condyle)

Flexor digitorum profundus m.
(medial portion only; lateral
portion supplied by anterior
interosseous branch of median n.)

Flexor capri ulnaris m.
(drawn aside)

Dorsal branch

Palmar branch

Superficial branch

Deep branch

Palmaris brevis
Abductor digiti minimi
Flexor digiti minimi brevis
Opponens digiti minimi

Hypothenar
muscles

Common palmar digital n.

Anastomotic branch to median n.

Palmar and dorsal interossei mm.

3rd and 4th lumbrical mm. (turned down)

Proper palmar digital nn.
(dorsal digital nerves are from dorsal branch)

Branches to dorsum of middle and distal phalanges

FIGURE II.24: ULNAR NERVE

The ulnar nerve (C8-T1) supplies motor fibers to the (1) flexor carpi ulnaris, (2) flexor digitorum profundus, (3) adductor pollicis, (4) abductor digiti V, (5) opponens digiti V, (6) flexor digiti brevis V, (7) interosseus dorsal and palmar, and (8) lumbrical muscles to the fourth and little fingers. It supplies sensory innervation to the dorsal and palmar medial surfaces of the hand for the little finger and medial half of the fourth finger. A lesion results in wasting of hand muscles, weakness of wrist flexion and ulnar deviation of the hand, weakness of abduction and adduction of the fingers, "claw hand" (hyperextension of the fingers at metacarpophalangeal joints and flexion at the interphalangeal joints), and loss of sensation in the ulnar distribution in the hand.

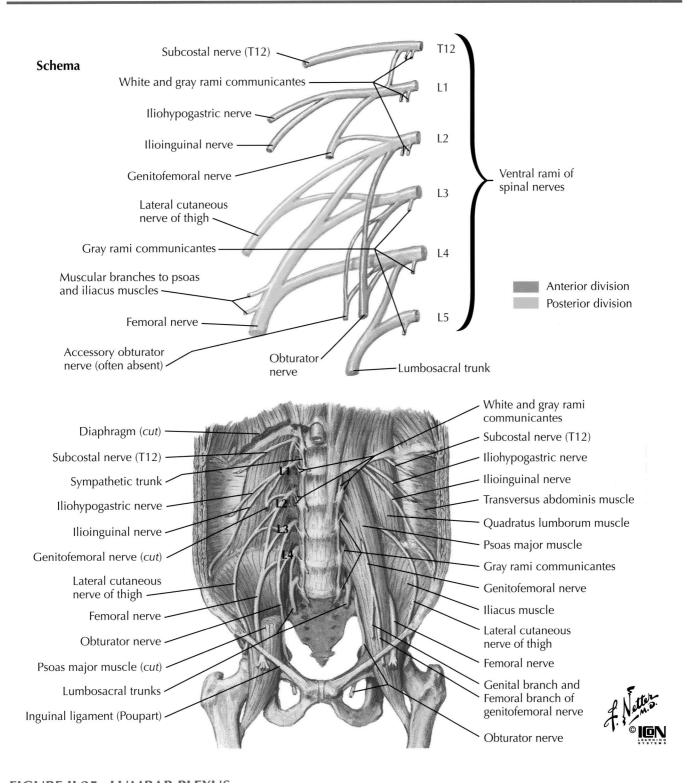

Schema

Subcostal nerve (T12)

White and gray rami communicantes

Iliohypogastric nerve

Ilioinguinal nerve

Genitofemoral nerve

Lateral cutaneous nerve of thigh

Gray rami communicantes

Muscular branches to psoas and iliacus muscles

Femoral nerve

Accessory obturator nerve (often absent)

Obturator nerve

Lumbosacral trunk

T12

L1

L2

L3

L4

L5

Ventral rami of spinal nerves

Anterior division
Posterior division

Diaphragm (cut)

Subcostal nerve (T12)

Sympathetic trunk

Iliohypogastric nerve

Ilioinguinal nerve

Genitofemoral nerve (cut)

Lateral cutaneous nerve of thigh

Femoral nerve

Obturator nerve

Psoas major muscle (cut)

Lumbosacral trunks

Inguinal ligament (Poupart)

White and gray rami communicantes

Subcostal nerve (T12)

Iliohypogastric nerve

Ilioinguinal nerve

Transversus abdominis muscle

Quadratus lumborum muscle

Psoas major muscle

Gray rami communicantes

Genitofemoral nerve

Iliacus muscle

Lateral cutaneous nerve of thigh

Femoral nerve

Genital branch and Femoral branch of genitofemoral nerve

Obturator nerve

FIGURE II.25: LUMBAR PLEXUS

The lumbar plexus is formed from the anterior primary rami of the L1, L2, L3, and L4 roots within the posterior substance of the psoas muscle. The L1 (and some of the L2) root forms the iliohypogastric and ilioinguinal nerves and the genitofemoral nerves. These nerves contribute innervation to the transverse and the oblique abdominal muscles. The remaining roots form the femoral, obturator, and lateral femoral cutaneous nerves. Lesions of the lumbar plexus are unusual because of the protection of the plexus within the psoas muscle. They result in weakness of flexion, weakness of adduction of the thigh and extension of the leg, and decreased sensation on the anterior thigh and leg.

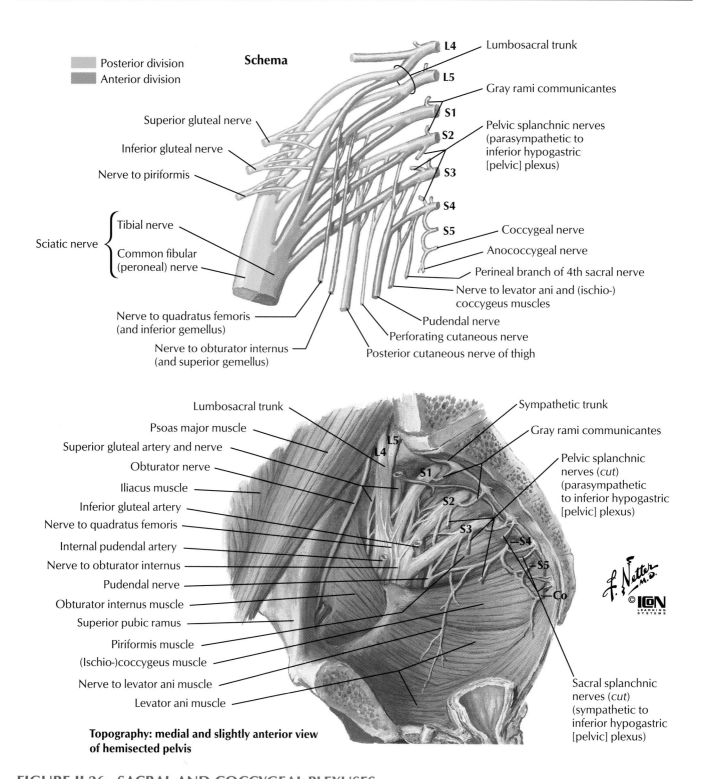

Schema

Posterior division
Anterior division

L4 — Lumbosacral trunk
L5
— Gray rami communicantes
S1
S2 — Pelvic splanchnic nerves (parasympathetic to inferior hypogastric [pelvic] plexus)
S3
S4
S5 — Coccygeal nerve
— Anococcygeal nerve
— Perineal branch of 4th sacral nerve
— Nerve to levator ani and (ischio-) coccygeus muscles
Pudendal nerve
Perforating cutaneous nerve
Posterior cutaneous nerve of thigh

Superior gluteal nerve
Inferior gluteal nerve
Nerve to piriformis

Sciatic nerve { Tibial nerve
Common fibular (peroneal) nerve

Nerve to quadratus femoris (and inferior gemellus)
Nerve to obturator internus (and superior gemellus)

Lumbosacral trunk
Psoas major muscle
Superior gluteal artery and nerve
Obturator nerve
Iliacus muscle
Inferior gluteal artery
Nerve to quadratus femoris
Internal pudendal artery
Nerve to obturator internus
Pudendal nerve
Obturator internus muscle
Superior pubic ramus
Piriformis muscle
(Ischio-)coccygeus muscle
Nerve to levator ani muscle
Levator ani muscle

Sympathetic trunk
Gray rami communicantes
Pelvic splanchnic nerves (cut) (parasympathetic to inferior hypogastric [pelvic] plexus)

L5
L4
S1
S2
S3
S4
S5
Co

Sacral splanchnic nerves (cut) (sympathetic to inferior hypogastric [pelvic] plexus)

Topography: medial and slightly anterior view of hemisected pelvis

FIGURE II.26: SACRAL AND COCCYGEAL PLEXUSES

The sacral and coccygeal plexuses are formed from the roots of the L4-S4 segments, located anterior to the piriformis muscle. The major branches include the superior (L4-S1) and inferior (L5-S2) gluteal nerves, the posterior femoral cutaneous nerve (S1-S3), the sciatic nerve (L4-S3) and its tibial and common peroneal divisions, and the pudendal nerve (S2-S4). The pudendal nerve supplies the perineal and sphincter muscles, which aid in closing the sphincters of the bladder and the rectum. Lesions of the sacral plexus result in weakness of the posterior thigh and the muscles of the leg and feet, with decreased sensation in the posterior thigh and a perianal/saddle location.

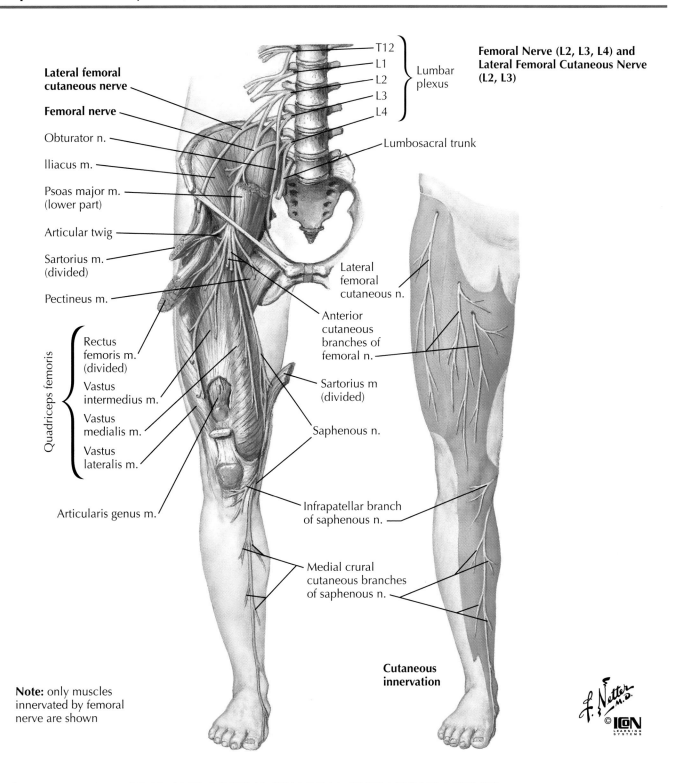

**Femoral Nerve (L2, L3, L4) and
Lateral Femoral Cutaneous Nerve
(L2, L3)**

Lateral femoral
cutaneous nerve

Femoral nerve

Obturator n.

Iliacus m.

Psoas major m.
(lower part)

Articular twig

Sartorius m.
(divided)

Pectineus m.

Rectus
femoris m.
(divided)

Vastus
intermedius m.

Vastus
medialis m.

Vastus
lateralis m.

Quadriceps femoris

Articularis genus m.

T12
L1
L2
L3
L4

Lumbar
plexus

Lumbosacral trunk

Lateral
femoral
cutaneous n.

Anterior
cutaneous
branches of
femoral n.

Sartorius m
(divided)

Saphenous n.

Infrapatellar branch
of saphenous n.

Medial crural
cutaneous branches
of saphenous n.

**Cutaneous
innervation**

Note: only muscles
innervated by femoral
nerve are shown

FIGURE II.27: FEMORAL AND LATERAL FEMORAL CUTANEOUS NERVES

The femoral nerve (mainly L2-L4) innervates the iliopsoas, sartorius, and quadriceps femoris muscles. It contributes to flexion and outward rotation of the hip, flexion and inward rotation of the lower leg, and extension of the lower leg around the knee joint. It supplies sensory fibers to the anterior thigh and to the anterior and medial surfaces of the leg and foot. A lesion results in weakness of extension of the leg and flexion of the hip and leg, with quadriceps atrophy, and in loss of sensation in territories of sensory distribution. The lateral femoral cutaneous nerve supplies sensation to the skin and fascia of the anterior and lateral surfaces of the thigh to the level of the knee; lesions result in loss of sensation in this distribution.

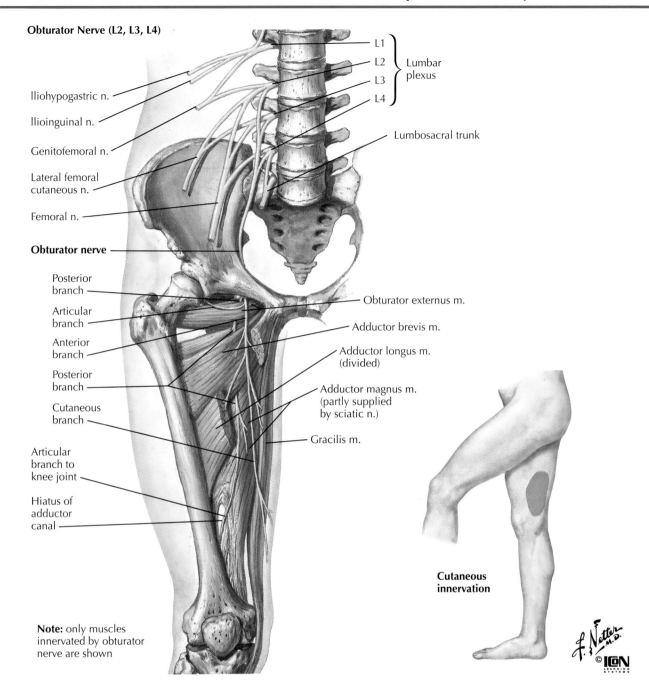

Obturator Nerve (L2, L3, L4)

Iliohypogastric n.

Ilioinguinal n.

Genitofemoral n.

Lateral femoral cutaneous n.

Femoral n.

Obturator nerve

Posterior branch

Articular branch

Anterior branch

Posterior branch

Cutaneous branch

Articular branch to knee joint

Hiatus of adductor canal

L1
L2
L3
L4

Lumbar plexus

Lumbosacral trunk

Obturator externus m.

Adductor brevis m.

Adductor longus m. (divided)

Adductor magnus m. (partly supplied by sciatic n.)

Gracilis m.

Note: only muscles innervated by obturator nerve are shown

Cutaneous innervation

FIGURE II.28: OBTURATOR NERVE

The obturator nerve (L2-L4) supplies the pectineus, adductor (longus, brevis, and magnus), gracilis, and external obturator muscles. This nerve regulates adduction and rotation of the thigh. A small cutaneous zone on the internal thigh is supplied by sensory fibers. A lesion of the obturator nerve results in weakness of adduction of the thigh, with a tendency to abduct the thigh in walking. There also is weakness of external rotation of the thigh. A small zone of anesthetic skin on the medial thigh is present.

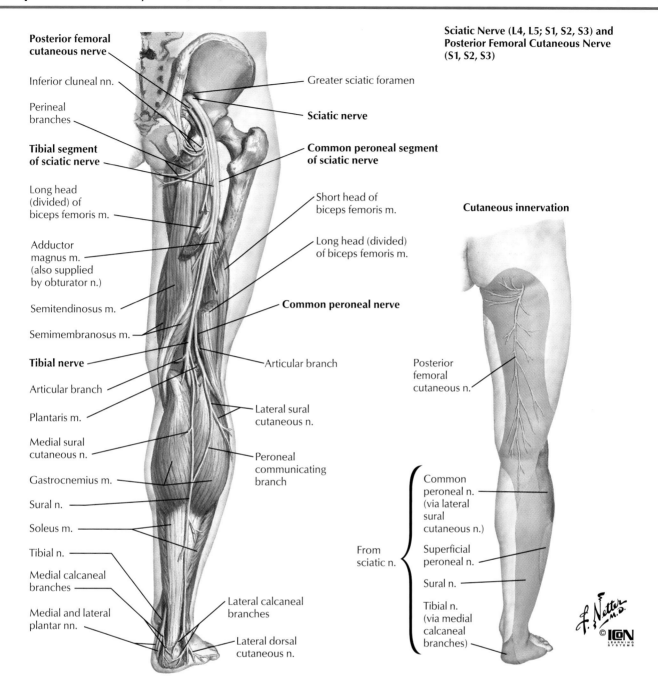

Sciatic Nerve (L4, L5; S1, S2, S3) and
Posterior Femoral Cutaneous Nerve
(S1, S2, S3)

Posterior femoral cutaneous nerve

Inferior cluneal nn.

Perineal branches

Tibial segment of sciatic nerve

Long head (divided) of biceps femoris m.

Adductor magnus m. (also supplied by obturator n.)

Semitendinosus m.

Semimembranosus m.

Tibial nerve

Articular branch

Plantaris m.

Medial sural cutaneous n.

Gastrocnemius m.

Sural n.

Soleus m.

Tibial n.

Medial calcaneal branches

Medial and lateral plantar nn.

Greater sciatic foramen

Sciatic nerve

Common peroneal segment of sciatic nerve

Short head of biceps femoris m.

Long head (divided) of biceps femoris m.

Common peroneal nerve

Articular branch

Lateral sural cutaneous n.

Peroneal communicating branch

Lateral calcaneal branches

Lateral dorsal cutaneous n.

Cutaneous innervation

Posterior femoral cutaneous n.

From sciatic n.

Common peroneal n. (via lateral sural cutaneous n.)

Superficial peroneal n.

Sural n.

Tibial n. (via medial calcaneal branches)

FIGURE II.29: SCIATIC AND POSTERIOR FEMORAL CUTANEOUS NERVES

The sciatic nerve is formed from the roots of the L4-S3 segments. The superior and inferior gluteal nerves branch proximally, just before the sciatic nerve's formation. The superior gluteal nerve (L4-S1) supplies the gluteus medius and minimus, tensor fascia lata, and piriformis muscles. It contributes to abduction and inward rotation and some outward rotation of the thigh and to flexion of the upper leg at the hip. The inferior gluteal nerve (L4-S1) supplies the gluteus maximus, obturator internus, gemellus, and quadratus muscles. It contributes to extension of the thigh at the hip and to outward rotation of the thigh. A lesion results in

difficulty climbing stairs or rising from a sitting position. The sciatic nerve proper supplies the biceps femoris, semitendinosus, and semimembranosus muscles (hamstrings); and it regulates flexion of the lower leg. Because it branches into the tibial and common peroneal nerves, major lesions of the sciatic nerve result in weakness of leg flexion, weakness of all muscles below the knee, and loss of sensation in the posterior thigh, posterior and lateral aspects of the leg, and sole of the foot. The posterior femoral cutaneous nerve (S1-S3) supplies sensory innervation to the posterior thigh, lateral part of the perineum, and lower portion of the buttock.

Tibial Nerve (L4, L5; S1, S2, S3)

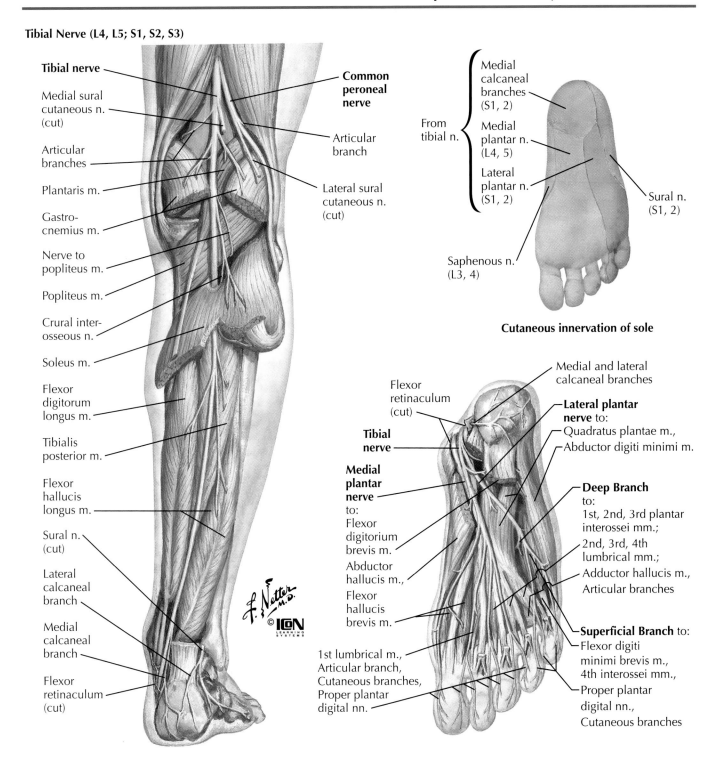

Cutaneous innervation of sole

FIGURE II.30: TIBIAL NERVE

The tibial nerve (L4-S2) supplies innervation to the (1) gastrocnemius and soleus (main plantar flexors of the foot), (2) tibialis posterior (plantar flexor and invertor), (3) flexor digitorum longus (plantar flexor and toe flexor), and (4) flexor hallucis longus (plantar flexor and great toe flexor) muscles, and (5) muscles of the foot, including the abductor digiti minimi pedis, flexor digiti minimi, adductor hallucis, interosseus, and third and fourth lumbrical muscles. Sensory branches supply the skin over the lateral calf, foot, heel, and small toe (sural nerve), and the medial aspect of the heel and the sole of the foot. A lesion can result in weakness of plantar flexion and inversion of the foot, weakness of toe flexion, and loss of sensation on the lateral calf and the plantar region of the foot.

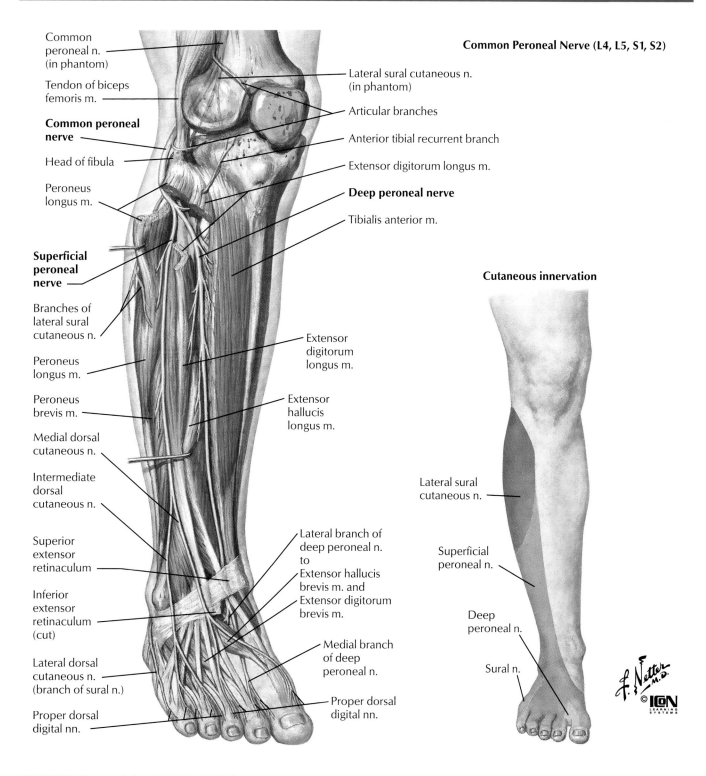

Common peroneal n. (in phantom)

Tendon of biceps femoris m.

Common peroneal nerve

Head of fibula

Peroneus longus m.

Superficial peroneal nerve

Branches of lateral sural cutaneous n.

Peroneus longus m.

Peroneus brevis m.

Medial dorsal cutaneous n.

Intermediate dorsal cutaneous n.

Superior extensor retinaculum

Inferior extensor retinaculum (cut)

Lateral dorsal cutaneous n. (branch of sural n.)

Proper dorsal digital nn.

Common Peroneal Nerve (L4, L5, S1, S2)

Lateral sural cutaneous n. (in phantom)

Articular branches

Anterior tibial recurrent branch

Extensor digitorum longus m.

Deep peroneal nerve

Tibialis anterior m.

Extensor digitorum longus m.

Extensor hallucis longus m.

Lateral branch of deep peroneal n. to Extensor hallucis brevis m. and Extensor digitorum brevis m.

Medial branch of deep peroneal n.

Proper dorsal digital nn.

Cutaneous innervation

Lateral sural cutaneous n.

Superficial peroneal n.

Deep peroneal n.

Sural n.

FIGURE II.31: COMMON PERONEAL NERVE

The common peroneal nerve (L4-S1) branches into the deep peroneal nerve, supplying the (1) tibialis anterior (foot dorsiflexion and inversion), (2) extensor hallucis longus (foot dorsiflexion and great toe extension), (3) extensor digitorum longus (extension of toes and foot dorsiflexion), (4) extensor digitorum brevis (extension of toes), and the superficial peroneal nerve, which supplies the peroneus longus and brevis muscles (plantar flexion and foot eversion). Sensory branches supply the lateral aspect of the leg below the knee and the skin on the dorsal surface of the foot. A lesion of this nerve can result in weakness of dorsiflexion of the foot, weakness of toe extension, and loss of sensation of the lateral aspect of the lower leg and the dorsum of the foot.

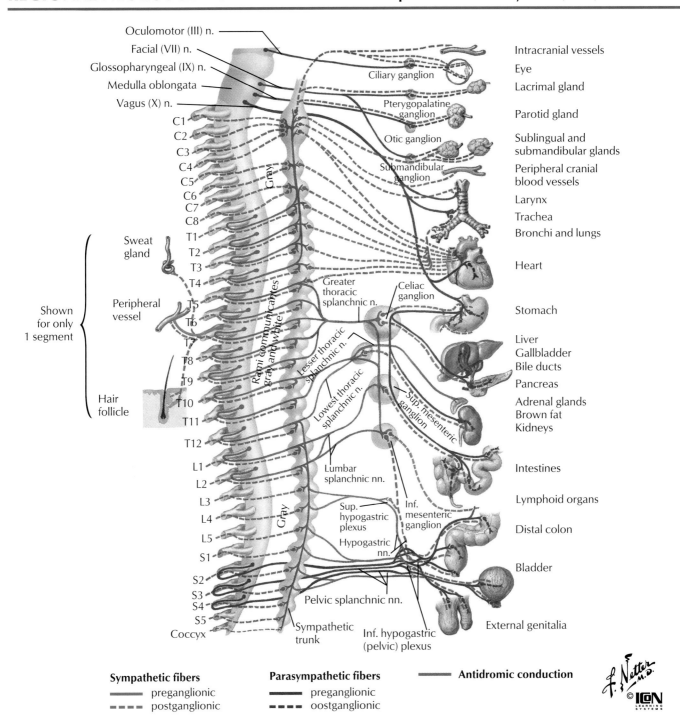

Oculomotor (III) n.
Facial (VII) n.
Glossopharyngeal (IX) n.
Medulla oblongata
Vagus (X) n.

C1
C2
C3
C4
C5
C6
C7
C8
T1
T2
T3
T4
T5
T6
T7
T8
T9
T10
T11
T12
L1
L2
L3
L4
L5
S1
S2
S3
S4
S5
Coccyx

Gray

Sweat gland

Shown for only 1 segment

Peripheral vessel

Hair follicle

Rami communicantes gray and white

Gray

Greater thoracic splanchnic n.
Lesser thoracic splanchnic n.
Lowest thoracic splanchnic n.
Lumbar splanchnic nn.
Sup. hypogastric plexus
Hypogastric nn.
Pelvic splanchnic nn.
Sympathetic trunk

Ciliary ganglion
Pterygopalatine ganglion
Otic ganglion
Submandibular ganglion

Celiac ganglion
Sup. mesenteric ganglion
Inf. mesenteric ganglion
Inf. hypogastric (pelvic) plexus

Intracranial vessels
Eye
Lacrimal gland
Parotid gland
Sublingual and submandibular glands
Peripheral cranial blood vessels
Larynx
Trachea
Bronchi and lungs
Heart
Stomach
Liver
Gallbladder
Bile ducts
Pancreas
Adrenal glands
Brown fat
Kidneys
Intestines
Lymphoid organs
Distal colon
Bladder
External genitalia

Sympathetic fibers
— preganglionic
- - - postganglionic

Parasympathetic fibers
— preganglionic
- - - oostganglionic

— **Antidromic conduction**

FIGURE II.32: GENERAL SCHEMA OF THE AUTONOMIC NERVOUS SYSTEM

The autonomic nervous system (ANS) is a 2-neuron chain. The preganglionic neuron arises from the brain stem or the spinal cord (CNS) and synapses on postganglionic neurons in the sympathetic chain, collateral ganglia (sympathetic), or an intramural ganglion (parasympathetic) near the organ innervated. The sympathetic division, derived from neurons in the T1-L2 (thoracolumbar) lateral horn, prepares the body for fight or flight—mobilization for emergency responses. The parasympathetic division is derived from neurons in the brain stem (cranial nerves [CNs] III, VII, IX, and X) and the sacral spinal cord (S2-S4 intermediate gray). This craniosacral system regulates reparative, homeostatic, and digestive functions. These autonomic systems achieve their actions through innervation of smooth muscle, cardiac muscle, secretory (exocrine) glands, metabolic cells (hepatocytes, brown fat), and cells of the immune system. Normally, both divisions work together to regulate visceral activities such as respiration, cardiovascular function, digestion, and some endocrine functions.

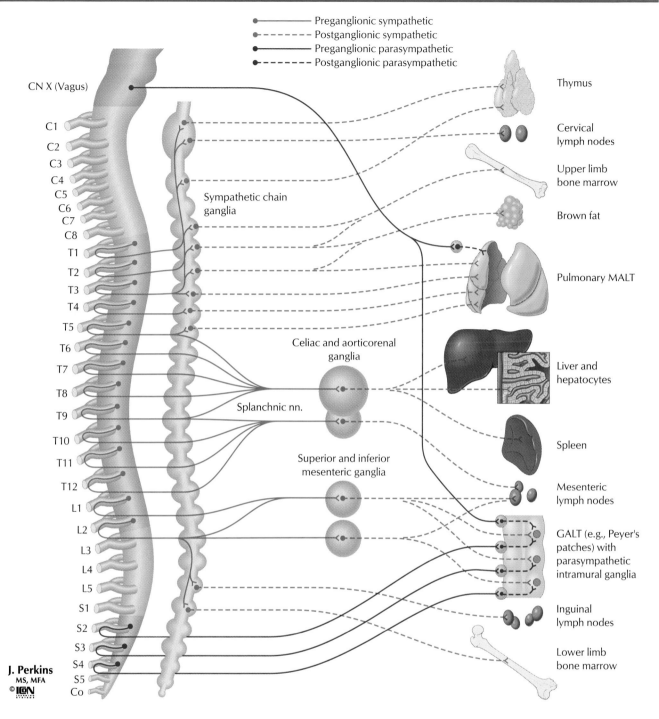

FIGURE II.33: INNERVATION OF ORGANS OF THE IMMUNE SYSTEM AND METABOLIC ORGANS

The ANS innervates the vasculature, the smooth muscle tissue, and the parenchyma of organs of the immune system mainly through the sympathetic division. In the bone marrow and the thymus, sympathetic fibers modulate cell proliferation, differentiation, and mobilization. In the spleen and the lymph nodes, they modulate innate immune reactivity and the magnitude and timing of acquired immune responses, particularly the choice of cell-mediated (Th1 cytokines) versus humoral (Th2 cytokines) immunity. Autonomic fibers regulate immune responses and inflammatory responses in the mucosal-associated lymphoid tissue of the gut and the lung and in the skin. Extensive neuropeptidergic innervation, derived from both the ANS and primary sensory neurons, is present in the parenchyma of lymphoid organs. Postganglionic sympathetic nerves also supply hepatocytes and fat cells.

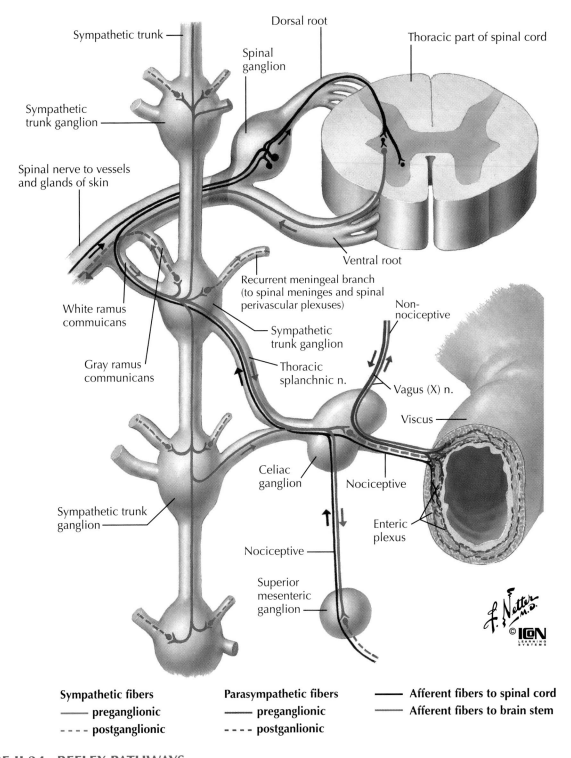

Dorsal root

Thoracic part of spinal cord

Sympathetic trunk

Spinal ganglion

Sympathetic trunk ganglion

Spinal nerve to vessels and glands of skin

Ventral root

Recurrent meningeal branch (to spinal meninges and spinal perivascular plexuses)

Non-nociceptive

White ramus commuicans

Sympathetic trunk ganglion

Gray ramus communicans

Thoracic splanchnic n.

Vagus (X) n.

Viscus

Celiac ganglion

Nociceptive

Sympathetic trunk ganglion

Enteric plexus

Nociceptive

Superior mesenteric ganglion

Sympathetic fibers	Parasympathetic fibers	—— Afferent fibers to spinal cord
—— preganglionic	—— preganglionic	—— Afferent fibers to brain stem
- - - postganglionic	- - - postganlionic	

FIGURE II.34: REFLEX PATHWAYS

Autonomic reflex pathways consist of a sensory (afferent) component, interneurons in the CNS, and autonomic efferent components that innervate the peripheral tissue responding to the afferent stimulus. The afferents can be autonomic (e.g., from the vagus nerve), processed by brain stem nuclei such as the nucleus solitarius; or they can be somatic (e.g., nociception), processed by spinal cord neurons. The preganglionic sympathetic or parasympathetic neurons are activated through interneurons to produce a reflex autonomic response (e.g., contraction of vascular smooth muscle to alter blood pressure, increase in heart rate and contractility). The efferent connectivity can be relayed via splanchnic or somatic nerves because of the complexity of autonomic efferent pathways.

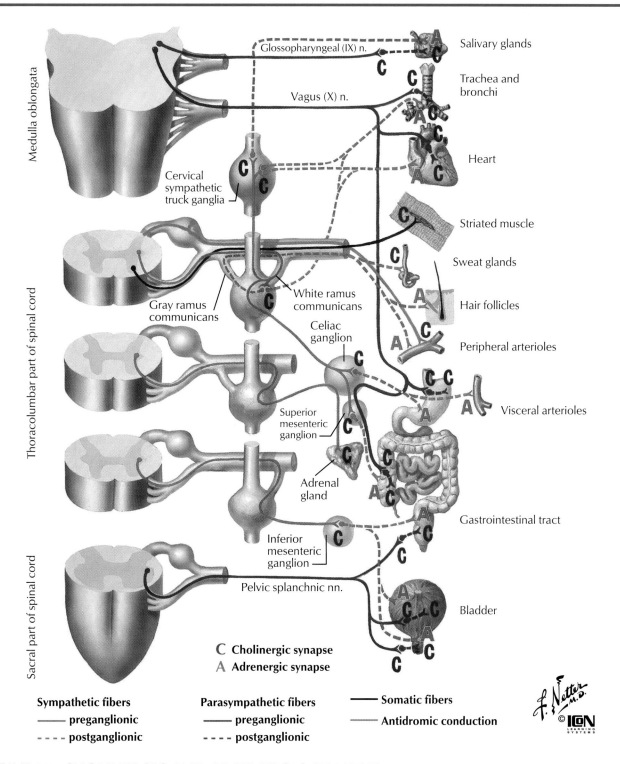

FIGURE II.35: CHOLINERGIC AND ADRENERGIC SYNAPSES

The ANS is a 2-neuron chain. All sympathetic and parasympathetic preganglionic neurons use acetylcholine (ACh) as the principal neurotransmitter in synapses on ganglion cells. These cholinergic (C) synapses activate mainly nicotinic (N) receptors on the ganglion cells. Postganglionic parasympathetic neurons use ACh at synapses (C) with target tissue to activate mainly muscarinic (M) receptors. Postganglionic sympathetic neurons mainly use norepinephrine (adrenergic responses [A]) to activate both alpha and beta receptors on target tissues. Although ACh and norepinephrine are the principal neurotransmitters in autonomic neurons, many co-localized neuropeptides and other neuromediators, including neuropeptide Y, substance P, somatostatin, enkephalins, histamine, and glutamate, are present.

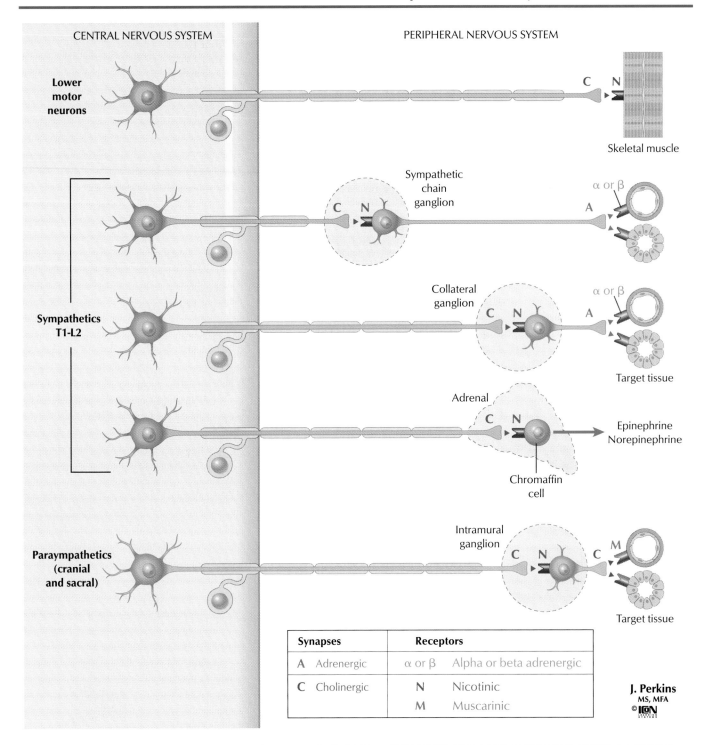

Synapses		Receptors	
A	Adrenergic	α or β	Alpha or beta adrenergic
C	Cholinergic	N	Nicotinic
		M	Muscarinic

J. Perkins
MS, MFA

FIGURE II.36: SCHEMATIC OF CHOLINERGIC AND ADRENERGIC DISTRIBUTION TO MOTOR AND AUTONOMIC STRUCTURES

All preganglionic neurons of both the sympathetic and parasympathetic nervous system use acetylcholine (ACh) as their neurotransmitter. All ganglion cells possess mainly nicotinic receptors for the fast response to cholinergic release from preganglionic axons. However, additional muscarinic receptors and dopamine receptors on ganglion cells help to mediate longer term excitability. The postganglionic sympathetic nerves use mainly norepinephrine (NE) as their neurotransmitter, and target structures in the periphery possess different subsets of alpha and beta adrenergic receptors for response to NE. Some postganglionic nerve fibers to sweat glands use ACh as their neurotransmitter. Postganglionic parasympathetic nerves use ACh as their neurotransmitter, and target structures in the periphery possess mainly muscarinic receptors for response to ACh.

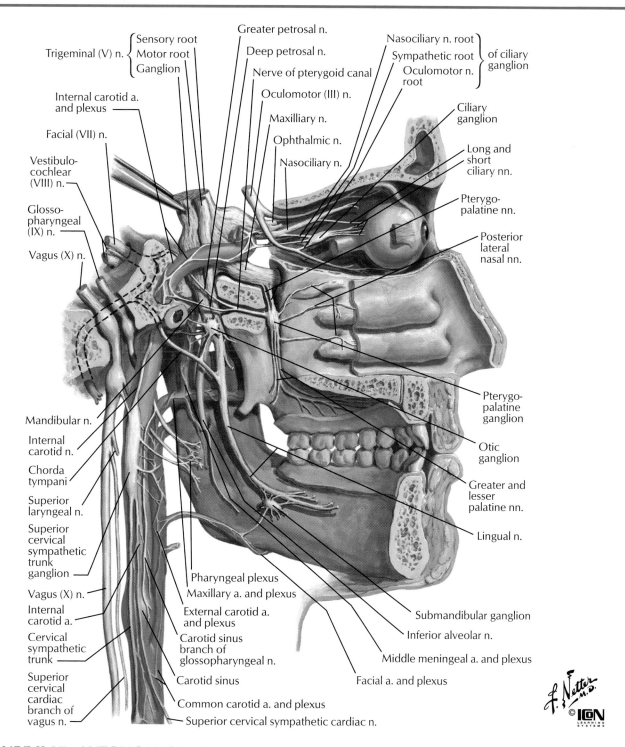

Greater petrosal n.

Trigeminal (V) n. { Sensory root / Motor root / Ganglion

Deep petrosal n.

Nerve of pterygoid canal

Internal carotid a. and plexus

Oculomotor (III) n.

Facial (VII) n.

Maxilliary n.

Vestibulo-cochlear (VIII) n.

Ophthalmic n.

Nasociliary n.

Glosso-pharyngeal (IX) n.

Vagus (X) n.

Nasociliary n. root
Sympathetic root } of ciliary ganglion
Oculomotor n. root

Ciliary ganglion

Long and short ciliary nn.

Pterygo-palatine nn.

Posterior lateral nasal nn.

Pterygo-palatine ganglion

Otic ganglion

Mandibular n.

Internal carotid n.

Chorda tympani

Superior laryngeal n.

Greater and lesser palatine nn.

Lingual n.

Superior cervical sympathetic trunk ganglion

Vagus (X) n.

Internal carotid a.

Cervical sympathetic trunk

Superior cervical cardiac branch of vagus n.

Pharyngeal plexus

Maxillary a. and plexus

External carotid a. and plexus

Carotid sinus branch of glossopharyngeal n.

Carotid sinus

Common carotid a. and plexus

Superior cervical sympathetic cardiac n.

Submandibular ganglion

Inferior alveolar n.

Middle meningeal a. and plexus

Facial a. and plexus

FIGURE II.37: AUTONOMIC DISTRIBUTION TO THE HEAD AND THE NECK: MEDIAL VIEW ____

Autonomic nerve distribution to the head and the neck includes components of both the parasympathetic and the sympathetic nervous systems. Parasympathetic components are associated with CNs III (ciliary ganglion), VII (pterygopalatine, submandibular ganglia), and IX (otic ganglion). The vagus nerve and its associated ganglia do not innervate effector tissue in the head and the neck, although they are present in the neck. Sympathetic components are associated with the superior cervical ganglion and, to a lesser extent, the middle cervical ganglion. The geniculate ganglion (CN VII), the petrosal ganglion (CN IX), and the nodose ganglion (CN X) process taste information. They are sometimes thought of as autonomic afferents, but they are not components of the autonomic efferent nervous system.

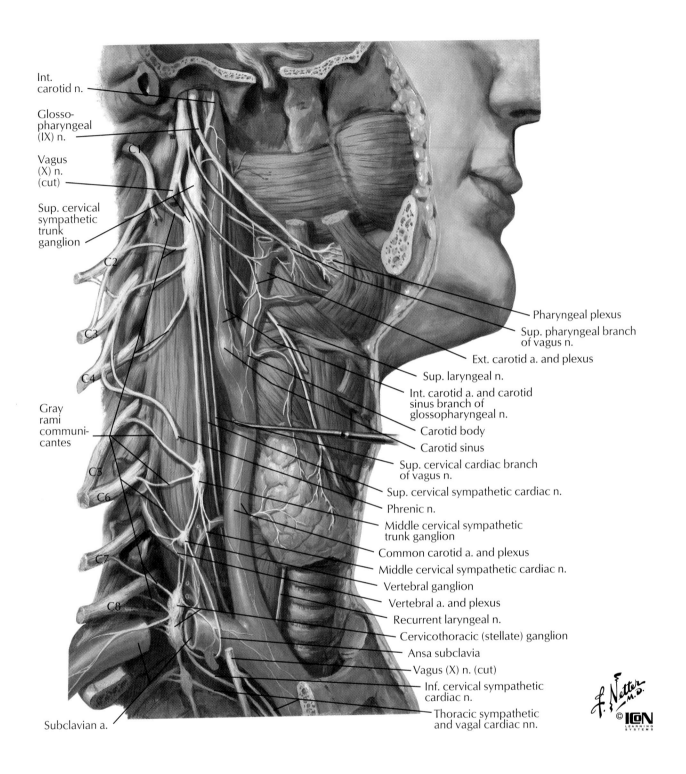

Int. carotid n.

Glosso-
pharyngeal
(IX) n.

Vagus
(X) n.
(cut)

Sup. cervical
sympathetic
trunk
ganglion

Gray
rami
communi-
cantes

C1
C2
C3
C4
C5
C6
C7
C8

Subclavian a.

Pharyngeal plexus
Sup. pharyngeal branch
of vagus n.
Ext. carotid a. and plexus
Sup. laryngeal n.
Int. carotid a. and carotid
sinus branch of
glossopharyngeal n.
Carotid body
Carotid sinus
Sup. cervical cardiac branch
of vagus n.
Sup. cervical sympathetic cardiac n.
Phrenic n.
Middle cervical sympathetic
trunk ganglion
Common carotid a. and plexus
Middle cervical sympathetic cardiac n.
Vertebral ganglion
Vertebral a. and plexus
Recurrent laryngeal n.
Cervicothoracic (stellate) ganglion
Ansa subclavia
Vagus (X) n. (cut)
Inf. cervical sympathetic
cardiac n.
Thoracic sympathetic
and vagal cardiac nn.

FIGURE II.38: AUTONOMIC DISTRIBUTION TO THE HEAD AND THE NECK: LATERAL VIEW

The parasympathetic nerve fibers to the head and the neck regulate pupillary constriction and accommodation for near vision (CN III, ciliary ganglion to pupillary constrictor muscle and ciliary muscle), tear production (CN VII, pterygopalatine ganglion to lacrimal glands), and salivation (CN VII, submandibular ganglion to submandibular and sublingual glands; CN IV, otic ganglion to parotid gland). The sympathetic nerve fibers to the head and the neck derive mainly from the superior cervical ganglion, with synapses to the pupillary dilator muscle, the sweat glands, the vascular smooth muscle, and the thymus gland.

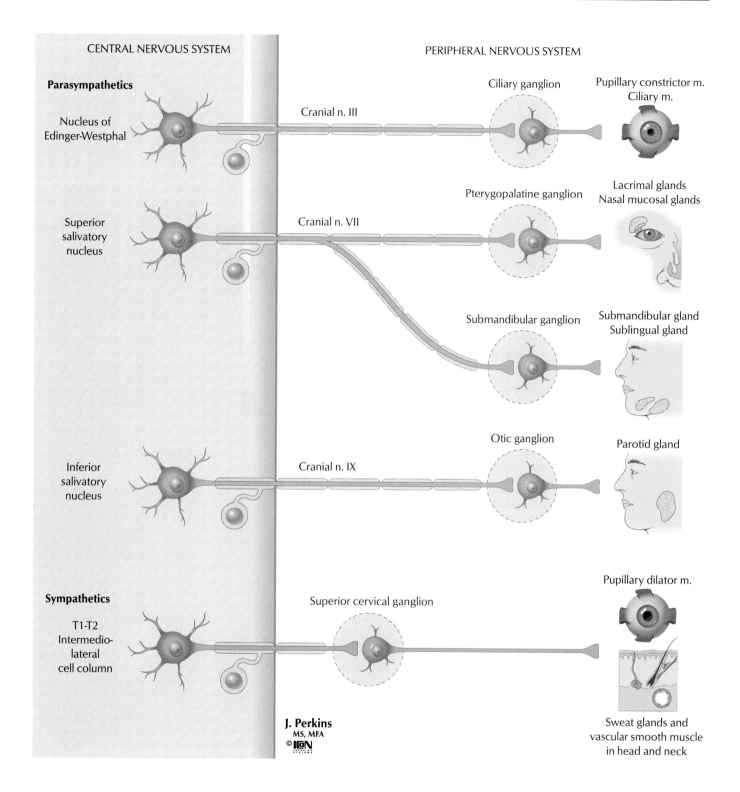

FIGURE II.39: SCHEMATIC OF AUTONOMIC DISTRIBUTION TO THE HEAD AND THE NECK ——

Autonomic innervation to the head and the neck is derived from parasympathetic neurons in the brain stem, including the Edinger-Westphal nucleus (CN III), the superior salivatory nucleus (CN VII), and the inferior salivatory nucleus (CN IX), and from sympathetic neurons in the T1-T2 intermediolateral cell column in the spinal cord. The associated ganglia and target (effector) tissue are also illustrated.

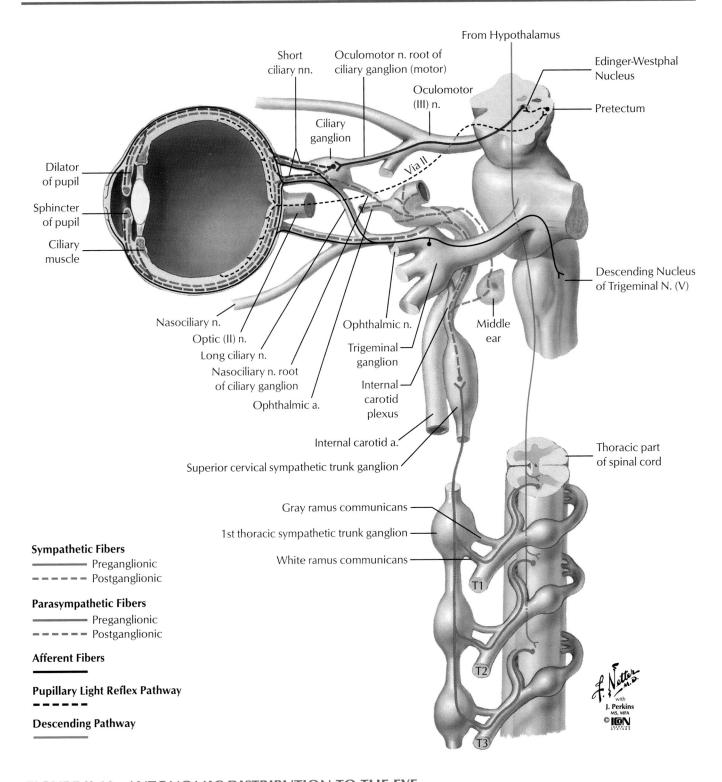

FIGURE II.40: AUTONOMIC DISTRIBUTION TO THE EYE

Parasympathetic preganglionic nerve fibers from the Edinger-Westphal nucleus innervate the ciliary ganglion, which supplies the ciliary muscle (aiding in accommodation to near vision), and the pupillary constrictor muscle (constricting the pupil). Sympathetic preganglionic nerve fibers from the T1-T2 intermediolateral cell column innervate the superior cervical ganglion, which supplies the dilator muscle of the pupil. The pupillary light reflex is a major reflex in neurological testing. The afferent limb is activated by light shone in either eye via CN II, processed through the pretectum to the Edinger-Westphal nucleus on both sides (via the posterior commissure); the efferent limb consists of automatic outflow to the pupillary constrictor muscles of both sides.

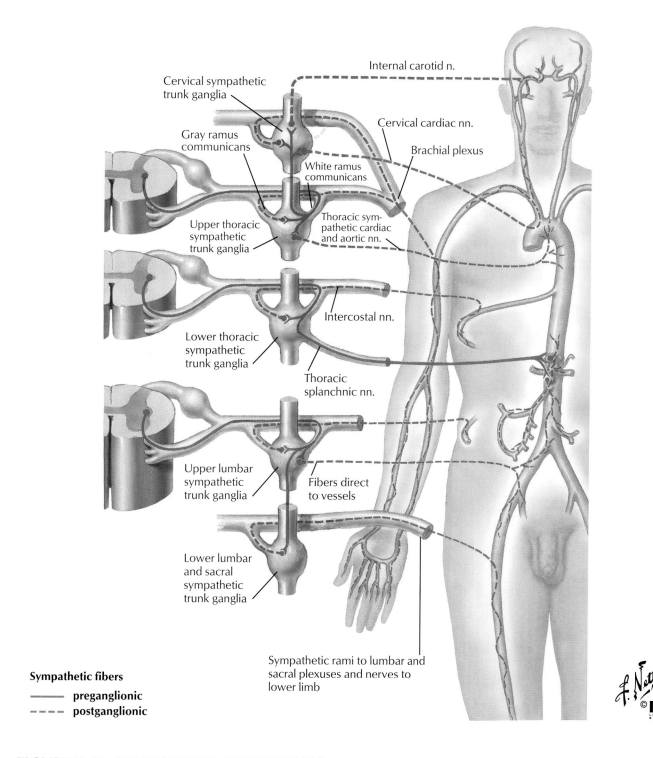

Internal carotid n.

Cervical sympathetic trunk ganglia

Cervical cardiac nn.

Gray ramus communicans

Brachial plexus

White ramus communicans

Upper thoracic sympathetic trunk ganglia

Thoracic sympathetic cardiac and aortic nn.

Intercostal nn.

Lower thoracic sympathetic trunk ganglia

Thoracic splanchnic nn.

Upper lumbar sympathetic trunk ganglia

Fibers direct to vessels

Lower lumbar and sacral sympathetic trunk ganglia

Sympathetic rami to lumbar and sacral plexuses and nerves to lower limb

Sympathetic fibers

——— preganglionic

– – – – postganglionic

FIGURE II.41: INNERVATION OF THE LIMBS

Autonomic innervation of the limbs derives from the sympathetic nervous system. Preganglionic sympathetic nerve fibers from the thoracolumbar intermediolateral cell column supply sympathetic chain ganglia. These ganglia send postganglionic noradrenergic nerve fibers through the gray rami communicantes into the peripheral nerves to supply vascular smooth muscle (vasomotor fibers), sweat glands (sudomotor fibers), and arrector pili muscles associated with hair follicles (pilomotor fibers).

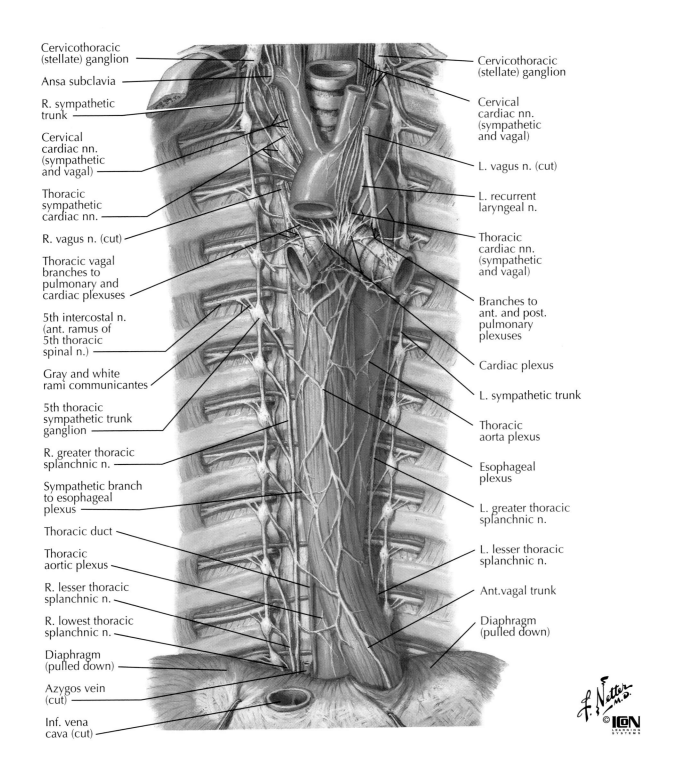

Cervicothoracic (stellate) ganglion

Ansa subclavia

R. sympathetic trunk

Cervical cardiac nn. (sympathetic and vagal)

Thoracic sympathetic cardiac nn.

R. vagus n. (cut)

Thoracic vagal branches to pulmonary and cardiac plexuses

5th intercostal n. (ant. ramus of 5th thoracic spinal n.)

Gray and white rami communicantes

5th thoracic sympathetic trunk ganglion

R. greater thoracic splanchnic n.

Sympathetic branch to esophageal plexus

Thoracic duct

Thoracic aortic plexus

R. lesser thoracic splanchnic n.

R. lowest thoracic splanchnic n.

Diaphragm (pulled down)

Azygos vein (cut)

Inf. vena cava (cut)

Cervicothoracic (stellate) ganglion

Cervical cardiac nn. (sympathetic and vagal)

L. vagus n. (cut)

L. recurrent laryngeal n.

Thoracic cardiac nn. (sympathetic and vagal)

Branches to ant. and post. pulmonary plexuses

Cardiac plexus

L. sympathetic trunk

Thoracic aorta plexus

Esophageal plexus

L. greater thoracic splanchnic n.

L. lesser thoracic splanchnic n.

Ant. vagal trunk

Diaphragm (pulled down)

FIGURE II.42: THORACIC SYMPATHETIC CHAIN AND SPLANCHNIC NERVES

The sympathetic chain is a collection of sympathetic ganglia that receive input from the thoracolumbar preganglionic nerve fibers derived from the spinal cord. The ganglia, interconnected by nerve trunks, are located in a paravertebral array from the neck to the coccygeal region. Postganglionic noradrenergic nerve fibers from the sympathetic chain supply effector tissue in the periphery. Some preganglionic nerve fibers do not synapse as they travel through the sympathetic chain. These fibers continue along the splanchnic nerves to synapse in collateral ganglia, which supply noradrenergic innervation to effector tissue in the viscera.

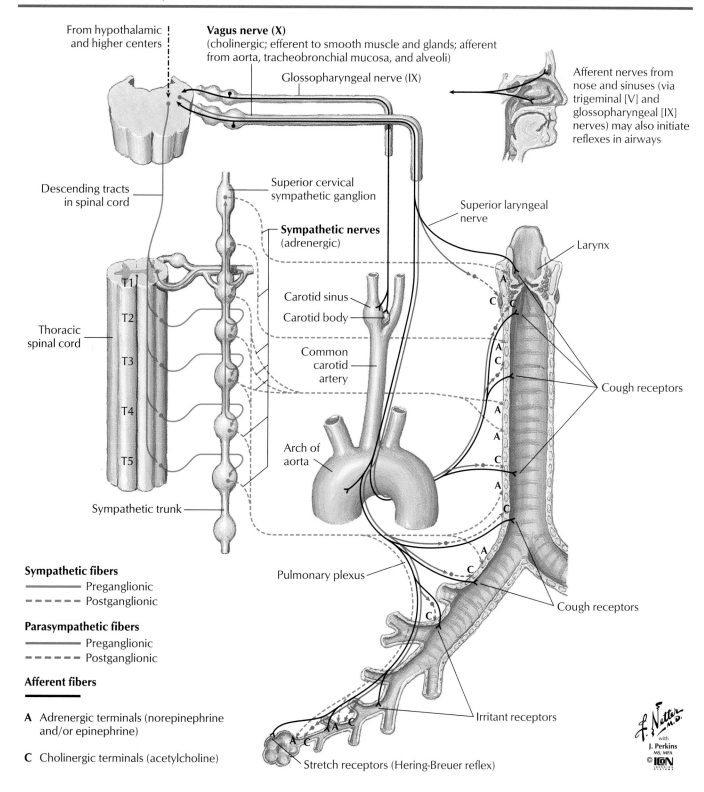

From hypothalamic and higher centers

Vagus nerve (X)
(cholinergic; efferent to smooth muscle and glands; afferent from aorta, tracheobronchial mucosa, and alveoli)

Glossopharyngeal nerve (IX)

Afferent nerves from nose and sinuses (via trigeminal [V] and glossopharyngeal [IX] nerves) may also initiate reflexes in airways

Descending tracts in spinal cord

Superior cervical sympathetic ganglion

Superior laryngeal nerve

Sympathetic nerves (adrenergic)

Larynx

T1

Thoracic spinal cord

T2

Carotid sinus

Carotid body

T3

Common carotid artery

T4

Cough receptors

T5

Arch of aorta

Sympathetic trunk

Sympathetic fibers

———— Preganglionic

- - - - Postganglionic

Parasympathetic fibers

———— Preganglionic

- - - - Postganglionic

Afferent fibers

————

A Adrenergic terminals (norepinephrine and/or epinephrine)

C Cholinergic terminals (acetylcholine)

Pulmonary plexus

Cough receptors

Irritant receptors

Stretch receptors (Hering-Breuer reflex)

FIGURE II.43: INNERVATION OF THE TRACHEOBRONCHIAL TREE

Both sympathetic (noradrenergic) and parasympathetic (cholinergic) innervation supply smooth muscle of the tracheobronchial tree. Sympathetics derive from the sympathetic chain, and parasympathetics derive from vagal autonomic input to local intramural ganglia. Sympathetic influences result in bronchodilation, and parasympathetic influences result in bronchoconstriction. Additional neuropeptidergic innervation, some as co-localized or independent autonomic fibers and some as primary afferent fibers, also distributes along the epithelium and among the alveoli, where it can influence innate immune reactivity and the production of inflammatory mediators.

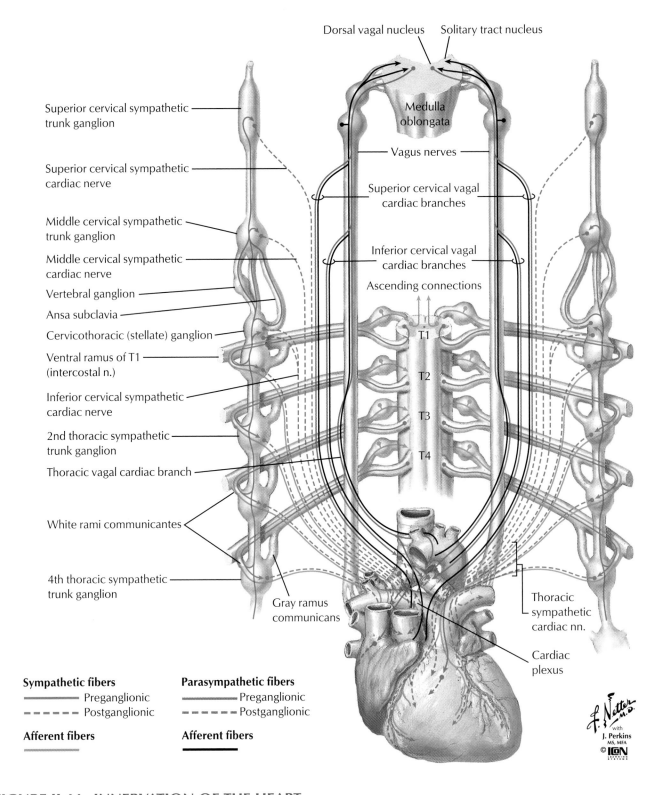

Dorsal vagal nucleus   Solitary tract nucleus

Medulla oblongata

Superior cervical sympathetic trunk ganglion

Vagus nerves

Superior cervical sympathetic cardiac nerve

Superior cervical vagal cardiac branches

Middle cervical sympathetic trunk ganglion

Inferior cervical vagal cardiac branches

Middle cervical sympathetic cardiac nerve

Ascending connections

Vertebral ganglion

Ansa subclavia

Cervicothoracic (stellate) ganglion

Ventral ramus of T1 (intercostal n.)

Inferior cervical sympathetic cardiac nerve

2nd thoracic sympathetic trunk ganglion

Thoracic vagal cardiac branch

White rami communicantes

T1

T2

T3

T4

4th thoracic sympathetic trunk ganglion

Gray ramus communicans

Thoracic sympathetic cardiac nn.

Cardiac plexus

Sympathetic fibers
——— Preganglionic
– – – – Postganglionic

Afferent fibers

Parasympathetic fibers
——— Preganglionic
– – – – Postganglionic

Afferent fibers

FIGURE II.44: INNERVATION OF THE HEART

Sympathetic noradrenergic nerve fibers (derived from chain ganglia) and parasympathetic cholinergic nerve fibers (derived from cardiac intramural ganglia innervated by the vagus nerve) supply the atria, the ventricles, the sinoatrial node, and the atrioventricular node and bundle. Sympathetic noradrenergic nerve fibers also distribute along the great vessels and the coronary arteries. Sympathetic fibers increase the force and rate of cardiac contraction, increase cardiac output, and dilate the coronary arteries. Parasympathetic fibers decrease the force and the rate of cardiac contraction and decrease cardiac output.

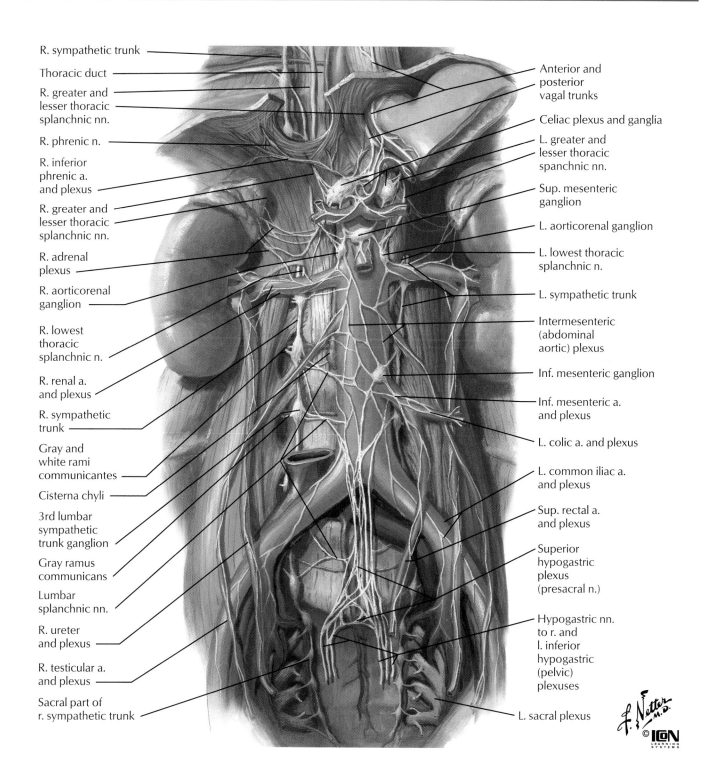

R. sympathetic trunk

Thoracic duct

R. greater and lesser thoracic splanchnic nn.

R. phrenic n.

R. inferior phrenic a. and plexus

R. greater and lesser thoracic splanchnic nn.

R. adrenal plexus

R. aorticorenal ganglion

R. lowest thoracic splanchnic n.

R. renal a. and plexus

R. sympathetic trunk

Gray and white rami communicantes

Cisterna chyli

3rd lumbar sympathetic trunk ganglion

Gray ramus communicans

Lumbar splanchnic nn.

R. ureter and plexus

R. testicular a. and plexus

Sacral part of r. sympathetic trunk

Anterior and posterior vagal trunks

Celiac plexus and ganglia

L. greater and lesser thoracic spanchnic nn.

Sup. mesenteric ganglion

L. aorticorenal ganglion

L. lowest thoracic splanchnic n.

L. sympathetic trunk

Intermesenteric (abdominal aortic) plexus

Inf. mesenteric ganglion

Inf. mesenteric a. and plexus

L. colic a. and plexus

L. common iliac a. and plexus

Sup. rectal a. and plexus

Superior hypogastric plexus (presacral n.)

Hypogastric nn. to r. and l. inferior hypogastric (pelvic) plexuses

L. sacral plexus

FIGURE II.45: ABDOMINAL NERVES AND GANGLIA

The abundance of sympathetic nerves in the abdomen and the pelvis is associated with innervation of the gastrointestinal (GI) and urogenital systems, associated vessels, the peritoneum, and the adrenal gland. The lumbar portion of the sympathetic chain and its branches and the splanchnic nerves and their collateral ganglia (celiac, superior and inferior mesenteric, hepatic, aorticorenal, adrenal, superior hypogastric, others) innervate smooth muscle, glands, lymphoid tissue, and metabolic cells in the abdomen and the pelvis. Most of the collateral ganglia (plexuses) also contain parasympathetic contributions from the vagus nerve and associated ganglia.

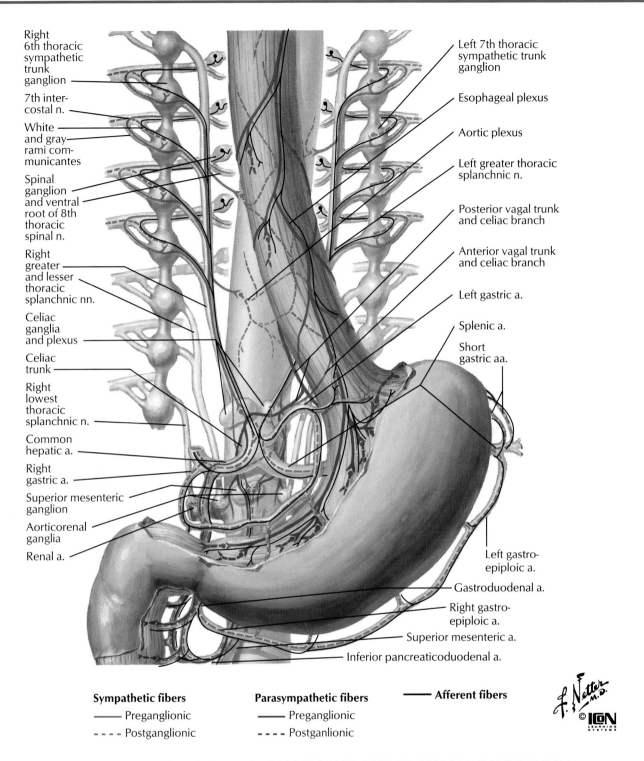

Right 6th thoracic sympathetic trunk ganglion

7th intercostal n.

White and gray rami communicantes

Spinal ganglion and ventral root of 8th thoracic spinal n.

Right greater and lesser thoracic splanchnic nn.

Celiac ganglia and plexus

Celiac trunk

Right lowest thoracic splanchnic n.

Common hepatic a.

Right gastric a.

Superior mesenteric ganglion

Aorticorenal ganglia

Renal a.

Left 7th thoracic sympathetic trunk ganglion

Esophageal plexus

Aortic plexus

Left greater thoracic splanchnic n.

Posterior vagal trunk and celiac branch

Anterior vagal trunk and celiac branch

Left gastric a.

Splenic a.

Short gastric aa.

Left gastroepiploic a.

Gastroduodenal a.

Right gastroepiploic a.

Superior mesenteric a.

Inferior pancreaticoduodenal a.

Sympathetic fibers	Parasympathetic fibers	── Afferent fibers
── Preganglionic	── Preganglionic	
- - - Postganglionic	- - - Postganlionic	

FIGURE II.46: INNERVATION OF THE STOMACH AND THE PROXIMAL DUODENUM

The stomach and the proximal duodenum receive sympathetic innervation in abundance from the celiac and superior mesenteric ganglia and to a lesser extent from the thoracic sympathetic trunk ganglia. The celiac and superior mesenteric ganglia receive preganglionic input from the greater and lesser thoracic splanchnic nerves. Parasympathetic fibers distribute to the stomach and the proximal duodenum from the celiac branches of the vagus nerve. Sympathetic fibers decrease peristalsis and secretomotor activities. Parasympathetics increase peristalsis and secretomotor activity (such as gastrin and HCl) and relax associated sphincters.

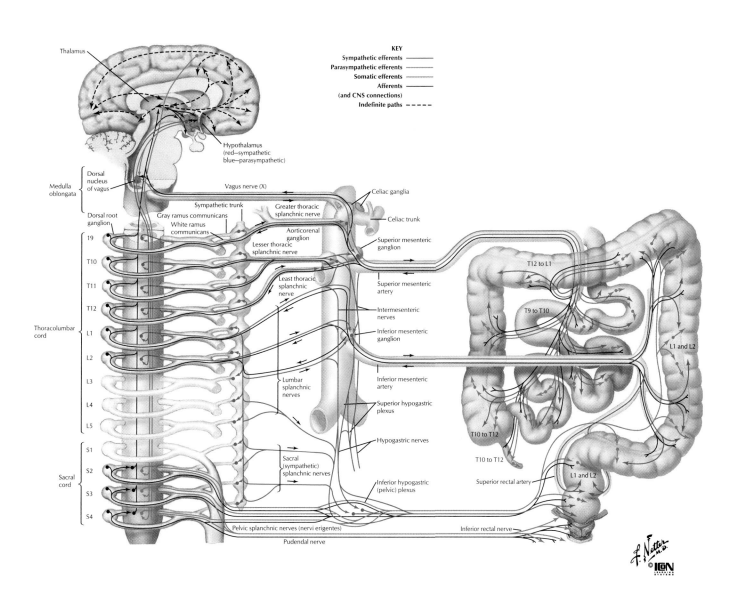

FIGURE II.47: INNERVATION OF THE SMALL AND LARGE INTESTINES

Autonomic innervation of the small and large intestines is supplied by extrinsic sympathetic and parasympathetic fibers. Sympathetic innervation derives from the T5-L2 intermediolateral cell column of the spinal cord, and it distributes to collateral ganglia (superior and inferior mesenteric, celiac). Parasympathetic innervation derives from the vagus nerve and from S2-S4 intermediate gray of the spinal cord, and it distributes to intramural ganglia and plexuses via CN X and pelvic splanchnic nerves. Sympathetics generally decrease peristalsis and secretomotor functions (i.e., decreased fluid secretion). Parasympathetics increase peristalsis, relax involuntary sphincters, and increase secretomotor activities. The extrinsic innervation of the intestines is integrated with the intrinsic (enteric) innervation:

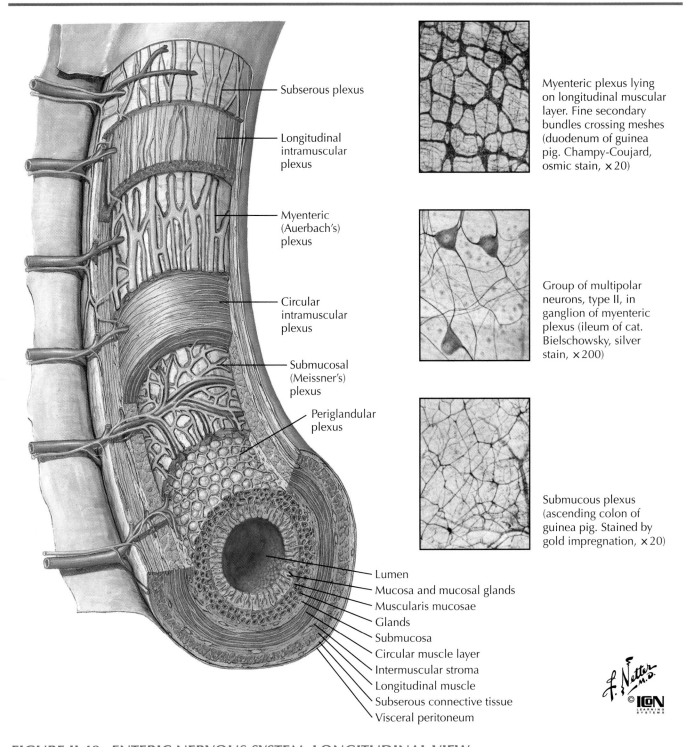

Myenteric plexus lying on longitudinal muscular layer. Fine secondary bundles crossing meshes (duodenum of guinea pig. Champy-Coujard, osmic stain, ×20)

Group of multipolar neurons, type II, in ganglion of myenteric plexus (ileum of cat. Bielschowsky, silver stain, ×200)

Submucous plexus (ascending colon of guinea pig. Stained by gold impregnation, ×20)

Subserous plexus
Longitudinal intramuscular plexus
Myenteric (Auerbach's) plexus
Circular intramuscular plexus
Submucosal (Meissner's) plexus
Periglandular plexus
Lumen
Mucosa and mucosal glands
Muscularis mucosae
Glands
Submucosa
Circular muscle layer
Intermuscular stroma
Longitudinal muscle
Subserous connective tissue
Visceral peritoneum

FIGURE II.48: ENTERIC NERVOUS SYSTEM: LONGITUDINAL VIEW

The enteric nervous system provides intrinsic innervation to the small and large intestines. The myenteric (Auerbach's) and submucosal (Meissner's) plexuses are its main elements. The myenteric plexus mainly controls motility; the submucosal plexus mainly controls fluid secretion and absorption. Neurons of this system interconnect with one another and with neuronal processes of the ANS, although many neuronal components of this network are free of autonomic influence. More

than 20 distinct neurotransmitters have been identified in enteric neurons (e.g., ACh, substance P, serotonin, vasoactive intestinal peptide [VIP], somatostatin, nitric oxide [NO]). ACh and substance P are excitatory to smooth muscle, whereas VIP and NO are inhibitory. Optimal functioning of the GI tract requires coordinated interactions between endocrine, paracrine, and neurocrine mediators.

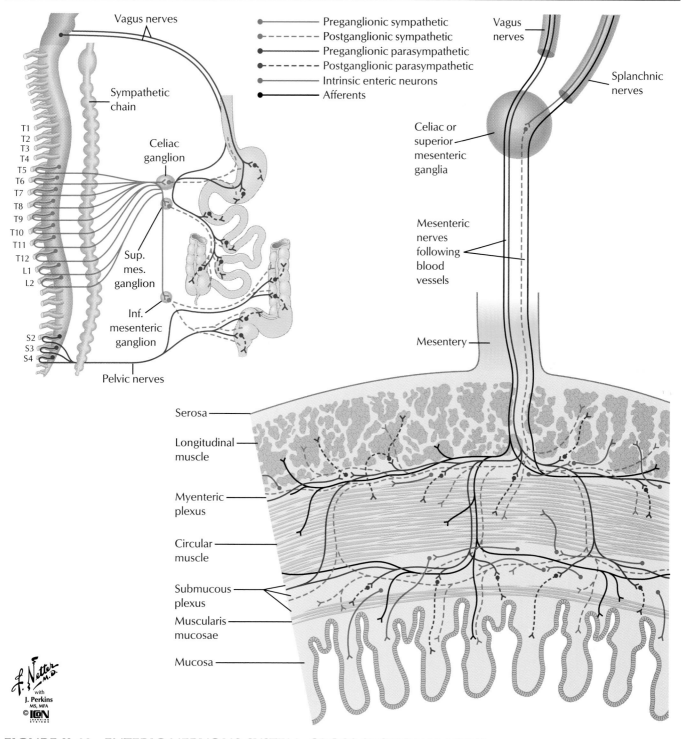

Legend:
- Preganglionic sympathetic
- Postganglionic sympathetic
- Preganglionic parasympathetic
- Postganglionic parasympathetic
- Intrinsic enteric neurons
- Afferents

Vagus nerves

Sympathetic chain

Celiac ganglion

T1, T2, T3, T4, T5, T6, T7, T8, T9, T10, T11, T12, L1, L2

Sup. mes. ganglion

Inf. mesenteric ganglion

S2, S3, S4

Pelvic nerves

Vagus nerves

Splanchnic nerves

Celiac or superior mesenteric ganglia

Mesenteric nerves following blood vessels

Mesentery

Serosa

Longitudinal muscle

Myenteric plexus

Circular muscle

Submucous plexus

Muscularis mucosae

Mucosa

J. Netter M.D.
with
J. Perkins
MS, MFA
©ICON

FIGURE II.49: ENTERIC NERVOUS SYSTEM: CROSS-SECTIONAL VIEW

In the myenteric and submucosal plexuses, some neurons are innervated by sympathetic nerve fibers from the sympathetic chain and collateral ganglia and by vagal or pelvic splanchnic parasympathetic nerve fibers; other neurons are independent of autonomic regulation. Autonomic postganglionic and intrinsic neuropeptidergic nerve fibers supply macrophages, T lymphocytes, plasma cells, and other cells of the immune system with innervation. This provides a regulatory network that modulates GI tract host defenses and immune reactivity of gut-associated lymphoid tissue (GALT).

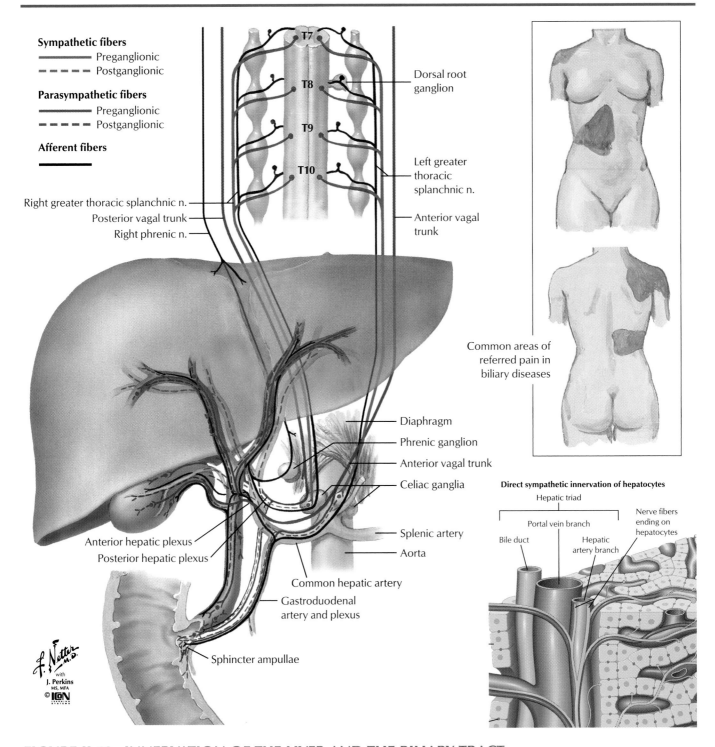

Sympathetic fibers
- Preganglionic
- Postganglionic

Parasympathetic fibers
- Preganglionic
- Postganglionic

Afferent fibers

T7
T8
T9
T10

Dorsal root ganglion

Left greater thoracic splanchnic n.

Anterior vagal trunk

Right greater thoracic splanchnic n.
Posterior vagal trunk
Right phrenic n.

Diaphragm
Phrenic ganglion
Anterior vagal trunk
Celiac ganglia
Splenic artery
Aorta

Anterior hepatic plexus
Posterior hepatic plexus

Common hepatic artery
Gastroduodenal artery and plexus

Sphincter ampullae

Common areas of referred pain in biliary diseases

Direct sympathetic innervation of hepatocytes
Hepatic triad
Portal vein branch
Bile duct
Hepatic artery branch
Nerve fibers ending on hepatocytes

FIGURE II.50: INNERVATION OF THE LIVER AND THE BILIARY TRACT

Sympathetic nerve fibers to the liver derive from T7-10 spinal cord and distribute mainly via the celiac ganglion and its associated plexus. Parasympathetic nerve fibers to the liver derive from the abdominal vagus nerve. Postganglionic noradrenergic sympathetic nerve fibers end directly adjacent to hepatocytes and initiate glycogenolysis, increase blood glucose for fight-or-flight responses, and induce gluconeogenesis. Autonomic innervation helps to regulate vascular, secretory, and phagocytic processes in the liver. The gallbladder, especially the sphincter ampullae and the sphincter of the choledochal duct, is also supplied by autonomic nerve fibers. The sympathetics cause contraction of the sphincters and dilation of the gallbladder; the parasympathetics cause opening of the sphincters and contraction of the gallbladder.

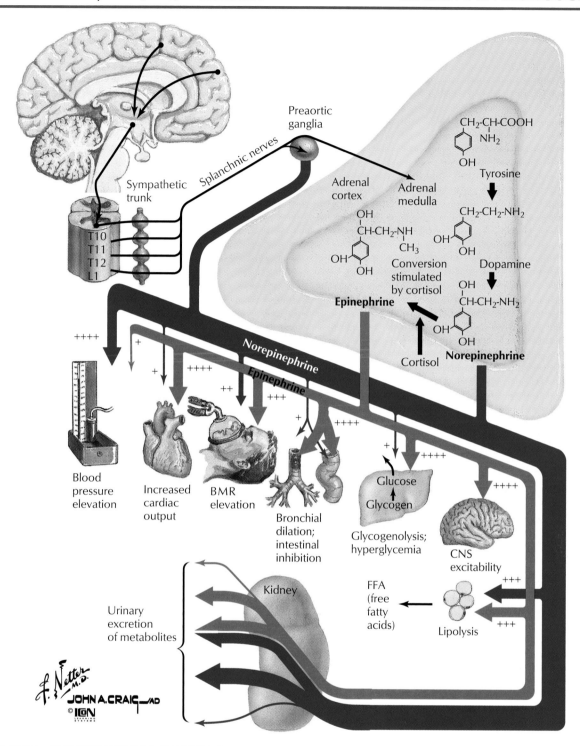

FIGURE II.51: INNERVATION OF THE ADRENAL GLAND

Sympathetic preganglionic nerve fibers from neurons in the T10-L1 intermediolateral cell column pass through the sympathetic chain and travel in splanchnic nerves to directly innervate adrenal medullary chromaffin cells, which function as sympathetic ganglion cells. An adrenal portal system conveys blood from the adrenal cortex directly to the adrenal medulla. Highly concentrated cortisol derived from action of the hypothalamo-pituitary-adrenal (HPA) axis bathes the chromaffin cells, inducing the enzyme phenylethanolamine N-methyl transferase (PNMT), which is responsible for the synthesis of epinephrine. Approximately 70% to 80% of the adrenal medullary output of catecholamines is epinephrine; the remaining output is norepinephrine. Both epinephrine and norepinephrine can be taken up into sympathetic postganglionic noradrenergic nerve terminals by the high-affinity uptake carrier and subsequently released.

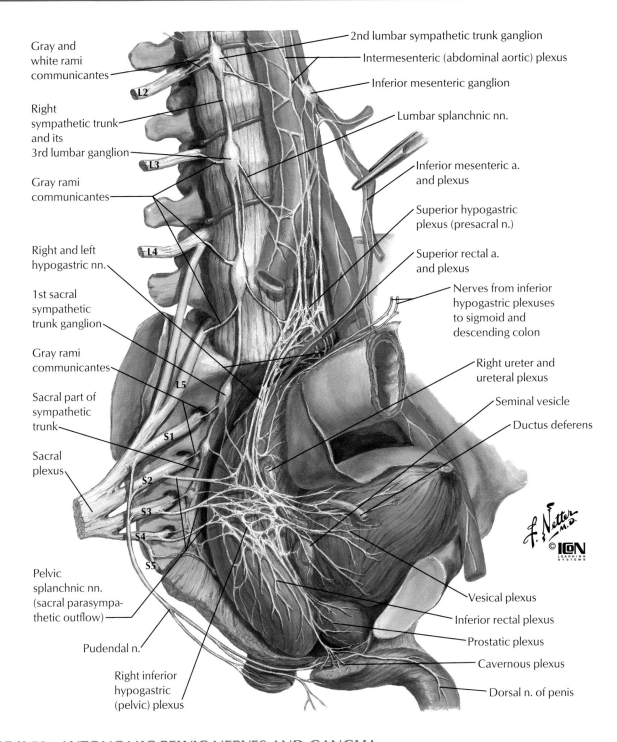

Gray and white rami communicantes

2nd lumbar sympathetic trunk ganglion

Intermesenteric (abdominal aortic) plexus

Inferior mesenteric ganglion

Right sympathetic trunk and its 3rd lumbar ganglion

Lumbar splanchnic nn.

Gray rami communicantes

Inferior mesenteric a. and plexus

Superior hypogastric plexus (presacral n.)

Right and left hypogastric nn.

Superior rectal a. and plexus

1st sacral sympathetic trunk ganglion

Nerves from inferior hypogastric plexuses to sigmoid and descending colon

Gray rami communicantes

Right ureter and ureteral plexus

Sacral part of sympathetic trunk

Seminal vesicle

Ductus deferens

Sacral plexus

Pelvic splanchnic nn. (sacral parasympathetic outflow)

Vesical plexus

Inferior rectal plexus

Pudendal n.

Prostatic plexus

Cavernous plexus

Right inferior hypogastric (pelvic) plexus

Dorsal n. of penis

L2, L3, L4, L5, S1, S2, S3, S4, S5

FIGURE II.52: AUTONOMIC PELVIC NERVES AND GANGLIA

The sympathetic nerve fibers supply the pelvis through the sympathetic trunk ganglia and the superior hypogastric plexus. The fibers travel along visceral and vascular nerves to the colon, the ureters, and the great vessels such as the inferior mesenteric and common iliac vessels.

Parasympathetic nerve fibers arise from the S2-S4 intermediate gray of the spinal cord and travel via the pelvic splanchnic nerves to distribute with the branches of the inferior hypogastric plexuses. The intramural parasympathetic ganglia are in, or adjacent to, the wall of the organ innervated.

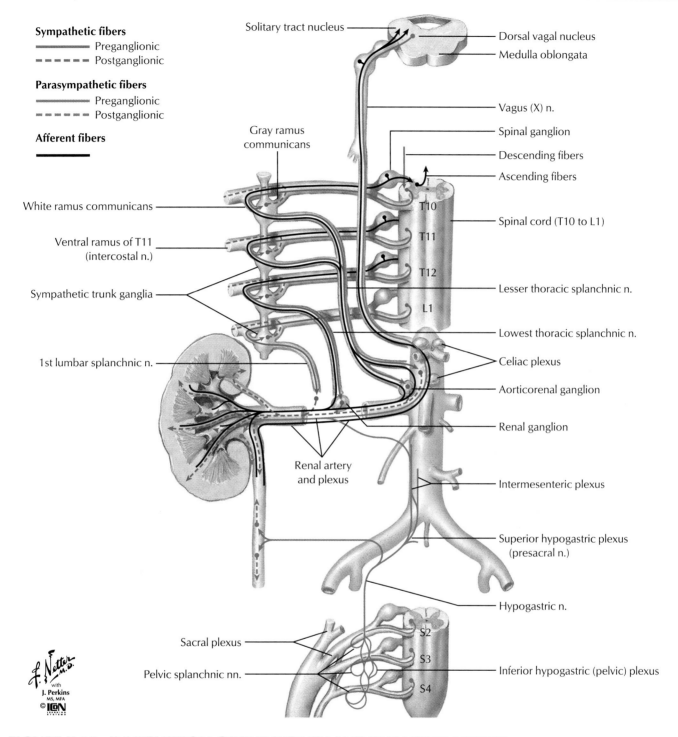

Sympathetic fibers
——————— Preganglionic
- - - - - - Postganglionic

Parasympathetic fibers
——————— Preganglionic
- - - - - - Postganglionic

Afferent fibers
———————

Solitary tract nucleus
Dorsal vagal nucleus
Medulla oblongata
Vagus (X) n.
Spinal ganglion
Descending fibers
Ascending fibers
Gray ramus communicans
White ramus communicans
Spinal cord (T10 to L1)
Ventral ramus of T11 (intercostal n.)
Sympathetic trunk ganglia
Lesser thoracic splanchnic n.
Lowest thoracic splanchnic n.
1st lumbar splanchnic n.
Celiac plexus
Aorticorenal ganglion
Renal ganglion
Renal artery and plexus
Intermesenteric plexus
Superior hypogastric plexus (presacral n.)
Hypogastric n.
Sacral plexus
Pelvic splanchnic nn.
Inferior hypogastric (pelvic) plexus

T10
T11
T12
L1

S2
S3
S4

FIGURE II.53: INNERVATION OF THE KIDNEY AND THE UPPER URETER

Sympathetic innervation of the kidney and the upper ureters arises from the T10-L1 intermediolateral cell column preganglionic neurons in the spinal cord and travels through the lower thoracic and upper lumbar splanchnic nerves to synapse in the celiac or aorticorenal ganglia. Postganglionic fibers travel in fascicles that accompany the upper ureteric, renal, pelvic, calyceal, and segmental branches of the renal vessels. Parasympathetics are distributed to renal ganglia by the vagus nerve and pelvic splanchnic nerves via a longer course through other plexuses. The sympathetic nerve fibers stimulate renin secretion (and the renin-angiotensin-aldosterone system), decrease the glomerular filtration rate (GFR), stimulate proximal tubule and collecting duct NaCl reabsorption, and stimulate contraction of the ureters. Parasympathetic nerve fibers cause relaxation of smooth muscle in the pelvis, the calyces, and the upper ureters.

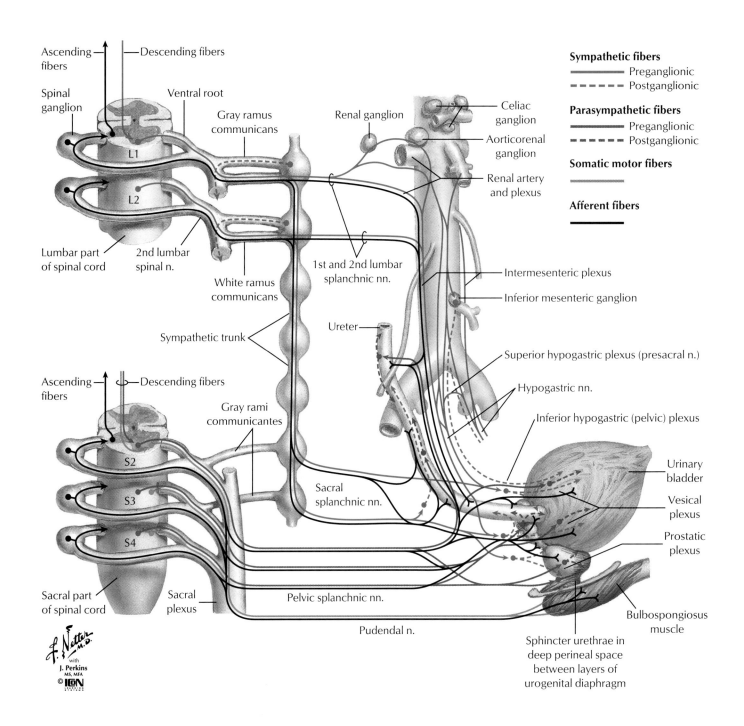

FIGURE II.54: INNERVATION OF THE URINARY BLADDER AND THE LOWER URETER

Sympathetic innervation of the bladder and the lower ureters derives mainly from the L1-L2 preganglionic neurons in the spinal cord and travels through sacral splanchnic nerves to the hypogastric plexus. Parasympathetic innervation derives from the S2-S4 intermediate gray of the spinal cord and distributes to intramural ganglia in the wall of the bladder via pelvic splanchnic nerves. Sympathetic nerves relax the detrusor muscle and contract the trigone and the internal sphincter. Parasympathetic nerves contract the detrusor muscle and relax the trigone and the internal sphincter, thus stimulating emptying of the bladder.

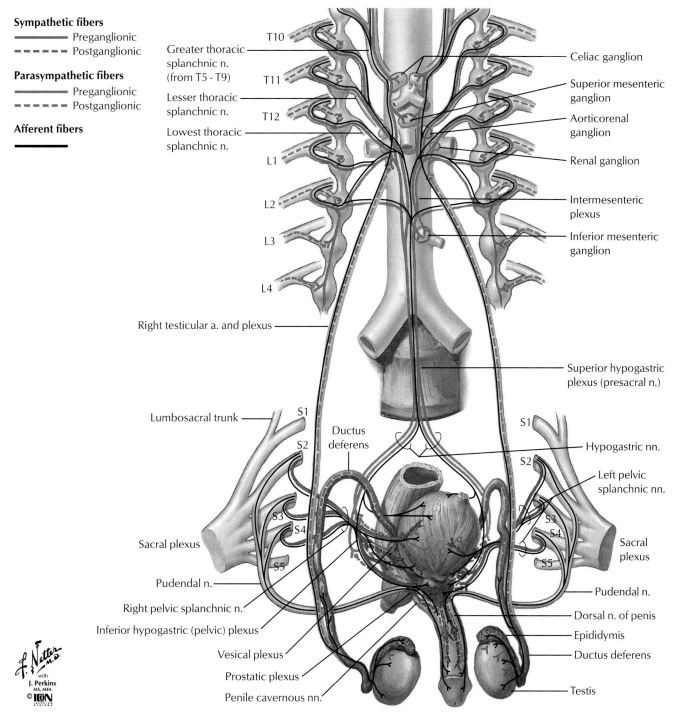

Sympathetic fibers
——— Preganglionic
– – – – Postganglionic

Parasympathetic fibers
——— Preganglionic
– – – – Postganglionic

Afferent fibers
———

T10
T11
T12
L1
L2
L3
L4

Greater thoracic splanchnic n. (from T5 - T9)
Lesser thoracic splanchnic n.
Lowest thoracic splanchnic n.
Right testicular a. and plexus

Celiac ganglion
Superior mesenteric ganglion
Aorticorenal ganglion
Renal ganglion
Intermesenteric plexus
Inferior mesenteric ganglion
Superior hypogastric plexus (presacral n.)

Lumbosacral trunk
S1
S2
Ductus deferens
S3
S4
S5
Sacral plexus
Pudendal n.
Right pelvic splanchnic n.
Inferior hypogastric (pelvic) plexus
Vesical plexus
Prostatic plexus
Penile cavernous nn.

S1
S2
Hypogastric nn.
Left pelvic splanchnic nn.
S3
S4
S5
Sacral plexus
Pudendal n.
Dorsal n. of penis
Epididymis
Ductus deferens
Testis

f. Netter m.d. with J. Perkins MS, MFA ©ICN

FIGURE II.55: INNERVATION OF THE MALE REPRODUCTIVE ORGANS

Sympathetic innervation of the male reproductive organs derives from T10-L2 intermediolateral cell column neurons and reaches the superior hypogastric plexus via thoracic and upper lumbar splanchnic nerves. Parasympathetic innervation derives from the S2-4 intermediate gray of the spinal cord and travels to the inferior hypogastric plexus via pelvic splanchnic nerves. Sympathetic nerves cause contraction of the vas deferens and the prostatic capsule, and contract the sphincter to the bladder, which prevents retrograde ejaculation. Sympathetics also contribute to vascular responses in the penile corpora cavernosa related to erection; beta-receptor blockade can result in erectile dysfunction. Parasympathetic nerves regulate the vascular dilation that initiates and maintains penile erection. Sympathetics and parasympathetics must work together to optimize sexual and reproductive function.

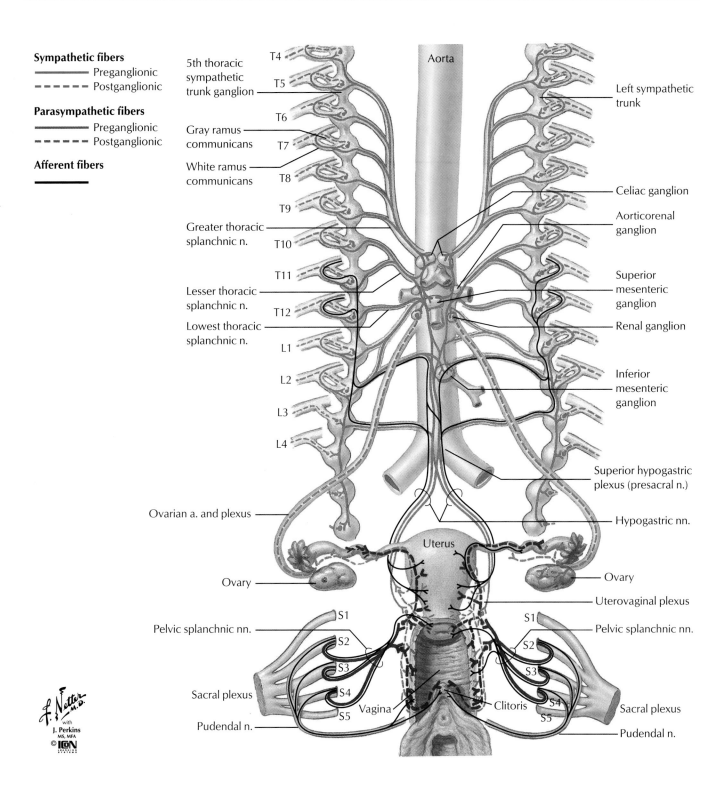

FIGURE II.56: INNERVATION OF THE FEMALE REPRODUCTIVE ORGANS

Autonomic nerves supplying the female reproductive organs have a similar origin to those supplying their male counterparts. Sympathetic nerves stimulate contraction of the uterus, but the extent of this action depends also on hormonal receptor responsiveness and neurotransmitter receptor expression. Sympathetics supply the vaginal arteries, the vestibular glands, and the erectile tissue. Parasympathetics supply the muscular and mucous coats of the vagina and the urethra, stimulate erectile tissue of the vestibular bulb and the corpora cavernosa of the clitoris, and supply the vestibular glands.

Nuclear cell columns   **Laminae of Rexed**

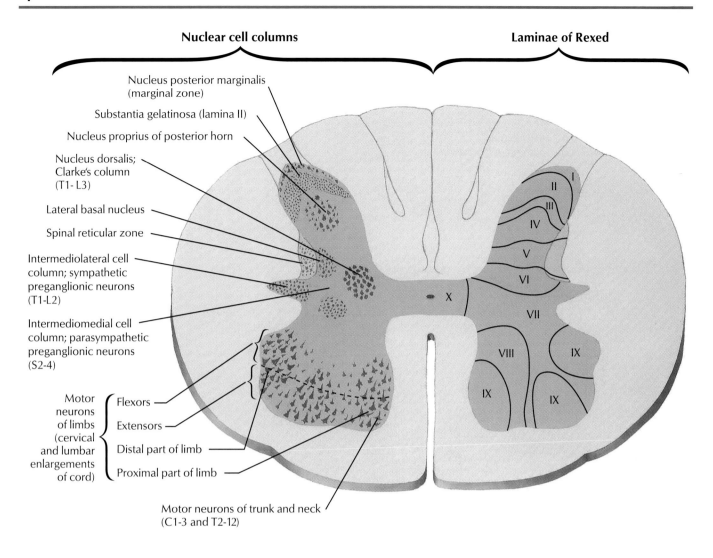

Nucleus posterior marginalis
(marginal zone)

Substantia gelatinosa (lamina II)

Nucleus proprius of posterior horn

Nucleus dorsalis;
Clarke's column
(T1- L3)

Lateral basal nucleus

Spinal reticular zone

Intermediolateral cell
column; sympathetic
preganglionic neurons
(T1-L2)

Intermediomedial cell
column; parasympathetic
preganglionic neurons
(S2-4)

Motor
neurons
of limbs
(cervical
and lumbar
enlargements
of cord)
{
Flexors

Extensors

Distal part of limb

Proximal part of limb
}

Motor neurons of trunk and neck
(C1-3 and T2-12)

FIGURE II.57: CYTOARCHITECTURE OF THE SPINAL CORD GRAY MATTER

The spinal cord gray matter is found in the interior of the spinal cord in a "butterfly" pattern. It is subdivided into 3 horns: (1) dorsal horn—site of major sensory processing, (2) intermediate gray with a lateral horn—site where preganglionic sympathetic (thoracolumbar) and parasympathetic (sacral) cell bodies reside and interneuronal processing occurs, and (3) ventral horn—site where lower motor neurons (LMNs) reside and where converging reflex and descending control of LMNs occur. Neuronal cell groups appear homogeneous in some regions of gray matter, with some discrete nuclei (e.g., Clarke's nucleus, substantia gelatinosa). Laminae of Rexed, an alternate system of cytoarchitectural

classification established in the 1950s, subdivides the spinal cord gray into 10 laminae. This system is used extensively for the dorsal horn and the intermediate gray, laminae I to VII, particularly in conjunction with anatomical details of nociceptive processing, and for some reflex and cerebellar processing. Although these laminae have distinctive characteristics at each segmental level, they show some similarities across segments. The absolute amount of spinal cord gray is more extensive in the cervical and lumbosacral enlargements of the spinal cord, which correspond to zones associated with limb innervation, than in the upper cervical, thoracic, and sacral regions.

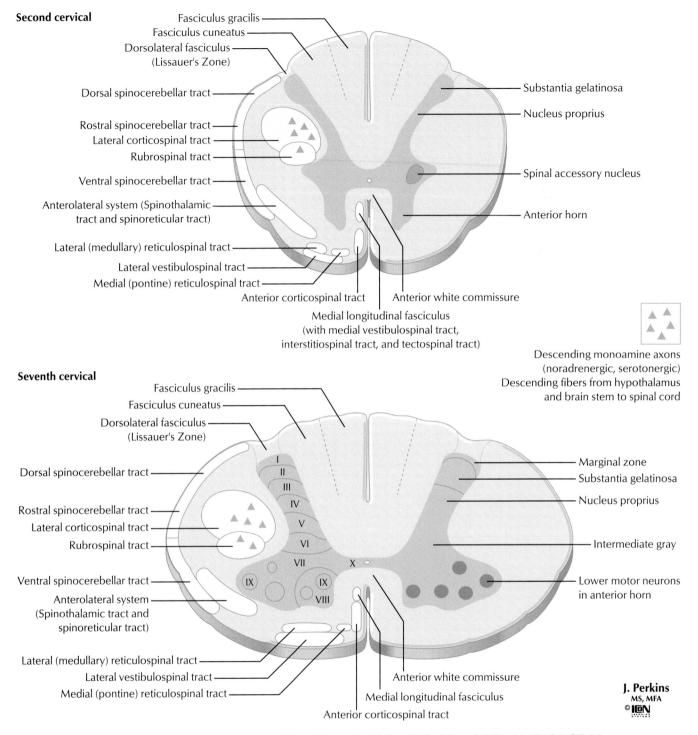

Second cervical

Fasciculus gracilis
Fasciculus cuneatus
Dorsolateral fasciculus (Lissauer's Zone)
Dorsal spinocerebellar tract
Rostral spinocerebellar tract
Lateral corticospinal tract
Rubrospinal tract
Ventral spinocerebellar tract
Anterolateral system (Spinothalamic tract and spinoreticular tract)
Lateral (medullary) reticulospinal tract
Lateral vestibulospinal tract
Medial (pontine) reticulospinal tract
Anterior corticospinal tract
Medial longitudinal fasciculus (with medial vestibulospinal tract, interstitiospinal tract, and tectospinal tract)

Substantia gelatinosa
Nucleus proprius
Spinal accessory nucleus
Anterior horn
Anterior white commissure

Descending monoamine axons (noradrenergic, serotonergic) Descending fibers from hypothalamus and brain stem to spinal cord

Seventh cervical

Fasciculus gracilis
Fasciculus cuneatus
Dorsolateral fasciculus (Lissauer's Zone)
Dorsal spinocerebellar tract
Rostral spinocerebellar tract
Lateral corticospinal tract
Rubrospinal tract
Ventral spinocerebellar tract
Anterolateral system (Spinothalamic tract and spinoreticular tract)
Lateral (medullary) reticulospinal tract
Lateral vestibulospinal tract
Medial (pontine) reticulospinal tract
Anterior corticospinal tract
Medial longitudinal fasciculus
Anterior white commissure

Marginal zone
Substantia gelatinosa
Nucleus proprius
Intermediate gray
Lower motor neurons in anterior horn

I, II, III, IV, V, VI, VII, IX, VIII, X

J. Perkins
MS, MFA
© I◎N

FIGURE II.58: SPINAL CORD LEVELS: CERVICAL, THORACIC, LUMBAR, AND SACRAL

The organization of the gray matter into laminae of Rexed is retained throughout the spinal cord. The dorsal and ventral horns are larger and wider at the levels of the cervical and lumbosacral enlargements. The lateral horn is present from L1 to T2. Some nuclei, such as the intermediolateral cell column with preganglionic sympathetic neurons (T1-L2 lateral horn), Clarke's nucleus (C8-L2), and the parasympathetic preganglionic nucleus (S2-4), are found only in circumscribed regions. The white matter increases in absolute amount from caudal to rostral. The dorsal columns contain only fasciculus gracilis below T6; fasciculus cuneatus is added laterally above T6. The spinothalamic/spinoreticular anterolateral system increases from caudal to rostral. The descending upper motor neuron (UMN) pathways diminish from rostral to caudal. The lateral corticospinal tract loses more than half of its axons as they synapse in the cervical segments; this tract then diminishes in size as it extends caudally.

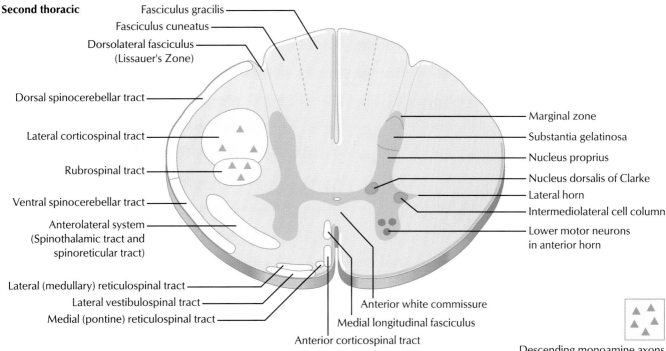

Second thoracic

- Fasciculus gracilis
- Fasciculus cuneatus
- Dorsolateral fasciculus (Lissauer's Zone)
- Dorsal spinocerebellar tract
- Lateral corticospinal tract
- Rubrospinal tract
- Ventral spinocerebellar tract
- Anterolateral system (Spinothalamic tract and spinoreticular tract)
- Lateral (medullary) reticulospinal tract
- Lateral vestibulospinal tract
- Medial (pontine) reticulospinal tract
- Anterior corticospinal tract
- Medial longitudinal fasciculus
- Anterior white commissure
- Marginal zone
- Substantia gelatinosa
- Nucleus proprius
- Nucleus dorsalis of Clarke
- Lateral horn
- Intermediolateral cell column
- Lower motor neurons in anterior horn

Descending monoamine axons (noradrenergic, serotonergic)
Descending fibers from hypothalamus and brain stem to spinal cord

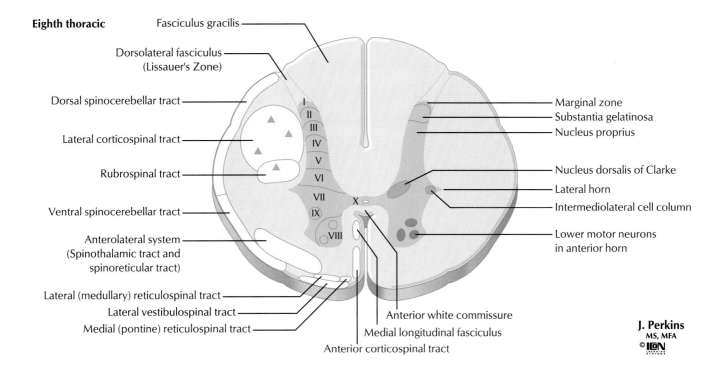

Eighth thoracic

- Fasciculus gracilis
- Dorsolateral fasciculus (Lissauer's Zone)
- Dorsal spinocerebellar tract
- Lateral corticospinal tract
- Rubrospinal tract
- Ventral spinocerebellar tract
- Anterolateral system (Spinothalamic tract and spinoreticular tract)
- Lateral (medullary) reticulospinal tract
- Lateral vestibulospinal tract
- Medial (pontine) reticulospinal tract
- Anterior corticospinal tract
- Medial longitudinal fasciculus
- Anterior white commissure
- Marginal zone
- Substantia gelatinosa
- Nucleus proprius
- Nucleus dorsalis of Clarke
- Lateral horn
- Intermediolateral cell column
- Lower motor neurons in anterior horn

J. Perkins
MS, MFA
© ICN

143

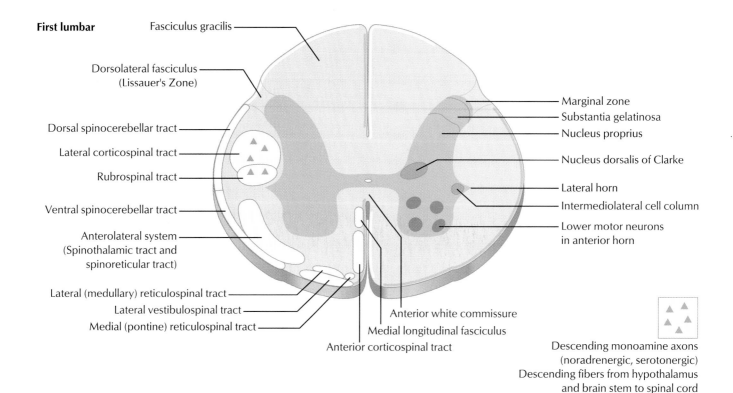

First lumbar

Fasciculus gracilis

Dorsolateral fasciculus (Lissauer's Zone)

Dorsal spinocerebellar tract

Lateral corticospinal tract

Rubrospinal tract

Ventral spinocerebellar tract

Anterolateral system (Spinothalamic tract and spinoreticular tract)

Lateral (medullary) reticulospinal tract

Lateral vestibulospinal tract

Medial (pontine) reticulospinal tract

Anterior corticospinal tract

Medial longitudinal fasciculus

Anterior white commissure

Marginal zone

Substantia gelatinosa

Nucleus proprius

Nucleus dorsalis of Clarke

Lateral horn

Intermediolateral cell column

Lower motor neurons in anterior horn

Descending monoamine axons (noradrenergic, serotonergic) Descending fibers from hypothalamus and brain stem to spinal cord

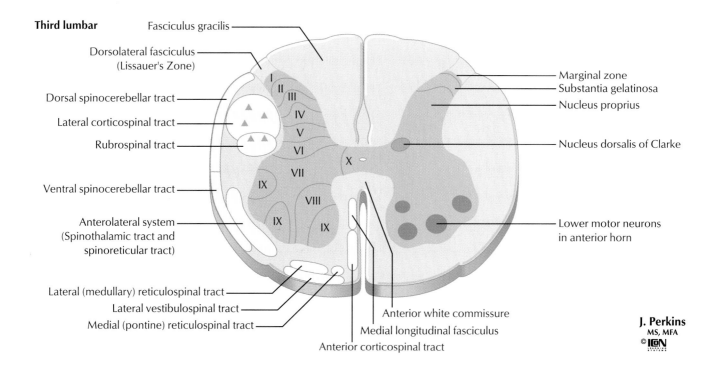

Third lumbar

Fasciculus gracilis

Dorsolateral fasciculus (Lissauer's Zone)

Dorsal spinocerebellar tract

Lateral corticospinal tract

Rubrospinal tract

Ventral spinocerebellar tract

Anterolateral system (Spinothalamic tract and spinoreticular tract)

Lateral (medullary) reticulospinal tract

Lateral vestibulospinal tract

Medial (pontine) reticulospinal tract

Anterior corticospinal tract

Medial longitudinal fasciculus

Anterior white commissure

Marginal zone

Substantia gelatinosa

Nucleus proprius

Nucleus dorsalis of Clarke

Lower motor neurons in anterior horn

J. Perkins
MS, MFA
©I◎N

First sacral

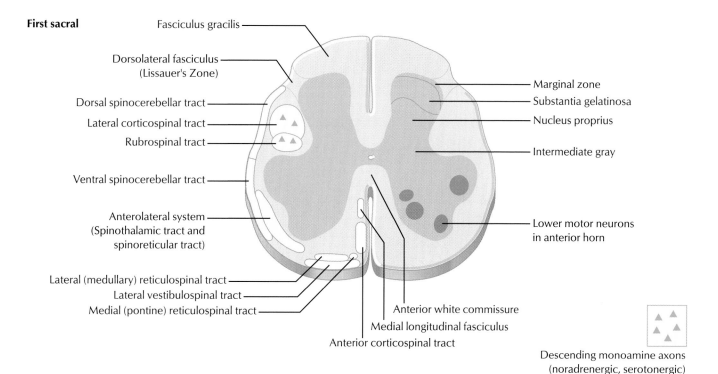

Fasciculus gracilis

Dorsolateral fasciculus
(Lissauer's Zone)

Dorsal spinocerebellar tract

Lateral corticospinal tract

Rubrospinal tract

Ventral spinocerebellar tract

Anterolateral system
(Spinothalamic tract and
spinoreticular tract)

Lateral (medullary) reticulospinal tract

Lateral vestibulospinal tract

Medial (pontine) reticulospinal tract

Marginal zone

Substantia gelatinosa

Nucleus proprius

Intermediate gray

Lower motor neurons
in anterior horn

Anterior white commissure

Medial longitudinal fasciculus

Anterior corticospinal tract

Descending monoamine axons
(noradrenergic, serotonergic)
Descending fibers from hypothalamus
and brain stem to spinal cord

Third sacral

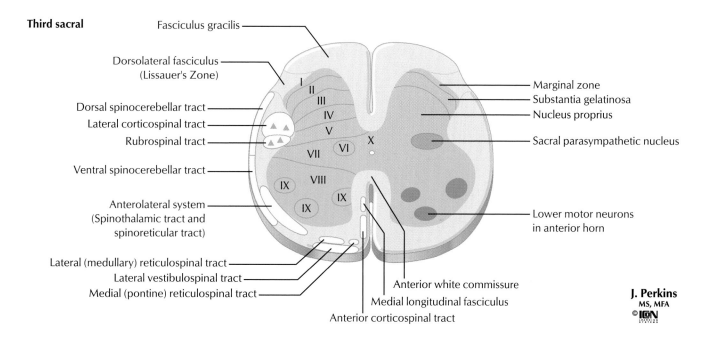

Fasciculus gracilis

Dorsolateral fasciculus
(Lissauer's Zone)

Dorsal spinocerebellar tract

Lateral corticospinal tract

Rubrospinal tract

Ventral spinocerebellar tract

Anterolateral system
(Spinothalamic tract and
spinoreticular tract)

Lateral (medullary) reticulospinal tract

Lateral vestibulospinal tract

Medial (pontine) reticulospinal tract

I
II
III
IV
V
VI
VII
VIII
IX
IX
IX
X

Marginal zone

Substantia gelatinosa

Nucleus proprius

Sacral parasympathetic nucleus

Lower motor neurons
in anterior horn

Anterior white commissure

Medial longitudinal fasciculus

Anterior corticospinal tract

J. Perkins
MS, MFA
©I**C**N

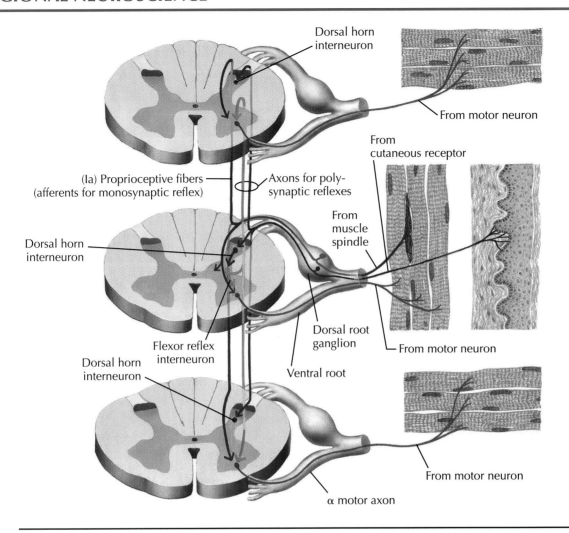

(Ia) Proprioceptive fibers
(afferents for monosynaptic reflex)

Axons for poly-
synaptic reflexes

Dorsal horn
interneuron

Dorsal horn
interneuron

From motor neuron

From
cutaneous receptor

From
muscle
spindle

Dorsal horn
interneuron

Flexor reflex
interneuron

Dorsal root
ganglion

From motor neuron

Ventral root

α motor axon

From motor neuron

Schematic representation of motor neurons

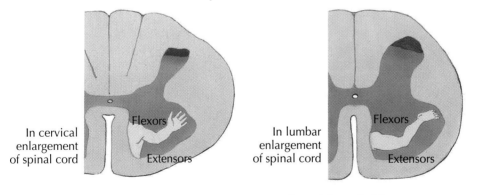

In cervical
enlargement
of spinal cord

Flexors

Extensors

In lumbar
enlargement
of spinal cord

Flexors

Extensors

FIGURE II.59: SPINAL CORD LOWER MOTOR NEURON CONTROL

Lower motor neurons are localized in the cervical, thoracic, lumbar, and sacral segments in the ventral (anterior) horn of the spinal cord. LMNs also have a medial to lateral and dorsal to ventral organization. LMNs supplying trunk musculature are found medially and ventrally; LMNs innervating more distal musculature are found dorsally and laterally. This organization also is apparent in the topography of UMN control of LMNs. UMNs regulating fine hand and finger movements are sent from the corticospinal system to terminate on dorsal and lateral LMNs. UMNs regulating basic truncal tone and posture are sent from the reticulospinal and vestibulospinal systems to terminate on ventral and medial LMNs. Reflex pathways regulate LMN activity through monosynaptic (muscle stretch reflex Ia afferents) or polysynaptic (flexor or cutaneous reflex afferents) pathways. Superimposed on this organization is the descending UMN control and coordination of LMNs.

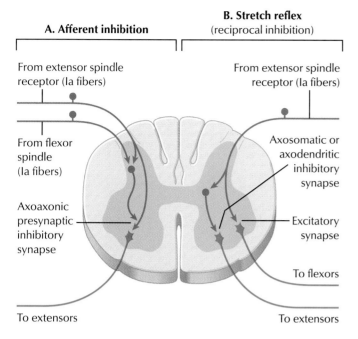

A. Afferent inhibition

From extensor spindle receptor (Ia fibers)

From flexor spindle (Ia fibers)

Axoaxonic presynaptic inhibitory synapse

To extensors

B. Stretch reflex
(reciprocal inhibition)

From extensor spindle receptor (Ia fibers)

Axosomatic or axodendritic inhibitory synapse

Excitatory synapse

To flexors

To extensors

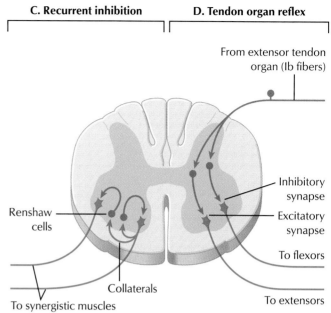

C. Recurrent inhibition

Renshaw cells

To synergistic muscles

Collaterals

D. Tendon organ reflex

From extensor tendon organ (Ib fibers)

Inhibitory synapse

Excitatory synapse

To flexors

To extensors

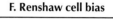

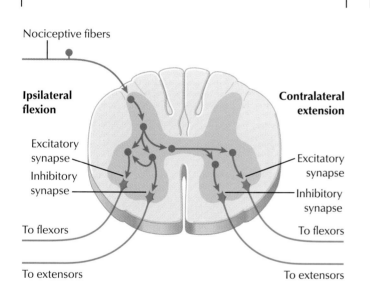

E. Flexor withdrawal reflex

Nociceptive fibers

Ipsilateral flexion

Excitatory synapse

Inhibitory synapse

To flexors

To extensors

Contralateral extension

Excitatory synapse

Inhibitory synapse

To flexors

To extensors

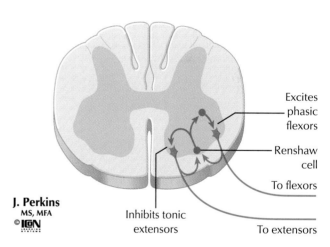

F. Renshaw cell bias

Excites phasic flexors

Renshaw cell

To flexors

Inhibits tonic extensors

To extensors

J. Perkins
MS, MFA
© ICN

FIGURE II.60: SPINAL SOMATIC REFLEX PATHWAYS

In the muscle stretch reflex, Ia afferents excite the homonymous LMN pool directly and inhibit the antagonist LMN pool reciprocally via Ia inhibitory interneurons. The Golgi tendon organ (GTO) reflex inhibits the homonymous LMN pool disynaptically and excites the antagonist LMN pool reciprocally. Flexor reflex responses excite a larger pool of LMNs, with reciprocal inhibition of the antagonist LMNs, to bring about a protective withdrawal response from a noxious stimulus. These reflexes can extend throughout the spinal cord. When an LMN fires an action potential, it excites a Renshaw cell, which inhibits the LMN, thereby ensuring a clean slate for the next set of inputs to it. Renshaw cells receive input from axon collaterals of both flexor and extensor LMNs to exert an inhibitory bias that is mainly directed toward inhibition of extensor LMNs and reciprocal excitation of flexor LMNs. Thus, the Renshaw cells favor flexor movements and help to inhibit extensor movements.

147

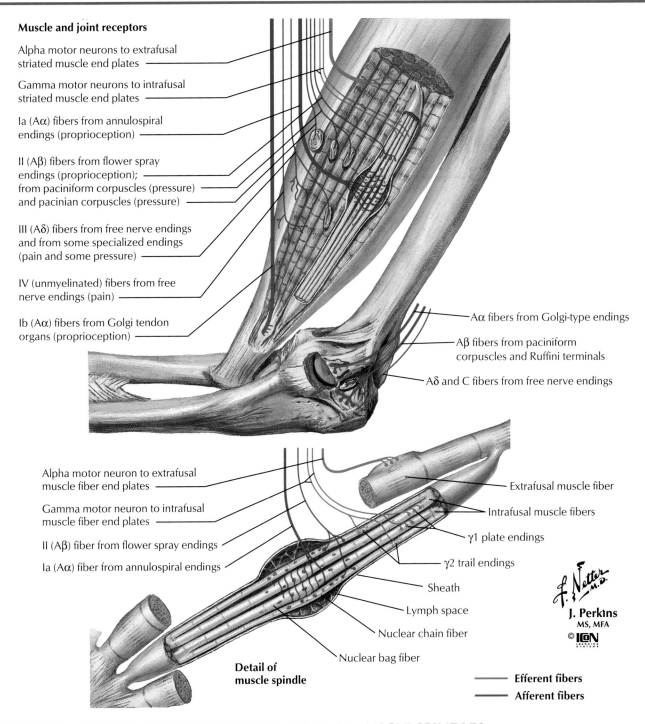

Muscle and joint receptors

Alpha motor neurons to extrafusal striated muscle end plates

Gamma motor neurons to intrafusal striated muscle end plates

Ia (Aα) fibers from annulospiral endings (proprioception)

II (Aβ) fibers from flower spray endings (proprioception); from paciniform corpuscles (pressure) and pacinian corpuscles (pressure)

III (Aδ) fibers from free nerve endings and from some specialized endings (pain and some pressure)

IV (unmyelinated) fibers from free nerve endings (pain)

Ib (Aα) fibers from Golgi tendon organs (proprioception)

Aα fibers from Golgi-type endings

Aβ fibers from paciniform corpuscles and Ruffini terminals

Aδ and C fibers from free nerve endings

Alpha motor neuron to extrafusal muscle fiber end plates

Gamma motor neuron to intrafusal muscle fiber end plates

II (Aβ) fiber from flower spray endings

Ia (Aα) fiber from annulospiral endings

Extrafusal muscle fiber

Intrafusal muscle fibers

γ1 plate endings

γ2 trail endings

Sheath

Lymph space

Nuclear chain fiber

Nuclear bag fiber

Detail of muscle spindle

J. Perkins MS, MFA

Efferent fibers
Afferent fibers

FIGURE II.61: MUSCLE AND JOINT RECEPTORS AND MUSCLE SPINDLES

Joints are innervated by a host of afferent receptors: bare nerve endings, Golgi-type endings, paciniform endings, Ruffini-like endings, and other encapsulated endings. GTOs innervate tendons and respond to stretch with increased discharge, causing disynaptic inhibition of the LMNs that contract the homonymous muscles. The muscle spindles, complex sensory receptors within the muscle, are arranged in parallel with the extrafusal (skeletal) muscle fibers. These receptors contain small intrafusal muscle fibers that are stretched when the muscle is stretched. The Ia afferent from the muscle spindle excites the homonymous LMN pool monosynaptically and responds to both the length and the velocity (change in length with respect to time) of the extrafusal muscle fiber. These muscle reflexes assist in maintaining homeostasis during contraction and help to regulate muscle tone during movement.

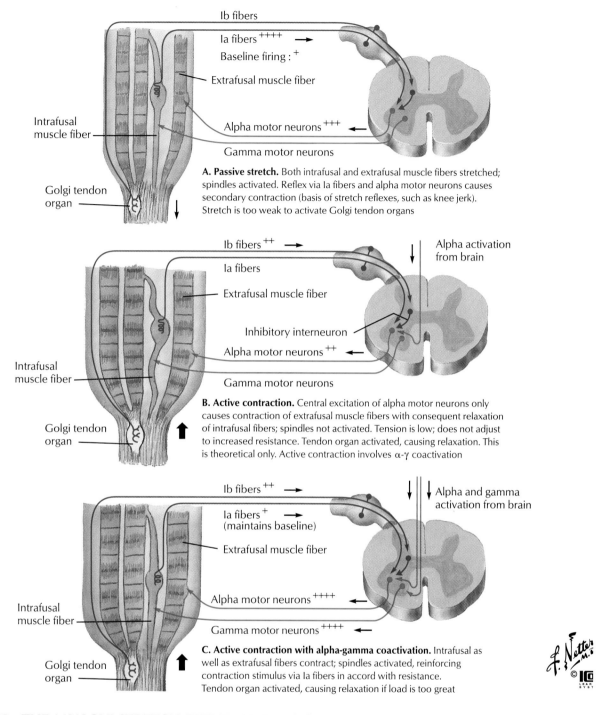

Ib fibers

Ia fibers $^{++++}$ →

Baseline firing : $^{+}$

Extrafusal muscle fiber

Intrafusal muscle fiber

Alpha motor neurons $^{+++}$ ←

Gamma motor neurons

Golgi tendon organ

A. Passive stretch. Both intrafusal and extrafusal muscle fibers stretched; spindles activated. Reflex via Ia fibers and alpha motor neurons causes secondary contraction (basis of stretch reflexes, such as knee jerk). Stretch is too weak to activate Golgi tendon organs

Ib fibers $^{++}$ →

Alpha activation from brain

Ia fibers

Extrafusal muscle fiber

Inhibitory interneuron

Intrafusal muscle fiber

Alpha motor neurons $^{++}$ ←

Gamma motor neurons

Golgi tendon organ

B. Active contraction. Central excitation of alpha motor neurons only causes contraction of extrafusal muscle fibers with consequent relaxation of intrafusal fibers; spindles not activated. Tension is low; does not adjust to increased resistance. Tendon organ activated, causing relaxation. This is theoretical only. Active contraction involves α-γ coactivation

Ib fibers $^{++}$ →

Alpha and gamma activation from brain

Ia fibers $^{+}$ → (maintains baseline)

Extrafusal muscle fiber

Intrafusal muscle fiber

Alpha motor neurons $^{++++}$ ←

Gamma motor neurons $^{++++}$ ←

Golgi tendon organ

C. Active contraction with alpha-gamma coactivation. Intrafusal as well as extrafusal fibers contract; spindles activated, reinforcing contraction stimulus via Ia fibers in accord with resistance. Tendon organ activated, causing relaxation if load is too great

FIGURE II.62: THE MUSCLE STRETCH REFLEX AND ITS CENTRAL CONTROL VIA GAMMA MOTOR NEURONS

During passive stretch, a muscle stretch reflex excites homonymous LMNs, which results in muscle contraction to restore homeostasis. If active contraction occurs without γ-LMN activation, the muscle spindle "unloads" and the tension in the intrafusal fibers is reduced, resulting in diminished firing of both Ia and group II afferents. However, when LMNs contract because of brain stem UMN activity or voluntary corticospinal activity, α-LMNs and γ-LMNs are activated together. This process,

α-γ-coactivation, ensures that the tension on the muscle spindle (through the intrafusal innervation by γ-fibers) adjusts immediately, that is, as the extrafusal muscle contraction (through α-fiber innervation) occurs. In normal physiological circumstances, α-LMNs and γ-LMNs are coactivated, although they can be modulated separately by central neuronal circuits. If γ-LMNs are differentially activated in pathological circumstances, increased muscle tone and spasticity ensue.

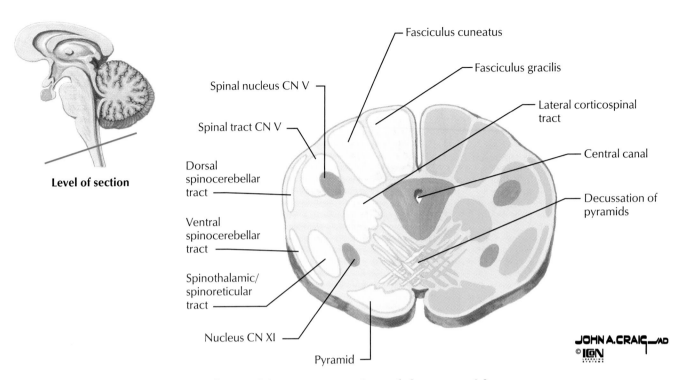

Fasciculus cuneatus

Fasciculus gracilis

Spinal nucleus CN V

Spinal tract CN V

Lateral corticospinal tract

Dorsal spinocerebellar tract

Central canal

Decussation of pyramids

Ventral spinocerebellar tract

Spinothalamic/ spinoreticular tract

Nucleus CN XI

Pyramid

Level of section

Section 1: Medulla-Spinal Cord Transition—Decussation of the Pyramids

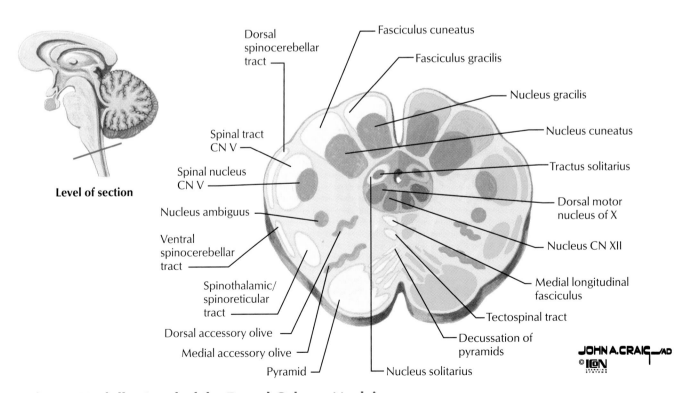

Dorsal spinocerebellar tract

Fasciculus cuneatus

Fasciculus gracilis

Nucleus gracilis

Nucleus cuneatus

Spinal tract CN V

Tractus solitarius

Spinal nucleus CN V

Dorsal motor nucleus of X

Nucleus ambiguus

Nucleus CN XII

Ventral spinocerebellar tract

Medial longitudinal fasciculus

Spinothalamic/ spinoreticular tract

Tectospinal tract

Dorsal accessory olive

Decussation of pyramids

Medial accessory olive

Pyramid

Nucleus solitarius

Level of section

Section 2: Medulla—Level of the Dorsal Column Nuclei

FIGURE II.63: BRAIN STEM CROSS-SECTIONAL ANATOMY _____

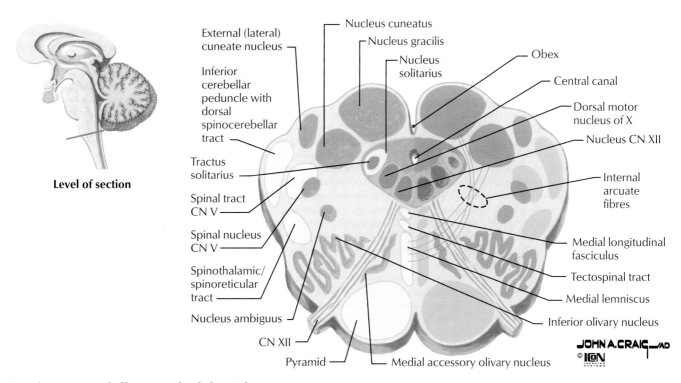

Level of section

External (lateral) cuneate nucleus

Inferior cerebellar peduncle with dorsal spinocerebellar tract

Tractus solitarius

Spinal tract CN V

Spinal nucleus CN V

Spinothalamic/ spinoreticular tract

Nucleus ambiguus

CN XII

Pyramid

Nucleus cuneatus

Nucleus gracilis

Nucleus solitarius

Obex

Central canal

Dorsal motor nucleus of X

Nucleus CN XII

Internal arcuate fibres

Medial longitudinal fasciculus

Tectospinal tract

Medial lemniscus

Inferior olivary nucleus

Medial accessory olivary nucleus

JOHN A. CRAIG _AD
© ICN

Section 3: Medulla—Level of the Obex

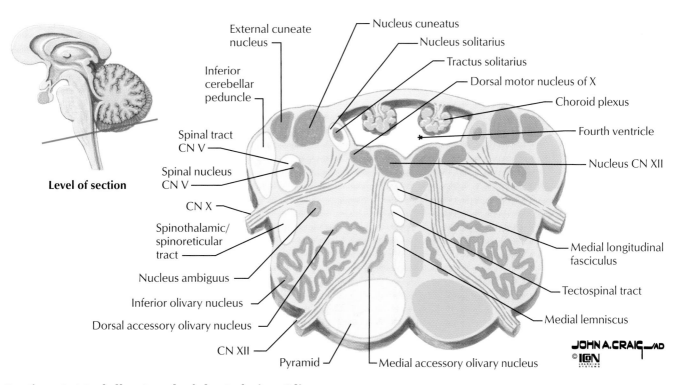

Level of section

External cuneate nucleus

Inferior cerebellar peduncle

Spinal tract CN V

Spinal nucleus CN V

CN X

Spinothalamic/ spinoreticular tract

Nucleus ambiguus

Inferior olivary nucleus

Dorsal accessory olivary nucleus

CN XII

Pyramid

Nucleus cuneatus

Nucleus solitarius

Tractus solitarius

Dorsal motor nucleus of X

Choroid plexus

Fourth ventricle

Nucleus CN XII

Medial longitudinal fasciculus

Tectospinal tract

Medial lemniscus

Medial accessory olivary nucleus

JOHN A. CRAIG _AD
© ICN

Section 4: Medulla—Level of the Inferior Olive

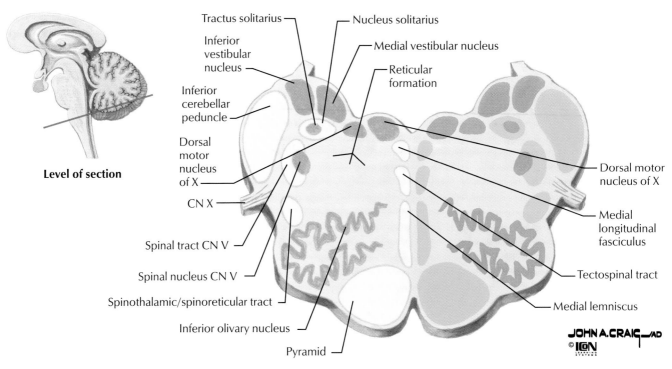

Level of section

Tractus solitarius

Nucleus solitarius

Inferior vestibular nucleus

Medial vestibular nucleus

Inferior cerebellar peduncle

Reticular formation

Dorsal motor nucleus of X

Dorsal motor nucleus of X

CN X

Medial longitudinal fasciculus

Spinal tract CN V

Spinal nucleus CN V

Tectospinal tract

Spinothalamic/spinoreticular tract

Medial lemniscus

Inferior olivary nucleus

Pyramid

Section 5: Medulla—Level of CN X and the Vestibular Nuclei

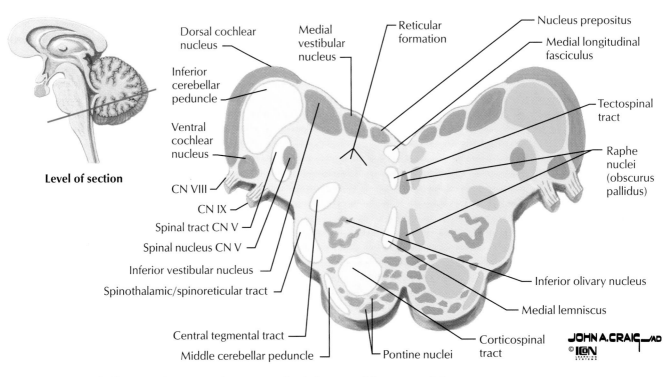

Level of section

Dorsal cochlear nucleus

Medial vestibular nucleus

Reticular formation

Nucleus prepositus

Inferior cerebellar peduncle

Medial longitudinal fasciculus

Ventral cochlear nucleus

Tectospinal tract

CN VIII

Raphe nuclei (obscurus pallidus)

CN IX

Spinal tract CN V

Spinal nucleus CN V

Inferior vestibular nucleus

Spinothalamic/spinoreticular tract

Inferior olivary nucleus

Medial lemniscus

Central tegmental tract

Corticospinal tract

Middle cerebellar peduncle

Pontine nuclei

Section 6: Medullo-Pontine Junction—Level of the Cochlear Nuclei

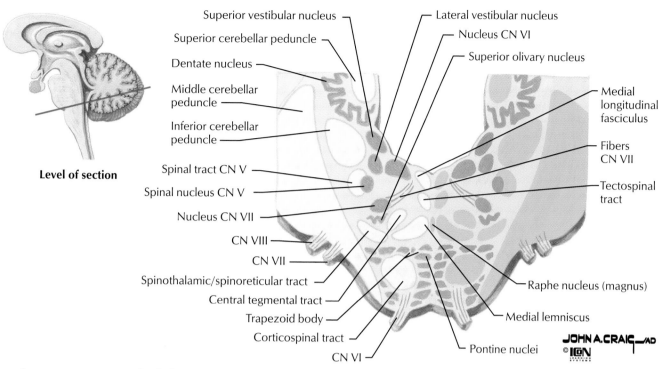

Level of section

Superior vestibular nucleus
Superior cerebellar peduncle
Dentate nucleus
Middle cerebellar peduncle
Inferior cerebellar peduncle
Spinal tract CN V
Spinal nucleus CN V
Nucleus CN VII
CN VIII
CN VII
Spinothalamic/spinoreticular tract
Central tegmental tract
Trapezoid body
Corticospinal tract
CN VI

Lateral vestibular nucleus
Nucleus CN VI
Superior olivary nucleus
Medial longitudinal fasciculus
Fibers CN VII
Tectospinal tract
Raphe nucleus (magnus)
Medial lemniscus
Pontine nuclei

JOHN A. CRAIG_AD
© ICN

Section 7: Pons—Level of the Facial Nucleus

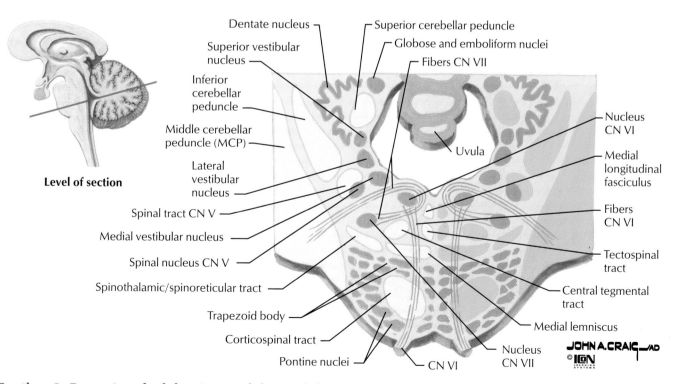

Level of section

Dentate nucleus
Superior vestibular nucleus
Inferior cerebellar peduncle
Middle cerebellar peduncle (MCP)
Lateral vestibular nucleus
Spinal tract CN V
Medial vestibular nucleus
Spinal nucleus CN V
Spinothalamic/spinoreticular tract
Trapezoid body
Corticospinal tract
Pontine nuclei

Superior cerebellar peduncle
Globose and emboliform nuclei
Fibers CN VII
Uvula
Nucleus CN VI
Medial longitudinal fasciculus
Fibers CN VI
Tectospinal tract
Central tegmental tract
Medial lemniscus
Nucleus CN VII
CN VI

JOHN A. CRAIG_AD
© ICN

Section 8: Pons—Level of the Genu of the Facial Nerve

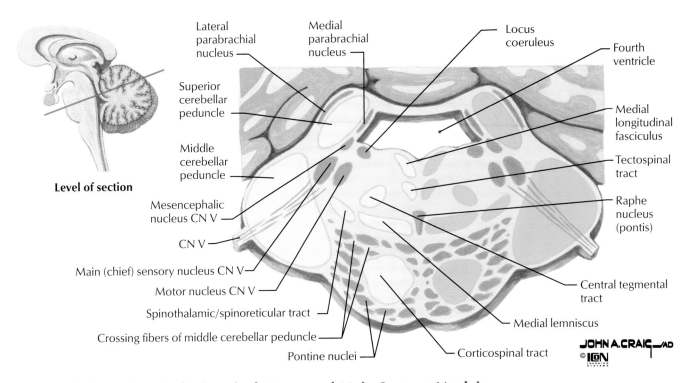

Lateral parabrachial nucleus

Medial parabrachial nucleus

Locus coeruleus

Fourth ventricle

Superior cerebellar peduncle

Medial longitudinal fasciculus

Middle cerebellar peduncle

Tectospinal tract

Mesencephalic nucleus CN V

Raphe nucleus (pontis)

CN V

Main (chief) sensory nucleus CN V

Motor nucleus CN V

Central tegmental tract

Spinothalamic/spinoreticular tract

Crossing fibers of middle cerebellar peduncle

Medial lemniscus

Pontine nuclei

Corticospinal tract

Level of section

JOHN A. CRAIG—AD
© ICN

Section 9: Pons—Level of Trigeminal Motor and Main Sensory Nuclei

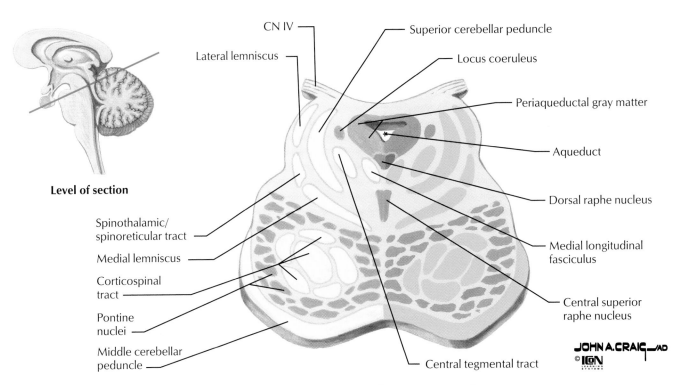

CN IV

Superior cerebellar peduncle

Lateral lemniscus

Locus coeruleus

Periaqueductal gray matter

Aqueduct

Dorsal raphe nucleus

Spinothalamic/ spinoreticular tract

Medial lemniscus

Medial longitudinal fasciculus

Corticospinal tract

Central superior raphe nucleus

Pontine nuclei

Middle cerebellar peduncle

Central tegmental tract

Level of section

JOHN A. CRAIG—AD
© ICN

Section 10: Pons-Midbrain Junction—Level of CN IV and Locus Coeruleus

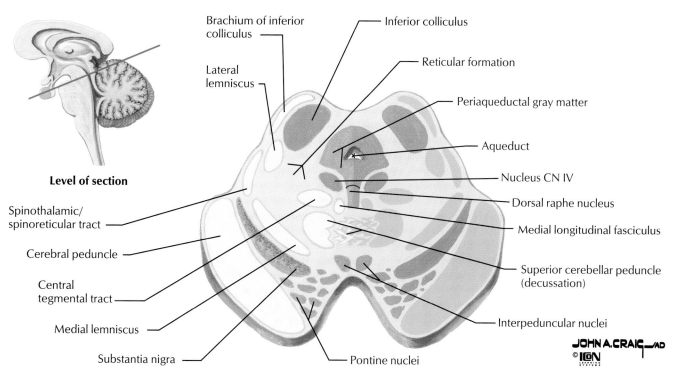

Level of section

Brachium of inferior colliculus

Lateral lemniscus

Inferior colliculus

Reticular formation

Periaqueductal gray matter

Aqueduct

Nucleus CN IV

Dorsal raphe nucleus

Medial longitudinal fasciculus

Superior cerebellar peduncle (decussation)

Interpeduncular nuclei

Spinothalamic/ spinoreticular tract

Cerebral peduncle

Central tegmental tract

Medial lemniscus

Substantia nigra

Pontine nuclei

Section 11: Midbrain—Level of the Inferior Colliculus

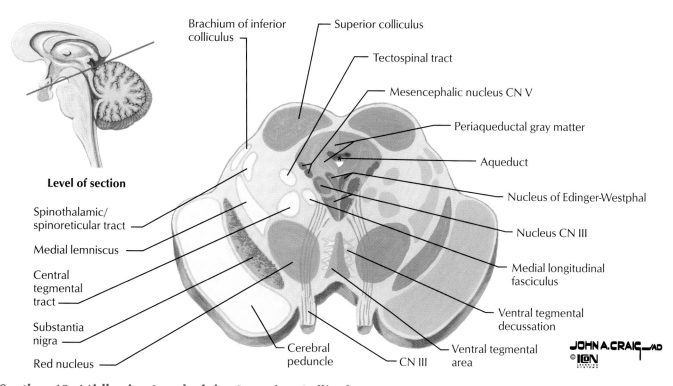

Level of section

Brachium of inferior colliculus

Superior colliculus

Tectospinal tract

Mesencephalic nucleus CN V

Periaqueductal gray matter

Aqueduct

Nucleus of Edinger-Westphal

Nucleus CN III

Medial longitudinal fasciculus

Ventral tegmental decussation

Ventral tegmental area

Spinothalamic/ spinoreticular tract

Medial lemniscus

Central tegmental tract

Substantia nigra

Red nucleus

Cerebral peduncle

CN III

Section 12: Midbrain—Level of the Superior Colliculus

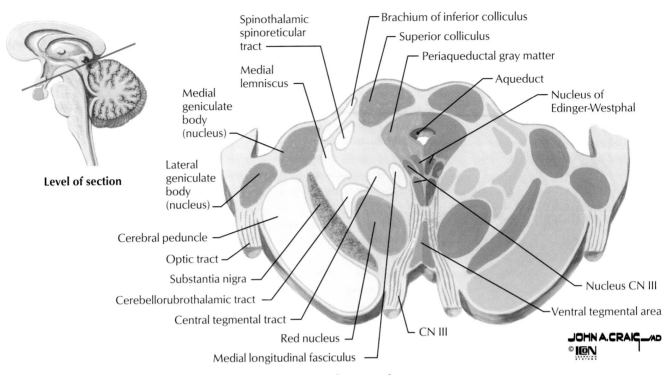

Spinothalamic spinoreticular tract

Medial lemniscus

Medial geniculate body (nucleus)

Lateral geniculate body (nucleus)

Cerebral peduncle

Optic tract

Substantia nigra

Cerebellorubrothalamic tract

Central tegmental tract

Red nucleus

Medial longitudinal fasciculus

Brachium of inferior colliculus

Superior colliculus

Periaqueductal gray matter

Aqueduct

Nucleus of Edinger-Westphal

Nucleus CN III

Ventral tegmental area

CN III

Level of section

JOHN A. CRAIG—AD
© ICN

Section 13: Midbrain—Level of the Medial Geniculate Body

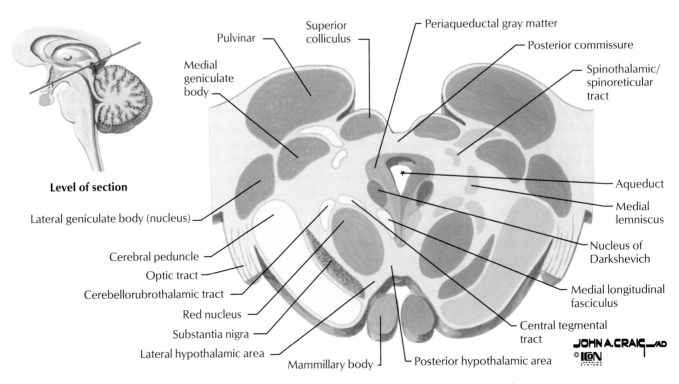

Pulvinar

Superior colliculus

Medial geniculate body

Lateral geniculate body (nucleus)

Cerebral peduncle

Optic tract

Cerebellorubrothalamic tract

Red nucleus

Substantia nigra

Lateral hypothalamic area

Mammillary body

Periaqueductal gray matter

Posterior commissure

Spinothalamic/ spinoreticular tract

Aqueduct

Medial lemniscus

Nucleus of Darkshevich

Medial longitudinal fasciculus

Central tegmental tract

Posterior hypothalamic area

Level of section

JOHN A. CRAIG—AD
© ICN

Section 14: Midbrain-Diencephalon Junction—Level of the Posterior Commissure

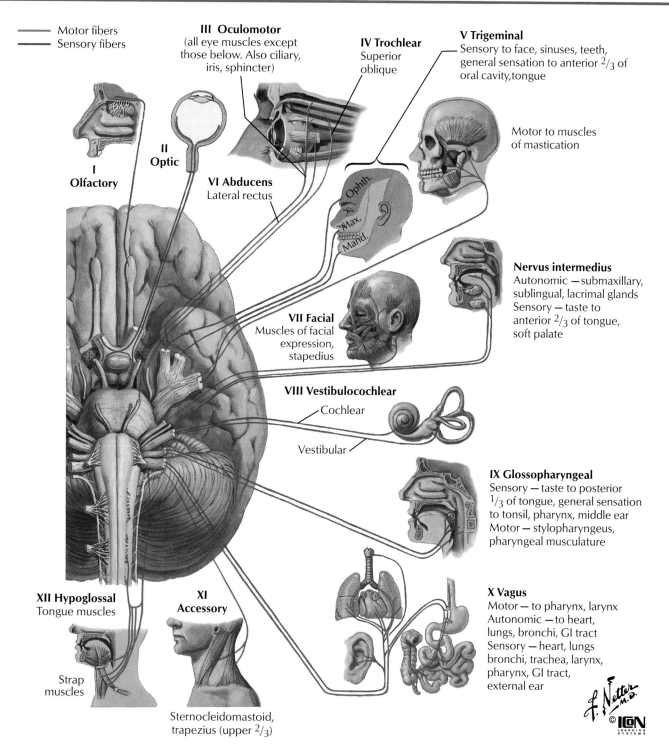

Motor fibers
Sensory fibers

III Oculomotor
(all eye muscles except
those below. Also ciliary,
iris, sphincter)

IV Trochlear
Superior
oblique

V Trigeminal
Sensory to face, sinuses, teeth,
general sensation to anterior $2/3$ of
oral cavity, tongue

II Optic

I Olfactory

VI Abducens
Lateral rectus

Motor to muscles
of mastication

Ophth.
Max.
Mand.

Nervus intermedius
Autonomic — submaxillary,
sublingual, lacrimal glands
Sensory — taste to
anterior $2/3$ of tongue,
soft palate

VII Facial
Muscles of facial
expression,
stapedius

VIII Vestibulocochlear

Cochlear

Vestibular

IX Glossopharyngeal
Sensory — taste to posterior
$1/3$ of tongue, general sensation
to tonsil, pharynx, middle ear
Motor — stylopharyngeus,
pharyngeal musculature

XII Hypoglossal
Tongue muscles

XI Accessory

X Vagus
Motor — to pharynx, larynx
Autonomic — to heart,
lungs, bronchi, GI tract
Sensory — heart, lungs
bronchi, trachea, larynx,
pharynx, GI tract,
external ear

Strap
muscles

Sternocleidomastoid,
trapezius (upper $2/3$)

FIGURE II.64: CRANIAL NERVES: SCHEMATIC OF DISTRIBUTION OF SENSORY, MOTOR, AND AUTONOMIC FIBERS

Cranial nerves (CNs) I and II, both sensory, are CNS tracts derived from the neural tube. CNs III-XII emerge from the brain stem and supply sensory (CNs V, VII-X), motor (CNs III-VII, IX-XII), and autonomic (CNs III, VII, IX, X) nerve fibers to structures in the head and the neck. All the cranial nerves that emerge from the brain stem distribute ipsilaterally to their target structures. The cranial nerve nuclei,

except CN nucleus IV (trochlear) and some motor components of CN nucleus III (oculomotor), are located ipsilateral to the point of emergence of the cranial nerve. The spinal accessory portion of CN XI emerges from motor neurons in the rostral spinal cord, but it ascends through the foramen magnum and then exits with CNs IX and X; thus, it is considered a cranial nerve.

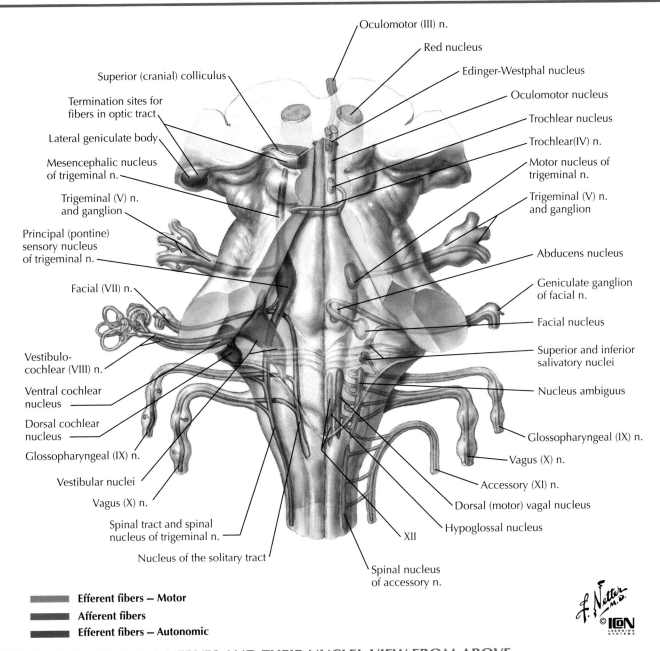

Efferent fibers — Motor
Afferent fibers
Efferent fibers — Autonomic

FIGURE II.65: CRANIAL NERVES AND THEIR NUCLEI: VIEW FROM ABOVE

Lower motor neurons (LMNs) of the brain stem are localized in a medial column (CNs III, IV, VI, XII) and a lateral column (CNs V and VII, nucleus ambiguus [CNs IX, X], CN XI). Preganglionic parasympathetic nuclei are found medially in the Edinger-Westphal nucleus (CN III) and the dorsal vagal nucleus (CN X) and laterally in the superior (CN VII) and inferior (CN IX) salivatory nuclei. Secondary sensory nuclei include the main sensory and descending nuclei of CN V, the vestibular nuclei and the cochlear nuclei (CN VIII), and the nucleus solitarius (CNs VII, IX, and X). The superior colliculus and the lateral geniculate body receive secondary sensory axonal projections from the optic tract; the inferior colliculus receives input from the cochlear nuclei and other accessory auditory nuclei. The nuclei gracilis and cuneatus, located in the medulla, receive input from dorsal root ganglion cells, which convey epicritic somatosensory modalities (fine discriminative touch, vibratory sensation, joint position sense).

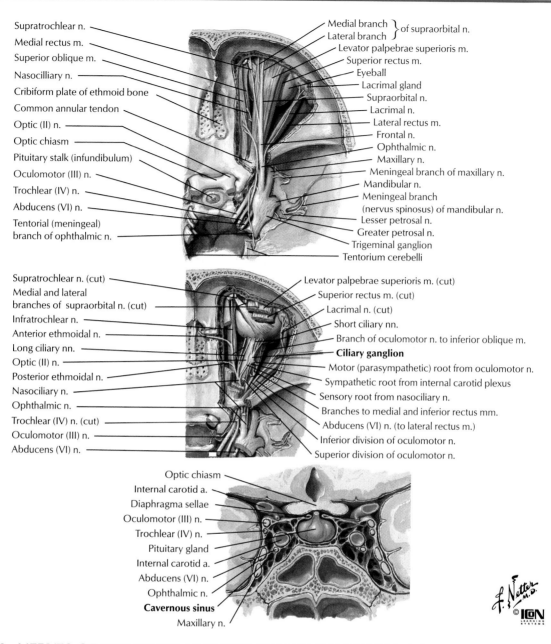

Supratrochlear n.
Medial rectus m.
Superior oblique m.
Nasocilliary n.
Cribiform plate of ethmoid bone
Common annular tendon
Optic (II) n.
Optic chiasm
Pituitary stalk (infundibulum)
Oculomotor (III) n.
Trochlear (IV) n.
Abducens (VI) n.
Tentorial (meningeal) branch of ophthalmic n.

Medial branch } of supraorbital n.
Lateral branch }
Levator palpebrae superioris m.
Superior rectus m.
Eyeball
Lacrimal gland
Supraorbital n.
Lacrimal n.
Lateral rectus m.
Frontal n.
Ophthalmic n.
Maxillary n.
Meningeal branch of maxillary n.
Mandibular n.
Meningeal branch (nervus spinosus) of mandibular n.
Lesser petrosal n.
Greater petrosal n.
Trigeminal ganglion
Tentorium cerebelli

Supratrochlear n. (cut)
Medial and lateral branches of supraorbital n. (cut)
Infratrochlear n.
Anterior ethmoidal n.
Long ciliary nn.
Optic (II) n.
Posterior ethmoidal n.
Nasociliary n.
Ophthalmic n.
Trochlear (IV) n. (cut)
Oculomotor (III) n.
Abducens (VI) n.

Levator palpebrae superioris m. (cut)
Superior rectus m. (cut)
Lacrimal n. (cut)
Short ciliary nn.
Branch of oculomotor n. to inferior oblique m.
Ciliary ganglion
Motor (parasympathetic) root from oculomotor n.
Sympathetic root from internal carotid plexus
Sensory root from nasociliary n.
Branches to medial and inferior rectus mm.
Abducens (VI) n. (to lateral rectus m.)
Inferior division of oculomotor n.
Superior division of oculomotor n.

Optic chiasm
Internal carotid a.
Diaphragma sellae
Oculomotor (III) n.
Trochlear (IV) n.
Pituitary gland
Internal carotid a.
Abducens (VI) n.
Ophthalmic n.
Cavernous sinus
Maxillary n.

FIGURE II.66: NERVES OF THE ORBIT AND THE CILIARY GANGLION: DORSAL VIEW AND CROSS-SECTION THROUGH THE CAVERNOUS SINUS

CN II carries visual information from the ipsilateral retina. Axons from the temporal hemiretinas remain ipsilateral, whereas axons from the nasal hemiretinas cross the midline in the optic chiasm. All axons then enter the optic tract. CNs III (from oculomotor nuclei), IV, and VI innervate the extrinsic muscles of the eye. Sensory portions of the ophthalmic division of CN V supply general sensation to the cornea and the eyeball and provide the afferent limb of the corneal reflex. Motor fibers of CN VII innervate the orbicularis oculi muscle, closing the eye; these fibers constitute the efferent limb of the corneal reflex. Parasympathetic preganglionic fibers from the Edinger-Westphal nucleus distribute

to the ciliary ganglion, which supplies the pupillary constrictor muscle and the ciliary muscle (accommodation for near vision). Preganglionic parasympathetic axons from the superior salivatory nucleus distribute to the pterygopalatine ganglion, which supplies the lacrimal gland (tear production). Sympathetic postganglionic nerve fibers from the superior cervical ganglion supply the pupillary dilator muscle and the superior tarsal muscle (damage results in mild ptosis). CNs III, IV, VI, and the ophthalmic and maxillary divisions of CN V traverse the cavernous sinus and are vulnerable to damage from cavernous sinus thrombosis.

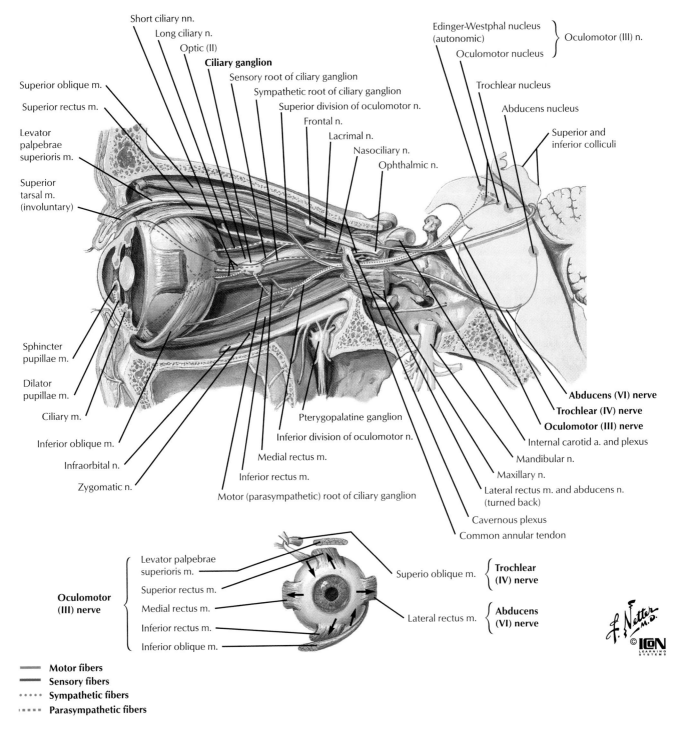

Short ciliary nn.
Long ciliary n.
Optic (II)
Ciliary ganglion
Sensory root of ciliary ganglion
Sympathetic root of ciliary ganglion
Superior division of oculomotor n.
Frontal n.
Lacrimal n.
Nasociliary n.
Ophthalmic n.

Edinger-Westphal nucleus (autonomic) } Oculomotor (III) n.
Oculomotor nucleus
Trochlear nucleus
Abducens nucleus
Superior and inferior colliculi

Superior oblique m.
Superior rectus m.
Levator palpebrae superioris m.
Superior tarsal m. (involuntary)

Sphincter pupillae m.
Dilator pupillae m.
Ciliary m.
Inferior oblique m.
Infraorbital n.
Zygomatic n.

Abducens (VI) nerve
Trochlear (IV) nerve
Oculomotor (III) nerve
Internal carotid a. and plexus
Mandibular n.
Maxillary n.
Lateral rectus m. and abducens n. (turned back)
Cavernous plexus
Common annular tendon

Pterygopalatine ganglion
Inferior division of oculomotor n.
Medial rectus m.
Inferior rectus m.
Motor (parasympathetic) root of ciliary ganglion

Oculomotor (III) nerve {
Levator palpebrae superioris m.
Superior rectus m.
Medial rectus m.
Inferior rectus m.
Inferior oblique m.

Superio oblique m. { **Trochlear (IV) nerve**
Lateral rectus m. { **Abducens (VI) nerve**

——— **Motor fibers**
——— **Sensory fibers**
· · · · **Sympathetic fibers**
ı ▪ ▪ ▪ **Parasympathetic fibers**

FIGURE II.67: EXTRAOCULAR NERVES (III, IV, AND VI) AND THE CILIARY GANGLION: VIEW IN RELATION TO THE EYE

CN VI innervates the lateral rectus muscle; damage results in ipsilateral paralysis of lateral gaze. CN IV innervates the superior oblique muscle; damage results in inability to look in and down (most conspicuous when climbing stairs, stepping off a curb, reading in bed). CN III (oculomotor nuclei) innervates the medial rectus, superior rectus, inferior rectus, and inferior oblique muscles (damage results in paralysis of ipsilateral medial gaze), and the levator palpebrae superioris muscle (damage results in profound ptosis). The ciliary ganglion gives rise to postganglionic parasympathetic axons that supply the pupillary constrictor muscle and the ciliary muscle. Damage results in a fixed and dilated pupil that will not constrict for the pupillary light reflex and will not accommodate to near vision.

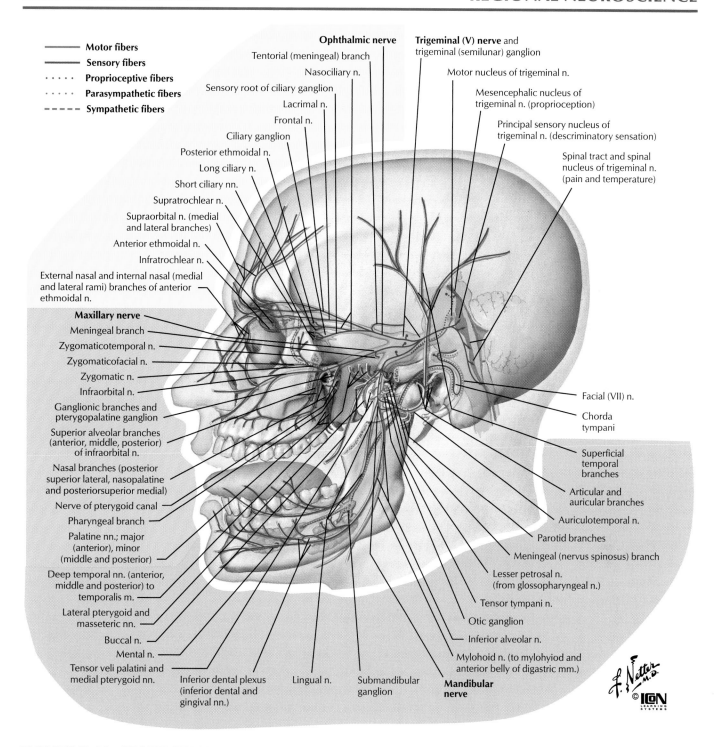

FIGURE II.68: TRIGEMINAL NERVE (V)

The trigeminal nerve (CN V) carries sensory information from the face, the sinuses, the teeth, and the anterior portion of the oral cavity. It has 3 subdivisions: (I) ophthalmic—sensory innervation, (II) maxillary—sensory innervation, and (III) mandibular—sensory innervation, and motor innervation of the masticatory and tensor tympani muscles. Primary sensory axons from trigeminal (semilunar, gasserian) ganglion cells that process fine discriminative touch (epicritic sensation) terminate in the

main sensory nucleus and the rostral descending nucleus of CN V. Those axons processing pain and temperature sensation (protopathic sensation) terminate in the caudal descending (spinal) nucleus of CN V. The trigeminal nerve also carries proprioceptive information from muscle spindles in the masticatory and extraocular muscles. The primary sensory cell bodies found in the mesencephalic nucleus of CN V are the only primary sensory neurons to reside in the CNS.

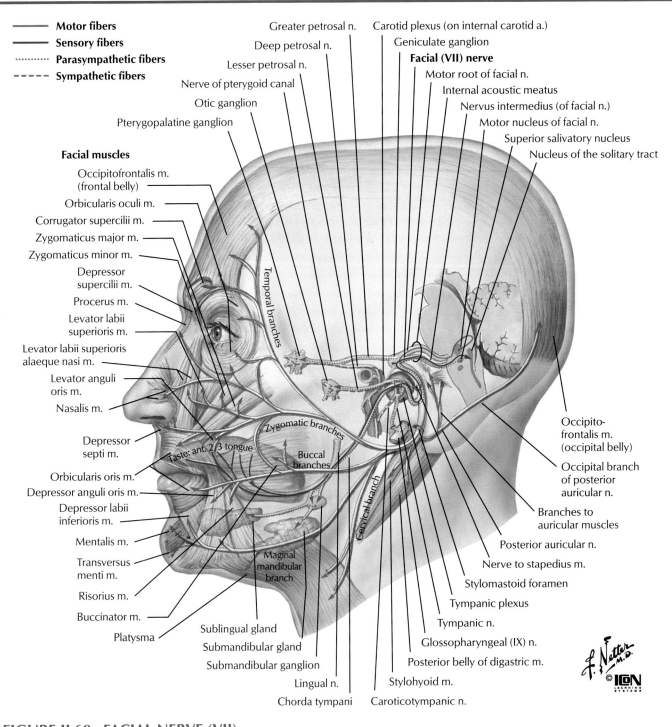

——— **Motor fibers**
——— **Sensory fibers**
·········· **Parasympathetic fibers**
----- **Sympathetic fibers**

Greater petrosal n.
Deep petrosal n.
Lesser petrosal n.
Nerve of pterygoid canal
Otic ganglion
Pterygopalatine ganglion

Carotid plexus (on internal carotid a.)
Geniculate ganglion
Facial (VII) nerve
Motor root of facial n.
Internal acoustic meatus
Nervus intermedius (of facial n.)
Motor nucleus of facial n.
Superior salivatory nucleus
Nucleus of the solitary tract

Facial muscles
Occipitofrontalis m. (frontal belly)
Orbicularis oculi m.
Corrugator supercilii m.
Zygomaticus major m.
Zygomaticus minor m.
Depressor supercilii m.
Procerus m.
Levator labii superioris m.
Levator labii superioris alaeque nasi m.
Levator anguli oris m.
Nasalis m.
Depressor septi m.
Orbicularis oris m.
Depressor anguli oris m.
Depressor labii inferioris m.
Mentalis m.
Transversus menti m.
Risorius m.
Buccinator m.
Platysma

Temporal branches
Zygomatic branches
Taste: ant. 2/3 tongue
Buccal branches
Cervical branch
Maginal mandibular branch
Sublingual gland
Submandibular gland
Submandibular ganglion
Lingual n.
Chorda tympani

Occipitofrontalis m. (occipital belly)
Occipital branch of posterior auricular n.
Branches to auricular muscles
Posterior auricular n.
Nerve to stapedius m.
Stylomastoid foramen
Tympanic plexus
Tympanic n.
Glossopharyngeal (IX) n.
Posterior belly of digastric m.
Stylohyoid m.
Caroticotympanic n.

FIGURE II.69: FACIAL NERVE (VII)

The facial nerve (CN VII) has motor, parasympathetic, and sensory components. The motor fibers distribute to the muscles of facial expression; the scalp, auricle, buccinator, stapedius, and stylohyoid muscles; and the posterior belly of the digastric muscle. Damage results in ipsilateral paralysis of facial expression, including the forehead (Bell's palsy). Activation of the stapedius dampens the ossicles in the presence of sustained loud noise; damage to CN VII also results in hyperacusis. Parasympathetic nerve fibers from the superior salivatory nucleus distribute to the pterygopalatine ganglion, which innervates the lacrimal glands, and to the submandibular ganglion, which innervates the submandibular and sublingual salivary glands. Special sensory taste fibers from the anterior two-thirds of the tongue (via the chorda tympani) and the soft palate (via the greater petrosal nerve), axons of the geniculate ganglion, convey information to the rostral portion of the nucleus solitarius in the medulla.

Vestibulocochlear (VIII) Nerve

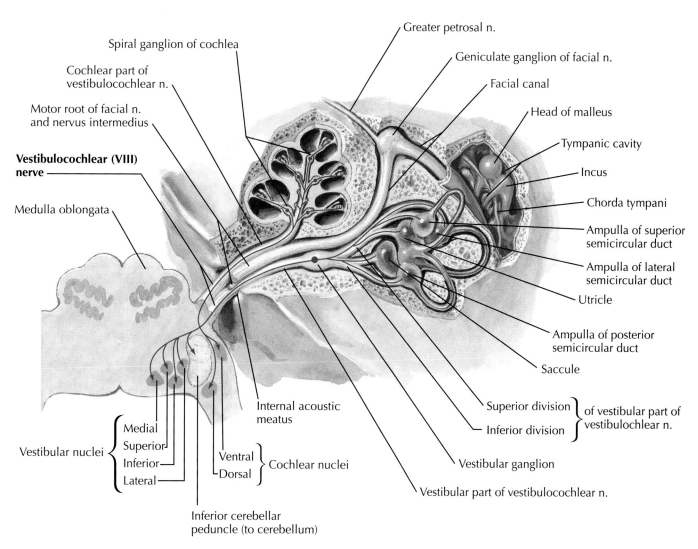

- Spiral ganglion of cochlea
- Cochlear part of vestibulocochlear n.
- Motor root of facial n. and nervus intermedius
- Vestibulocochlear (VIII) nerve
- Medulla oblongata
- Greater petrosal n.
- Geniculate ganglion of facial n.
- Facial canal
- Head of malleus
- Tympanic cavity
- Incus
- Chorda tympani
- Ampulla of superior semicircular duct
- Ampulla of lateral semicircular duct
- Utricle
- Ampulla of posterior semicircular duct
- Saccule
- Superior division } of vestibular part of vestibulochlear n.
- Inferior division
- Vestibular ganglion
- Vestibular part of vestibulocochlear n.
- Internal acoustic meatus
- Vestibular nuclei { Medial, Superior, Inferior, Lateral }
- Ventral, Dorsal } Cochlear nuclei
- Inferior cerebellar peduncle (to cerebellum)

FIGURE II.70: VESTIBULOCOCHLEAR NERVE (VIII)

The vestibulocochlear nerve (CN VIII) arises from bipolar primary sensory neurons in the vestibular (Scarpa's) ganglion and the spiral (cochlear) ganglion. The peripheral process of the vestibular ganglion neurons innervates hair cells in the utricle and the saccule that respond to linear acceleration (gravity) and in the ampullae of the semicircular ducts that respond to angular acceleration (movement). The utricle, the saccule, and the semicircular ducts provide neural signals for coordination and equilibration of position, and movements of the head and the neck. The central processes of vestibular ganglion cells terminate in the medial, lateral, superior, or inferior vestibular nuclei in the medulla and the pons and in the cerebellum. The peripheral processes of spiral ganglion cells innervate hair cells that lie along the cochlear duct in the organ of Corti. They convey hearing information into the dorsal and ventral cochlear nuclei via the central axonal processes. A lesion to CN VIII results in ipsilateral deafness and vertigo and loss of equilibrium.

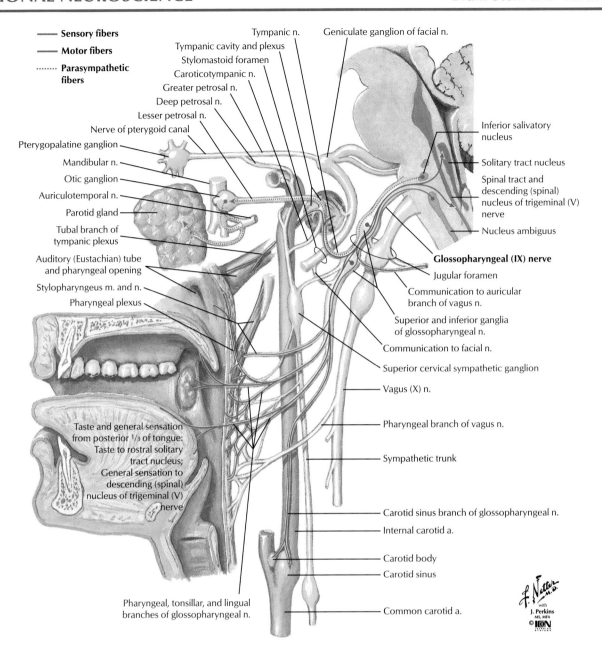

Sensory fibers
Motor fibers
Parasympathetic fibers

Tympanic n.
Tympanic cavity and plexus
Stylomastoid foramen
Caroticotympanic n.
Greater petrosal n.
Deep petrosal n.
Lesser petrosal n.
Nerve of pterygoid canal
Pterygopalatine ganglion
Mandibular n.
Otic ganglion
Auriculotemporal n.
Parotid gland
Tubal branch of tympanic plexus
Auditory (Eustachian) tube and pharyngeal opening
Stylopharyngeus m. and n.
Pharyngeal plexus

Geniculate ganglion of facial n.

Inferior salivatory nucleus
Solitary tract nucleus
Spinal tract and descending (spinal) nucleus of trigeminal (V) nerve
Nucleus ambiguus

Glossopharyngeal (IX) nerve
Jugular foramen
Communication to auricular branch of vagus n.
Superior and inferior ganglia of glossopharyngeal n.
Communication to facial n.
Superior cervical sympathetic ganglion
Vagus (X) n.
Pharyngeal branch of vagus n.
Sympathetic trunk

Taste and general sensation from posterior ⅓ of tongue: Taste to rostral solitary tract nucleus; General sensation to descending (spinal) nucleus of trigeminal (V) nerve

Carotid sinus branch of glossopharyngeal n.
Internal carotid a.
Carotid body
Carotid sinus

Pharyngeal, tonsillar, and lingual branches of glossopharyngeal n.

Common carotid a.

FIGURE II.71: GLOSSOPHARYNGEAL NERVE (IX)

The glossopharyngeal nerve (CN IX) is a mixed nerve with motor, parasympathetic, and sensory components. Motor fibers from the nucleus ambiguus supply the stylopharyngeus muscle and may assist in innervation of pharyngeal muscles, for swallowing. Preganglionic axons from the inferior salivatory nucleus travel with CN IX to the otic ganglion, whose neurons innervate the parotid gland and the mucous glands. Special sensory axons from the petrosal (inferior) ganglion convey information from taste buds on the posterior third of the tongue and on part of the soft palate. These axons terminate in the rostral portion of the nucleus solitarius. Axons from additional primary sensory neurons in the inferior ganglion carry general sensation from the posterior third of the tongue and from the pharynx, the fauces, the tonsil, the tympanic cavity, the eustachian tube, and the mastoid cells. The central axon branches terminate in the descending (spinal) nucleus of CN V. The general sensory fibers from the pharynx provide the afferent limb of the gag reflex. Additional primary sensory neurons innervate the carotid body (chemoreception of CO_2) and the carotid sinus (baroceptors) and convey the central axons to the caudal nucleus solitarius. Primary sensory neurons in the superior ganglion innervate a small region behind the ear and convey general sensation into the descending nucleus of CN V.

Nucleus solitarius = Solitary tract nucleus.

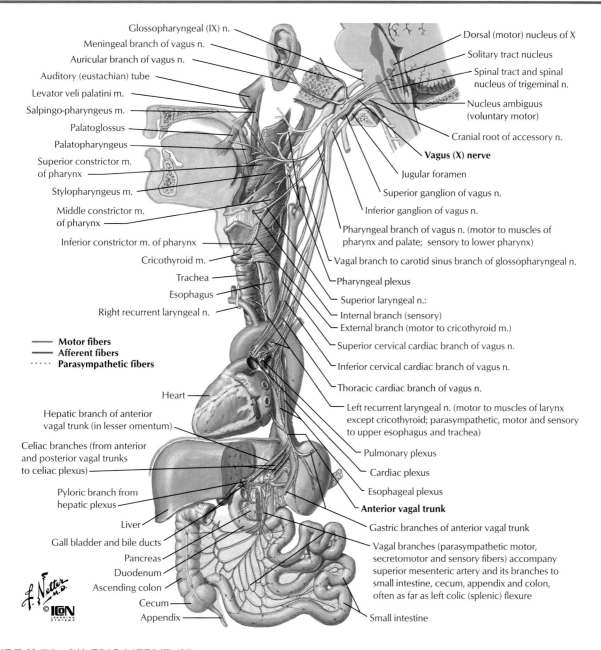

Glossopharyngeal (IX) n.
Meningeal branch of vagus n.
Auricular branch of vagus n.
Auditory (eustachian) tube
Levator veli palatini m.
Salpingo-pharyngeus m.
Palatoglossus
Palatopharyngeus
Superior constrictor m. of pharynx
Stylopharyngeus m.
Middle constrictor m. of pharynx
Inferior constrictor m. of pharynx
Cricothyroid m.
Trachea
Esophagus
Right recurrent laryngeal n.

—— **Motor fibers**
—— **Afferent fibers**
····· **Parasympathetic fibers**

Heart
Hepatic branch of anterior vagal trunk (in lesser omentum)
Celiac branches (from anterior and posterior vagal trunks to celiac plexus)
Pyloric branch from hepatic plexus
Liver
Gall bladder and bile ducts
Pancreas
Duodenum
Ascending colon
Cecum
Appendix

Dorsal (motor) nucleus of X
Solitary tract nucleus
Spinal tract and spinal nucleus of trigeminal n.
Nucleus ambiguus (voluntary motor)
Cranial root of accessory n.
Vagus (X) nerve
Jugular foramen
Superior ganglion of vagus n.
Inferior ganglion of vagus n.
Pharyngeal branch of vagus n. (motor to muscles of pharynx and palate; sensory to lower pharynx)
Vagal branch to carotid sinus branch of glossopharyngeal n.
Pharyngeal plexus
Superior laryngeal n.:
Internal branch (sensory)
External branch (motor to cricothyroid m.)
Superior cervical cardiac branch of vagus n.
Inferior cervical cardiac branch of vagus n.
Thoracic cardiac branch of vagus n.
Left recurrent laryngeal n. (motor to muscles of larynx except cricothyroid; parasympathetic, motor and sensory to upper esophagus and trachea)
Pulmonary plexus
Cardiac plexus
Esophageal plexus
Anterior vagal trunk
Gastric branches of anterior vagal trunk
Vagal branches (parasympathetic motor, secretomotor and sensory fibers) accompany superior mesenteric artery and its branches to small intestine, cecum, appendix and colon, often as far as left colic (splenic) flexure
Small intestine

FIGURE II.72: VAGUS NERVE (X)

The vagus nerve (CN X) is a mixed nerve with motor, parasympathetic, and sensory components. LMN axons from the nucleus ambiguus in the medulla supply muscles of the soft palate, the pharynx, and the larynx, which control speaking and swallowing. A lesion results in hoarseness, dysphagia, and decreased gag reflex (efferent limb). Preganglionic parasympathetic axons from neurons in the dorsal (motor) nucleus of CN X in the medulla distribute to intramural ganglia associated with thoracic and abdominal viscera to supply autonomic innervation to the heart, the lung, and the GI tract to the descending colon. Special sensory axons from the nodose (inferior) ganglion, which carry information from taste buds in the posterior pharynx (found mainly in children), send central branches to terminate in the rostral nucleus solitarius. Primary sensory axons from the inferior ganglion, which convey general sensation from the larynx, the pharynx, and the thoracic and abdominal viscera, terminate mainly in the caudal nucleus solitarius. Primary sensory axons from the superior (jugular) ganglion, which convey general sensation from the external auditory meatus, terminate in the descending (spinal) nucleus of CN V.

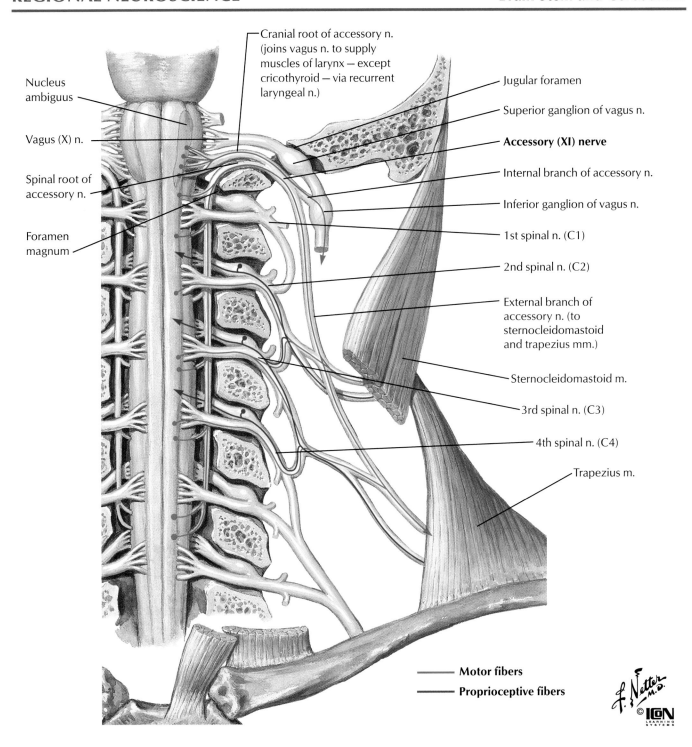

Nucleus ambiguus

Cranial root of accessory n. (joins vagus n. to supply muscles of larynx — except cricothyroid — via recurrent laryngeal n.)

Jugular foramen

Superior ganglion of vagus n.

Vagus (X) n.

Accessory (XI) nerve

Internal branch of accessory n.

Spinal root of accessory n.

Inferior ganglion of vagus n.

1st spinal n. (C1)

Foramen magnum

2nd spinal n. (C2)

External branch of accessory n. (to sternocleidomastoid and trapezius mm.)

Sternocleidomastoid m.

3rd spinal n. (C3)

4th spinal n. (C4)

Trapezius m.

——— Motor fibers

——— Proprioceptive fibers

FIGURE II.73: ACCESSORY NERVE (XI)

The accessory nerve (CN XI) is a motor nerve with cranial and spinal portions. The cranial portion arises from LMNs at the caudal end of the nucleus ambiguus; the axons travel through an internal branch that distributes with the pharyngeal and laryngeal branches of the vagus nerve (CN X) and the nerves to the soft palate. These axons are often considered to be part of CN X. The spinal portion arises from LMNs in the lateral part of the upper four or five segments of the cervical spinal cord.

The axons then emerge as rootlets from the lateral margin of the spinal cord, ascend behind the denticulate ligaments, and coalesce as a single nerve. This nerve then ascends through the foramen magnum and joins the vagus nerve to exit through the jugular foramen. The spinal accessory LMNs supply the sternocleidomastoid muscle and the upper two-thirds of the trapezius muscle. Damage to this division results in weakness of head rotation and shoulder elevation.

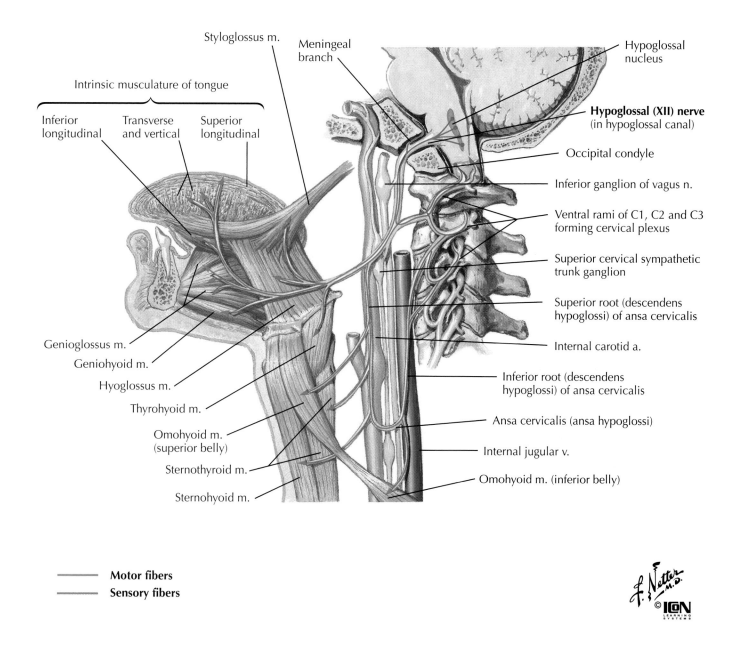

Styloglossus m.

Meningeal branch

Hypoglossal nucleus

Intrinsic musculature of tongue

Hypoglossal (XII) nerve (in hypoglossal canal)

Inferior longitudinal

Transverse and vertical

Superior longitudinal

Occipital condyle

Inferior ganglion of vagus n.

Ventral rami of C1, C2 and C3 forming cervical plexus

Superior cervical sympathetic trunk ganglion

Genioglossus m.

Geniohyoid m.

Hyoglossus m.

Thyrohyoid m.

Superior root (descendens hypoglossi) of ansa cervicalis

Internal carotid a.

Inferior root (descendens hypoglossi) of ansa cervicalis

Omohyoid m. (superior belly)

Ansa cervicalis (ansa hypoglossi)

Internal jugular v.

Sternothyroid m.

Sternohyoid m.

Omohyoid m. (inferior belly)

——— Motor fibers
——— Sensory fibers

FIGURE II.74: HYPOGLOSSAL NERVE (XII)

The hypoglossal nerve (CN XII) is a motor nerve. LMNs in the hypoglossal nucleus of the caudal medulla exit from the ventral surface of the medulla in the preolivary sulcus (between the medullary pyramid and the inferior olive) to innervate the extrinsic hyoglossus, styloglossus, chondroglossus, and genioglossus tongue muscles and the intrinsic superior and inferior longitudinal, transverse, and vertical lingual tongue muscles. Damage to this nerve leads to weakness of the ipsilateral tongue muscles; the protruded tongue deviates toward the weak side because of the unopposed action of the innervated contralateral genioglossus muscle.

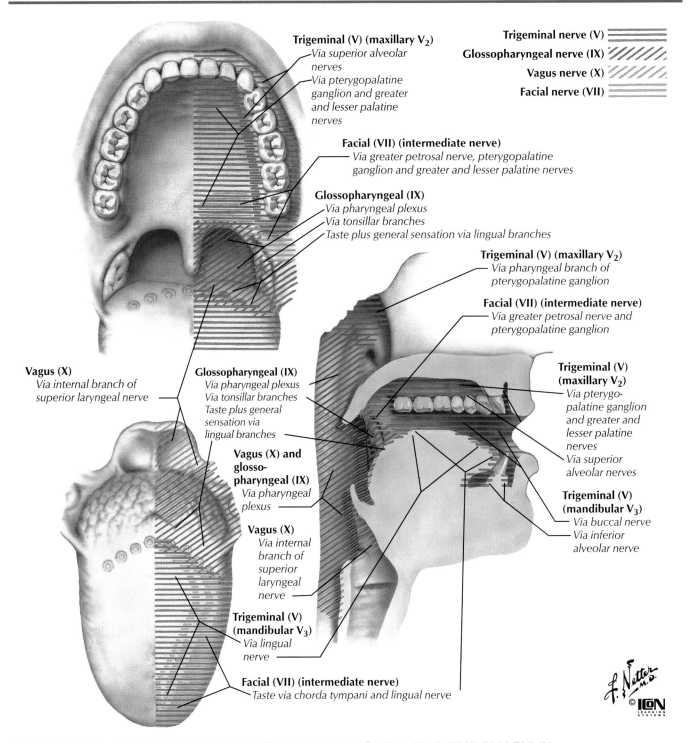

Trigeminal (V) (maxillary V₂)
Via superior alveolar nerves
Via pterygopalatine ganglion and greater and lesser palatine nerves

Trigeminal nerve (V)
Glossopharyngeal nerve (IX)
Vagus nerve (X)
Facial nerve (VII)

Facial (VII) (intermediate nerve)
Via greater petrosal nerve, pterygopalatine ganglion and greater and lesser palatine nerves

Glossopharyngeal (IX)
Via pharyngeal plexus
Via tonsillar branches
Taste plus general sensation via lingual branches

Trigeminal (V) (maxillary V₂)
Via pharyngeal branch of pterygopalatine ganglion

Facial (VII) (intermediate nerve)
Via greater petrosal nerve and pterygopalatine ganglion

Vagus (X)
Via internal branch of superior laryngeal nerve

Glossopharyngeal (IX)
Via pharyngeal plexus
Via tonsillar branches
Taste plus general sensation via lingual branches

Trigeminal (V) (maxillary V₂)
Via pterygo-palatine ganglion and greater and lesser palatine nerves
Via superior alveolar nerves

Vagus (X) and glosso-pharyngeal (IX)
Via pharyngeal plexus

Vagus (X)
Via internal branch of superior laryngeal nerve

Trigeminal (V) (mandibular V₃)
Via buccal nerve
Via inferior alveolar nerve

Trigeminal (V) (mandibular V₃)
Via lingual nerve

Facial (VII) (intermediate nerve)
Taste via chorda tympani and lingual nerve

FIGURE II.75: AFFERENT INNERVATION OF THE MOUTH AND THE PHARYNX

Primary sensory axons of the maxillary and mandibular divisions of CN V (trigeminal ganglion) provide general sensation to the mouth, the teeth, the gums, the sinuses, and the anterior two-thirds of the tongue. General sensation to the posterior third of the tongue, the pharynx, and the larynx is provided by primary sensory axons of CN IX (inferior or petrosal ganglion) and, to a lesser extent, by CN X (inferior or nodose ganglion) for the pharynx and the larynx. Chemosensation from taste buds is conveyed by CN VII (geniculate ganglion) for the anterior two-thirds of the tongue, CN IX (petrosal ganglion) for the posterior third of the tongue, and CN X (nodose ganglion) for the posterior pharynx.

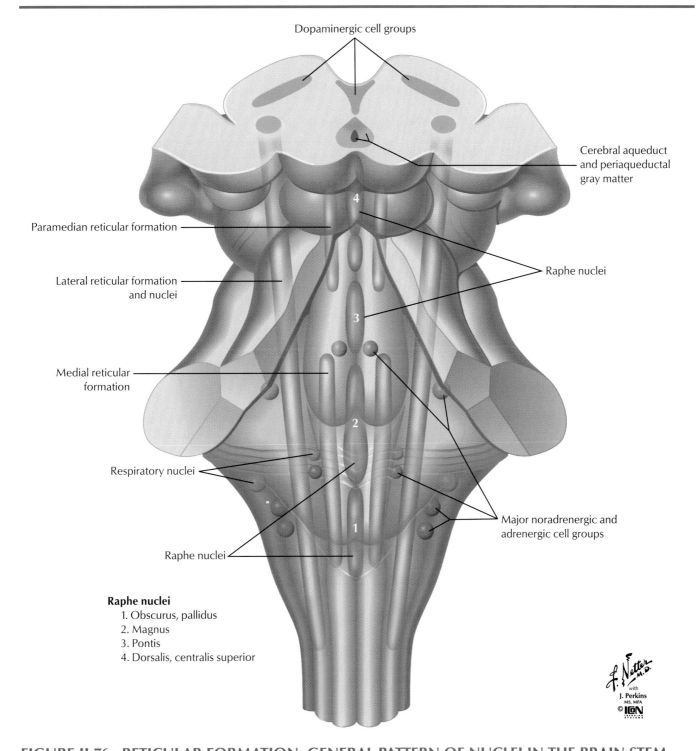

Dopaminergic cell groups

Cerebral aqueduct and periaqueductal gray matter

Paramedian reticular formation

Raphe nuclei

Lateral reticular formation and nuclei

Medial reticular formation

Respiratory nuclei

Major noradrenergic and adrenergic cell groups

Raphe nuclei

Raphe nuclei
1. Obscurus, pallidus
2. Magnus
3. Pontis
4. Dorsalis, centralis superior

FIGURE II.76: RETICULAR FORMATION: GENERAL PATTERN OF NUCLEI IN THE BRAIN STEM

The reticular formation (RF), the neuronal core of the brain stem, consists of neurons with characteristic isodendritic morphology. The RF extends from the rostral spinal cord through the hypothalamus into the septal region. RF neurons are large cells with axonal arborizations that terminate at a distance from their cell bodies and dendritic tree; they are not interneurons. The major nuclei are found in a lateral zone (sensory functions), a medial zone (motor functions), and a column of raphe nuclei (serotonergic neurons). The serotonergic neurons exert modulatory influences on their targets. The catecholaminergic neurons (locus coeruleus, tegmental noradrenergic and adrenergic groups) in several regions of the RF have widespread projections and exert mainly modulatory influences on their targets. The dopaminergic neurons of the midbrain are included in this illustration, although some experts question whether they are RF neurons.

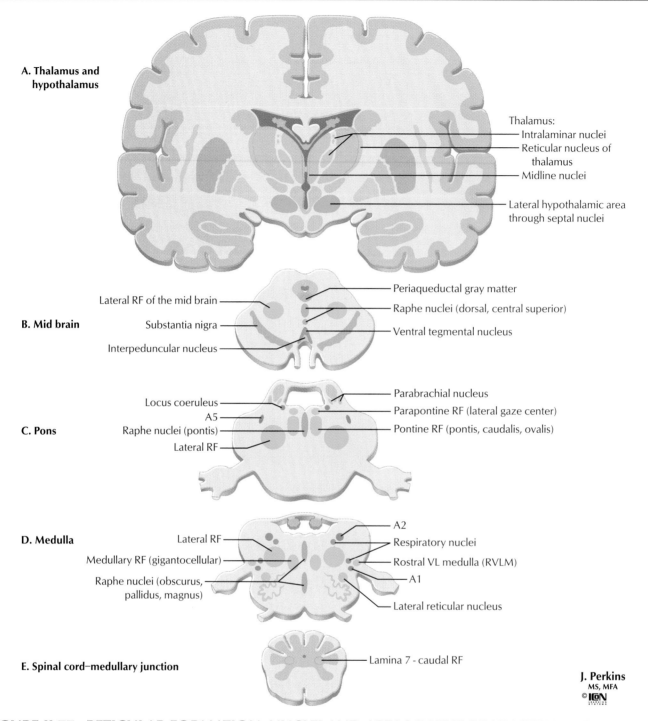

A. Thalamus and hypothalamus

Thalamus:
- Intralaminar nuclei
- Reticular nucleus of thalamus
- Midline nuclei

Lateral hypothalamic area through septal nuclei

B. Mid brain

- Lateral RF of the mid brain
- Substantia nigra
- Interpeduncular nucleus
- Periaqueductal gray matter
- Raphe nuclei (dorsal, central superior)
- Ventral tegmental nucleus

C. Pons

- Locus coeruleus
- A5
- Raphe nuclei (pontis)
- Lateral RF
- Parabrachial nucleus
- Parapontine RF (lateral gaze center)
- Pontine RF (pontis, caudalis, ovalis)

D. Medulla

- Lateral RF
- Medullary RF (gigantocellular)
- Raphe nuclei (obscurus, pallidus, magnus)
- A2
- Respiratory nuclei
- Rostral VL medulla (RVLM)
- A1
- Lateral reticular nucleus

E. Spinal cord–medullary junction

- Lamina 7 - caudal RF

J. Perkins
MS, MFA
© I©N

FIGURE II.77: RETICULAR FORMATION: NUCLEI AND AREAS IN THE BRAIN STEM AND DIENCEPHALON

Many of the named nuclei of the RF are present in the medulla, the pons, and the midbrain. Important medial RF groups include the medullary (giganto-cellular) and pontine (caudal and rostral) RF, which are involved in reticulospinal regulation of spinal cord LMNs; and the parapontine RF (PPRF), the horizontal (lateral) gaze center. Lateral RF areas and nuclei (such as the lateral reticular nucleus) are involved in polymodal sensory functions. RF respiratory and cardiovascular neurons are found in the medulla. Catecholaminergic neurons are found in the locus coeruleus and the tegmental groups. Raphe nuclei are found in the midline and in the wings of cells that extend laterally. The core of the RF continues rostrally from the lateral regions of the brain stem into the lateral hypothalamic area and extends through the hypothalamus to the septal nuclei. The intralaminar, midline, and reticular thalamic nuclei are classified as part of the RF.

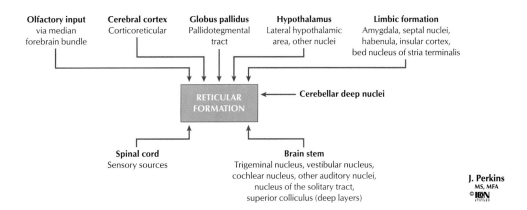

FIGURE II.78: MAJOR AFFERENT CONNECTIONS TO THE RETICULAR FORMATION

Extensive sensory information (particularly nociceptive) from spinal cord somatosensory sources and virtually all brain stem sensory modalities is sent to the lateral regions of the RF. Olfactory input arrives through olfactory tract projections into forebrain regions. Many limbic and hypothalamic structures provide input to the RF, particularly for visceral and autonomic regulatory functions. The cerebral cortex, the globus pallidus, and the cerebellum also provide input to the RF medial zones involved in motor regulation.

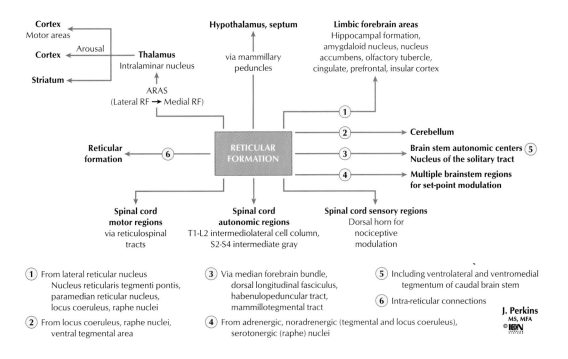

FIGURE II.79: MAJOR EFFERENT CONNECTIONS OF THE RETICULAR FORMATION

The ascending reticular activating system (ARAS) of the RF is responsible for consciousness and arousal. It projects through nonspecific nuclei of the thalamus to the cortex; lesions in this area lead to coma. The RF sends extensive axonal projections to sensory, motor, and autonomic regions of the spinal cord that modulate nociceptive input, preganglionic autonomic outflow, and LMN outflow, respectively. The RF sends extensive connections to brain stem nuclei (such as the nucleus tractus solitarius) and to autonomic regulatory centers and nuclei for modulation of visceral functions. Efferent RF projections to the hypothalamus, the septal nuclei, and the limbic forebrain areas help to modulate visceral autonomic functions, neuroendocrine outflow, and emotional responsiveness and behavior. Efferent RF projections to the cerebellum and the basal ganglia participate in modulating UMN control of LMNs.

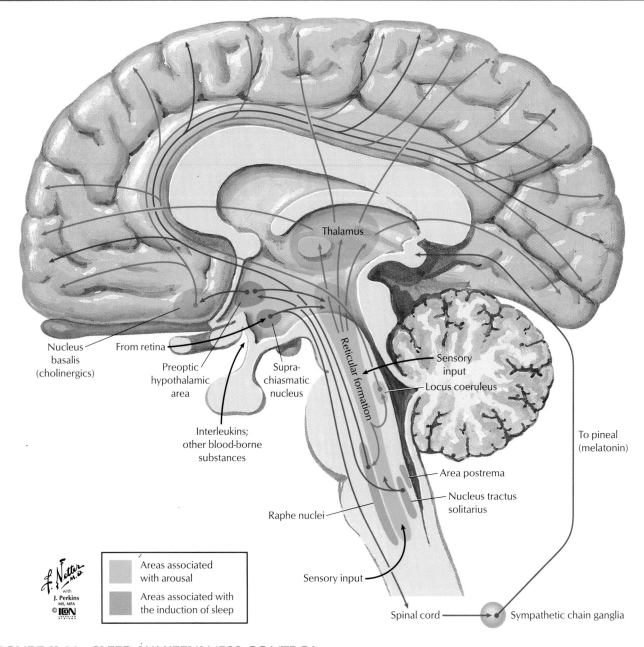

Nucleus basalis (cholinergics)

From retina

Preoptic hypothalamic area

Supra-chiasmatic nucleus

Thalamus

Reticular formation

Sensory input

Locus coeruleus

To pineal (melatonin)

Interleukins; other blood-borne substances

Area postrema

Nucleus tractus solitarius

Raphe nuclei

Sensory input

Areas associated with arousal

Areas associated with the induction of sleep

Spinal cord

Sympathetic chain ganglia

FIGURE II.80: SLEEP–WAKEFULNESS CONTROL

Sleep is a normal physiological state involving a cyclic temporary loss of consciousness; it is readily reversed by appropriate sensory stimuli. Sleep is an active process initiated by activity in several chemically specific collections of neurons of the brain: locus coeruleus of the pons (noradrenergic); raphe nuclei of the medulla and pons (serotonergic); nucleus solitarius of the medulla; cholinergic neurons of the brain stem tegmentum; lateral RF, particularly in the pons; anterior, posterior, and preoptic areas of the hypothalamus; and reticular nucleus of the thalamus. Many of these regions actively inhibit the lateral (sensory) portion of the RF, which is responsible for maintaining a waking state and consciousness. Circulating substances such as interleukin (IL)-1β can act on key sites in the hypothalamus and the brain stem to influence components of sleep. Illness behavior involves enhanced slow-wave sleep induced by IL-1β and other inflammatory mediators. Non-REM, or slow-wave, sleep, initiated by hypothalamic neurons and other regions, is accompanied by decreased activity of the locus coeruleus and the cholinergic tegmental neurons. During REM sleep, activity in the noradrenergic locus coeruleus neurons and the serotonergic raphe neurons diminishes, which prevents the cerebral cortex from attending to external stimuli. Dreams are likely the result of the cortex's attending to internal stimuli from stored memories.

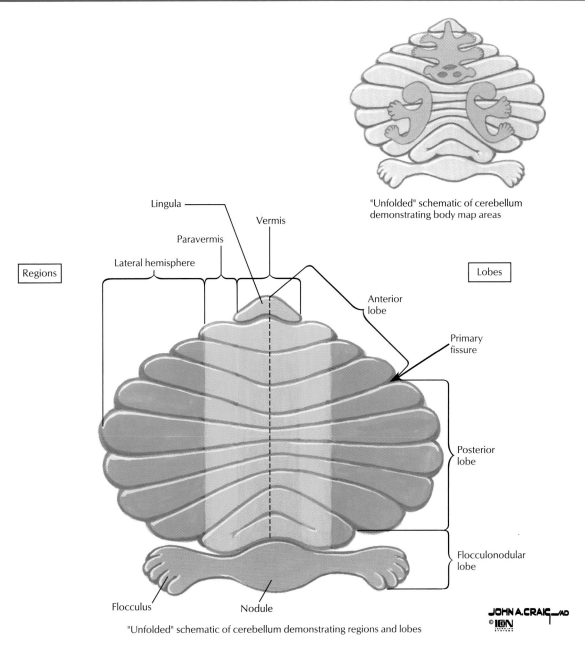

"Unfolded" schematic of cerebellum demonstrating body map areas

Lingula

Vermis

Paravermis

Lateral hemisphere

Regions

Lobes

Anterior lobe

Primary fissure

Posterior lobe

Flocculonodular lobe

Flocculus

Nodule

JOHN A.CRAIG—AD
© ICN

"Unfolded" schematic of cerebellum demonstrating regions and lobes

FIGURE II.81: CEREBELLAR ORGANIZATION: LOBES AND REGIONS

The cerebellum is organized anatomically into 3 major lobes: anterior, posterior, and flocculonodular. Distinct syndromes are associated with damage to each lobe. The functional organization of the cerebellum follows a vertical arrangement of hemispheres: (1) vermis (midline), (2) paravermis, and (3) lateral hemisphere. Each functional region is associated with specific deep nuclei (fastigial, globose and emboliform, and dentate, respectively) that help to regulate the activity of the reticulospinal and vestibulospinal tracts, the rubrospinal tract, and the corticospinal tract, respectively. At least 3 representations of the body are mapped onto the cerebellar cortex. The cerebellar cortex has multiple, orderly, small infoldings, or convolutions, called folia.

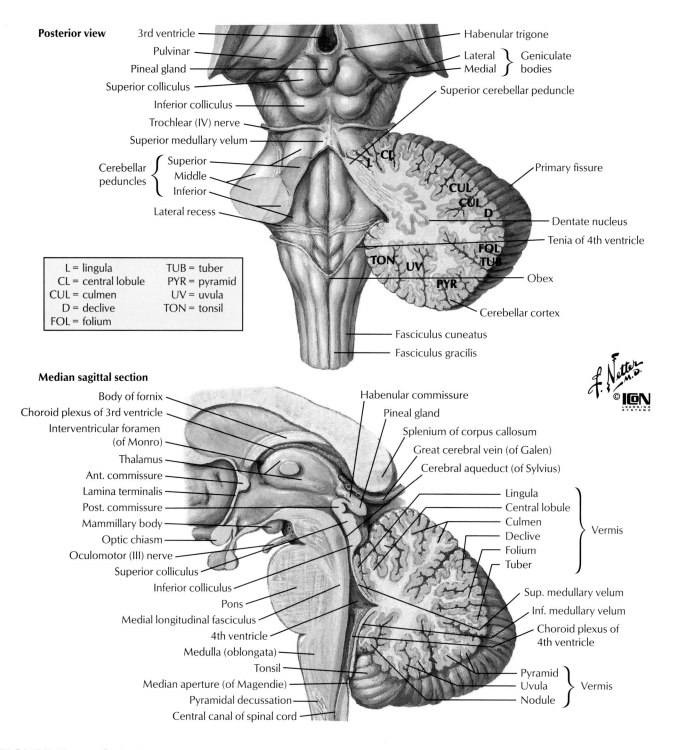

Posterior view

- 3rd ventricle
- Pulvinar
- Pineal gland
- Superior colliculus
- Inferior colliculus
- Trochlear (IV) nerve
- Superior medullary velum
- Cerebellar peduncles { Superior, Middle, Inferior }
- Lateral recess
- Habenular trigone
- Lateral / Medial } Geniculate bodies
- Superior cerebellar peduncle
- Primary fissure
- Dentate nucleus
- Tenia of 4th ventricle
- Obex
- Cerebellar cortex
- Fasciculus cuneatus
- Fasciculus gracilis

L = lingula
CL = central lobule
CUL = culmen
D = declive
FOL = folium
TUB = tuber
PYR = pyramid
UV = uvula
TON = tonsil

Median sagittal section

- Body of fornix
- Choroid plexus of 3rd ventricle
- Interventricular foramen (of Monro)
- Thalamus
- Ant. commissure
- Lamina terminalis
- Post. commissure
- Mammillary body
- Optic chiasm
- Oculomotor (III) nerve
- Superior colliculus
- Inferior colliculus
- Pons
- Medial longitudinal fasciculus
- 4th ventricle
- Medulla (oblongata)
- Tonsil
- Median aperture (of Magendie)
- Pyramidal decussation
- Central canal of spinal cord
- Habenular commissure
- Pineal gland
- Splenium of corpus callosum
- Great cerebral vein (of Galen)
- Cerebral aqueduct (of Sylvius)
- Lingula
- Central lobule
- Culmen
- Declive
- Folium
- Tuber } Vermis
- Sup. medullary velum
- Inf. medullary velum
- Choroid plexus of 4th ventricle
- Pyramid
- Uvula
- Nodule } Vermis

FIGURE II.82: CEREBELLAR ANATOMY: LOBULES

The 10 lobules of the cerebellar cortex are seen in both midline and cross-sectional views. Inputs to the 3 layers of the cerebellar cortex arrive mainly as mossy fibers; the inferior olivary nucleus sends climbing fibers to end on Purkinje cell dendrites, and the locus coeruleus sends diffuse varicose inputs to many regions of the cerebellar cortex. The deep nuclei provide the "coarse adjustment" upon which is superimposed the "fine adjustment" from the cerebellar cortex. The cerebellar cortex sends its output via inhibitory Purkinje cell projections (using GABA) to deep nuclei, which in turn project to UMNs. Afferents and efferents pass through the cerebellar peduncles, which connect the cerebellum with the brain stem and the diencephalon. The table lists the major afferent and efferent projections through the 3 cerebellar peduncles.

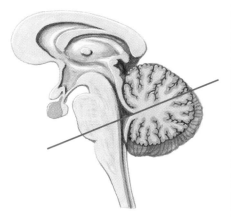

Level of section

Peduncle	Input (afferents)	Output (efferents)	
Inferior (restiform body)	Spinocerebellar Dorsal Rostral Cuneocerebellar Olive-cerebellar Reticulocerebellar Trigeminocerebellar Raphe-cerebellar	Fastigiobulbar, Uncinate fasciculus	To vestibular and reticular nuclei
		Direct cerebellovestibular (to LVN)	
Juxtarestiform body	Vestibulospinal (primary, secondary)		
Middle (brachium pontis)	Pontocerebellar		
Superior (brachium conjunctivum)	Ventral spinocerebellar Trigeminocerebellar Tectocerebellar Superior colliculus Inferior colliculus Coeruleo-cerebellar	Dentatothalamic Dentatorubral Dentatoreticular Interpositus-rubral connections (globose, emboliform)	

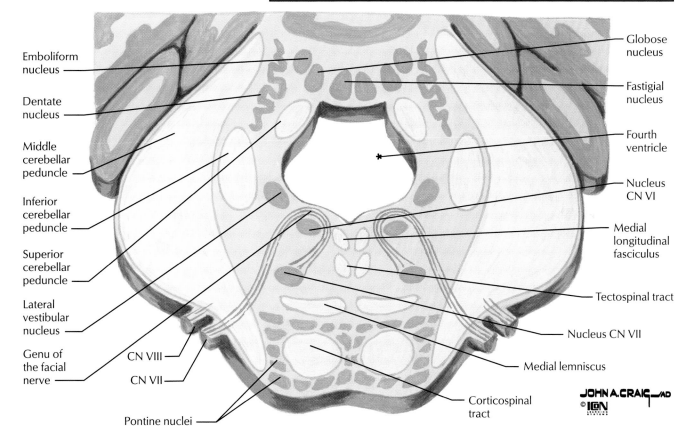

Emboliform nucleus

Dentate nucleus

Middle cerebellar peduncle

Inferior cerebellar peduncle

Superior cerebellar peduncle

Lateral vestibular nucleus

Genu of the facial nerve

CN VIII

CN VII

Pontine nuclei

Globose nucleus

Fastigial nucleus

Fourth ventricle

Nucleus CN VI

Medial longitudinal fasciculus

Tectospinal tract

Nucleus CN VII

Medial lemniscus

Corticospinal tract

JOHN A. CRAIG—AD
© ICN

FIGURE II.83: CEREBELLAR ANATOMY: DEEP NUCLEI AND CEREBELLAR PEDUNCLES

The deep cerebellar nuclei are found at the roof of the fourth ventricle in a cross-sectional view of the pons at the level of cranial motor nuclei for CNs VI and VII. The fastigial nucleus receives input from the vermis and sends projections to reticular and vestibular nuclei, the cells of origin for the reticulospinal and vestibulospinal tracts. Some vermal and flocculonodular Purkinje cells project directly to the lateral vestibular nuclei, which some authors consider a fifth deep cerebellar nucleus. The globose and emboliform nuclei receive input from the paravermis and project to the red nucleus (rubrospinal tract). The dentate nucleus receives input from the lateral hemispheres and projects to the ventrolateral and ventral anterior nuclei of the thalamus, which then project to the cells of origin for the corticospinal and corticobulbar tracts. The 3 cerebellar peduncles are seen in this cross section.

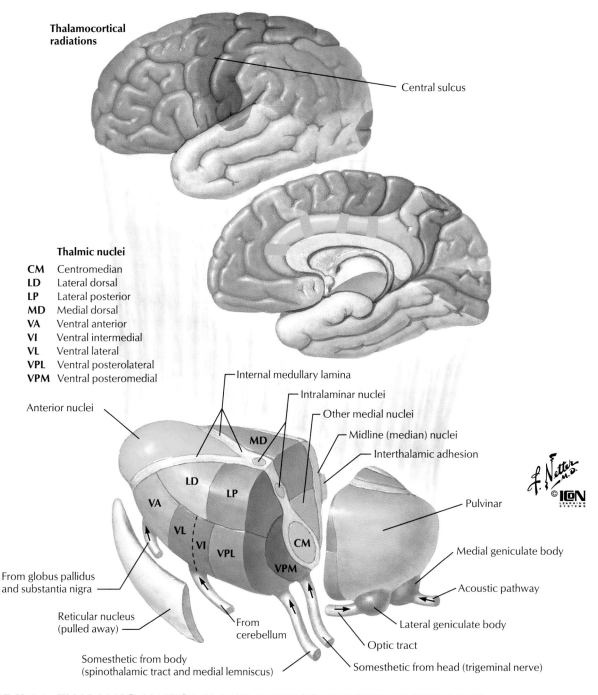

Thalamocortical radiations

Central sulcus

Thalamic nuclei

CM	Centromedian
LD	Lateral dorsal
LP	Lateral posterior
MD	Medial dorsal
VA	Ventral anterior
VI	Ventral intermedial
VL	Ventral lateral
VPL	Ventral posterolateral
VPM	Ventral posteromedial

Internal medullary lamina

Intralaminar nuclei

Other medial nuclei

Midline (median) nuclei

Interthalamic adhesion

Anterior nuclei

MD

LD

LP

VA

VL

VI VPL

CM

VPM

Pulvinar

Medial geniculate body

Acoustic pathway

Lateral geniculate body

Optic tract

From globus pallidus and substantia nigra

Reticular nucleus (pulled away)

From cerebellum

Somesthetic from body (spinothalamic tract and medial lemniscus)

Somesthetic from head (trigeminal nerve)

FIGURE II.84: THALAMIC ANATOMY AND INTERCONNECTIONS WITH THE CEREBRAL CORTEX

The thalamus conveys extensive sensory, motor, and autonomic information from the brain stem and the spinal cord to the cortex. Thalamic nuclei are reciprocally interconnected with regions of the cortex. Specific thalamic nuclei project to circumscribed regions of the cortex; these nuclei include (1) sensory projection nuclei (VPL—somatosensory; VPM—trigeminal; lateral geniculate body—visual; medial geniculate body—auditory), (2) motor-related nuclei (VL and VI—cerebellum; VA and VL—basal ganglia), (3) autonomic and limbic-related nuclei (anterior and LD—cingulate cortex; MD—frontal and cingulate cortices), and (4) nuclei related to association areas and LP—parietal cortex. Nonspecific thalamic nuclei (intralaminar nuclei [CM, parafascicular] and medial VA) send diffuse connections to widespread regions of the cerebral cortex and to other thalamic nuclei. The reticular nucleus of the thalamus helps to regulate the excitability of thalamic projection nuclei. Some thalamic lesions can lead to excruciating neuropathic pain, referred to as thalamic syndrome.

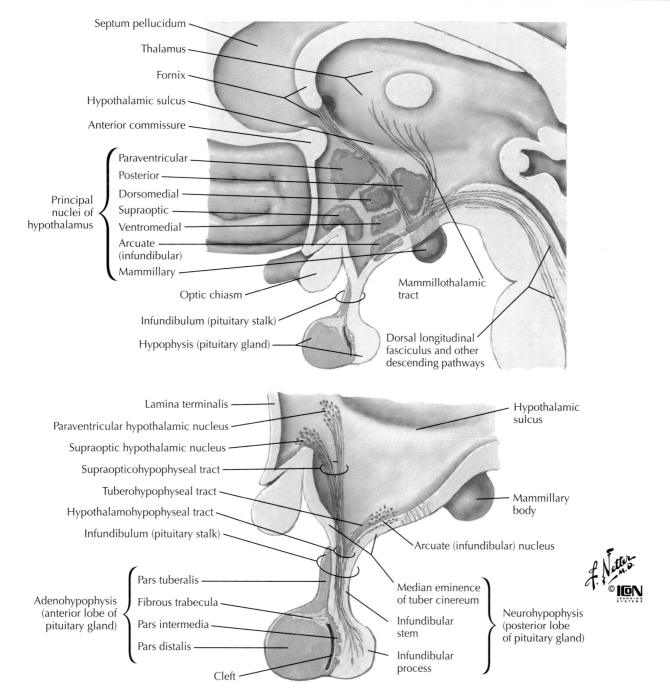

Septum pellucidum
Thalamus
Fornix
Hypothalamic sulcus
Anterior commissure

Principal nuclei of hypothalamus
- Paraventricular
- Posterior
- Dorsomedial
- Supraoptic
- Ventromedial
- Arcuate (infundibular)
- Mammillary

Optic chiasm
Infundibulum (pituitary stalk)
Hypophysis (pituitary gland)

Mammillothalamic tract
Dorsal longitudinal fasciculus and other descending pathways

Lamina terminalis
Paraventricular hypothalamic nucleus
Supraoptic hypothalamic nucleus
Supraopticohypophyseal tract
Tuberohypophyseal tract
Hypothalamohypophyseal tract
Infundibulum (pituitary stalk)

Adenohypophysis (anterior lobe of pituitary gland)
- Pars tuberalis
- Fibrous trabecula
- Pars intermedia
- Pars distalis

Cleft

Hypothalamic sulcus
Mammillary body
Arcuate (infundibular) nucleus

Median eminence of tuber cinereum
Infundibular stem
Infundibular process

Neurohypophysis (posterior lobe of pituitary gland)

FIGURE II.85: THE HYPOTHALAMUS AND THE PITUITARY GLAND

The hypothalamus is the major region of the CNS involved in neuroendocrine regulation and control of visceral functions, such as temperature regulation, food and appetite regulation, thirst and water balance, reproduction and sexual behavior, parturition and control of lactation, respiratory and cardiovascular regulation, gastrointestinal regulation, stress responses, and reparative states. It is subdivided into rostral-to-caudal zones (preoptic, anterior or supraoptic, tuberal, and mammillary or posterior) as well as medial-to-lateral zones (periventricular, medial, lateral). These zones contain some discrete nuclei and more diffuse "centers" or areas. The neuroendocrine portion of the hypothalamus consists of (1) magnocellular portions of the paraventricular nucleus (PVN) and the supraoptic nucleus (SON), which send axons directly to the posterior pituitary, (2) releasing-factor and inhibitory-factor neurons, which project axons to the hypophyseal portal vasculature in the median eminence, and (3) the tuberoinfundibular system.

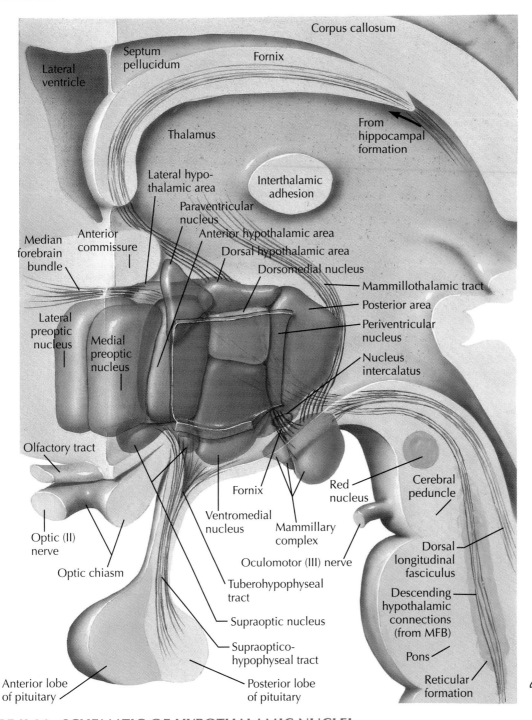

Corpus callosum

Septum pellucidum

Fornix

Lateral ventricle

Thalamus

From hippocampal formation

Lateral hypo-thalamic area

Interthalamic adhesion

Paraventricular nucleus

Anterior hypothalamic area

Median forebrain bundle

Anterior commissure

Dorsal hypothalamic area

Dorsomedial nucleus

Mammillothalamic tract

Posterior area

Periventricular nucleus

Lateral preoptic nucleus

Medial preoptic nucleus

Nucleus intercalatus

Olfactory tract

Fornix

Red nucleus

Cerebral peduncle

Optic (II) nerve

Ventromedial nucleus

Mammillary complex

Dorsal longitudinal fasciculus

Optic chiasm

Oculomotor (III) nerve

Descending hypothalamic connections (from MFB)

Tuberohypophyseal tract

Supraoptic nucleus

Pons

Supraoptico-hypophyseal tract

Reticular formation

Anterior lobe of pituitary

Posterior lobe of pituitary

FIGURE II.86: SCHEMATIC OF HYPOTHALAMIC NUCLEI

Hypothalamic nuclei and areas are associated with visceral and neuroendocrine functions. The magnocellular neurons supraoptic nucleus of the SON and PVN release oxytocin and vasopressin into the posterior pituitary general circulation. PVN parvocellular neurons containing CRH project to the hypophyseal portal system in the median eminence and induce the release of ACTH. Descending axons of the PVN project to brain stem and spinal cord preganglionic neurons and related nuclei to regulate outflow from the ANS. The anterior and posterior areas coordinate parasympathetic and sympathetic outflow, respectively. Nuclei DM and VM, and the lateral hypothalamic area regulate appetitive, drinking, and reproductive behavior. The preoptic area regulates cyclic neuroendocrine behavior and thermoregulation. The suprachiasmatic nucleus receives visual inputs from the optic tract and regulates circadian rhythms. Several hypothalamic regions are involved in the regulation of sleep.

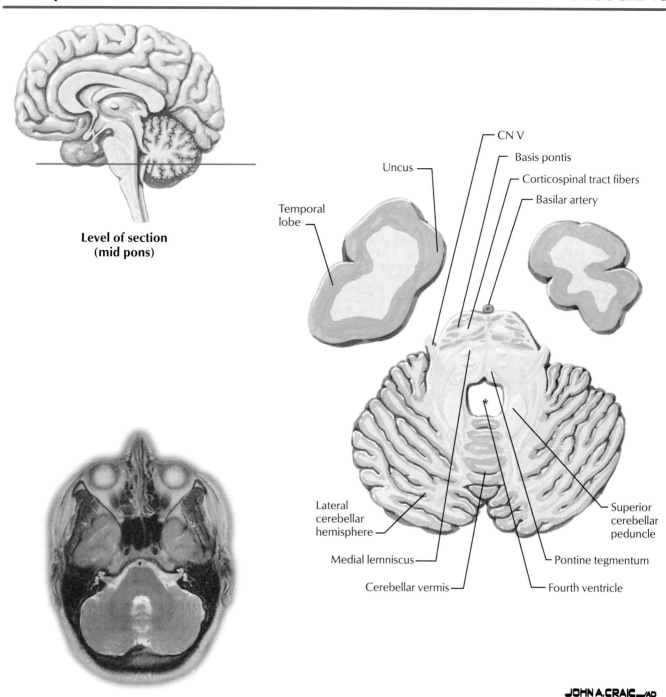

**Level of section
(mid pons)**

CN V
Uncus
Basis pontis
Corticospinal tract fibers
Temporal lobe
Basilar artery

Lateral cerebellar hemisphere
Superior cerebellar peduncle
Medial lemniscus
Pontine tegmentum
Cerebellar vermis
Fourth ventricle

JOHN A. CRAIG—AD
© ICN

FIGURE II.87: HORIZONTAL SECTIONS THROUGH THE FOREBRAIN

These plates compare anatomical sections, MR images, and CT scans. These are cut in the true horizontal plane, not in the older, 25° tilt. The most important anatomical relationships in these sections center around the internal capsule (IC). The head of the caudate nucleus, medial to the anterior limb of the IC, forms the lateral margin of the frontal pole of the lateral ventricle. The thalamus is medial to the posterior limb of the IC. The globus pallidus and the putamen are lateral to the wedge-shaped IC. The posterior limb carries the major descending corticospinal, corticorubral, and corticoreticular fibers, and the ascending sensory fibers for the somatosensory and trigeminal systems. The most posterior portions also carry the auditory and visual projections to their cortices. The genu carries the corticobulbar fibers. The anterior limb carries cortical projections to the striatum and the pontine nuclei (pontocerebellar system). The MR images for the horizontal sections are T2-weighted, with high signal intensity, so the ventricles (cerebrospinal fluid) appear bright.

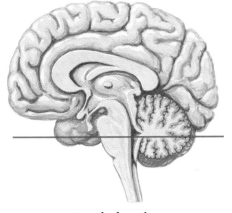

**Level of section
(rostral pons)**

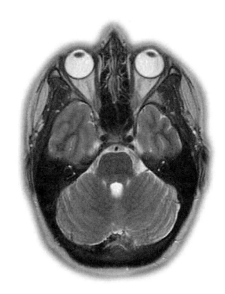

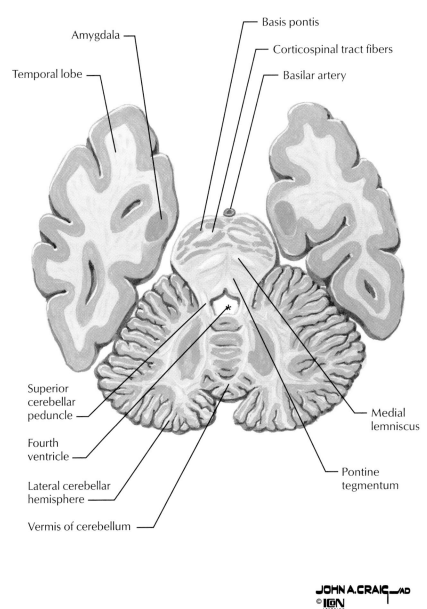

Amygdala

Temporal lobe

Basis pontis

Corticospinal tract fibers

Basilar artery

Superior
cerebellar
peduncle

Fourth
ventricle

Lateral cerebellar
hemisphere

Vermis of cerebellum

Medial
lemniscus

Pontine
tegmentum

JOHN A. CRAIG —AD
©I©N

Rostral Pons

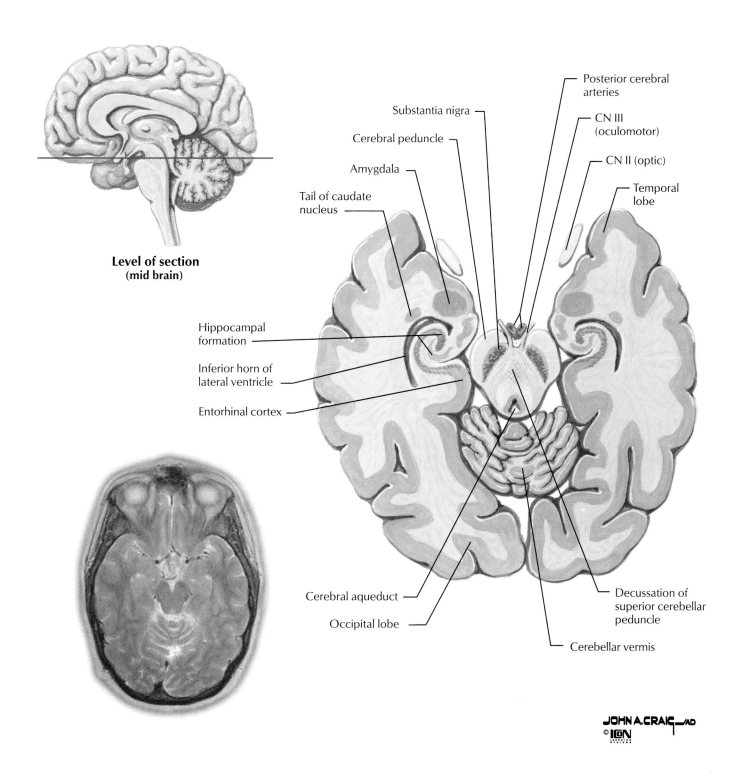

Level of section
(mid brain)

Substantia nigra

Cerebral peduncle

Amygdala

Tail of caudate
nucleus

Hippocampal
formation

Inferior horn of
lateral ventricle

Entorhinal cortex

Posterior cerebral
arteries

CN III
(oculomotor)

CN II (optic)

Temporal
lobe

Cerebral aqueduct

Occipital lobe

Decussation of
superior cerebellar
peduncle

Cerebellar vermis

JOHN A.CRAIG—AD
© ICN

Midbrain

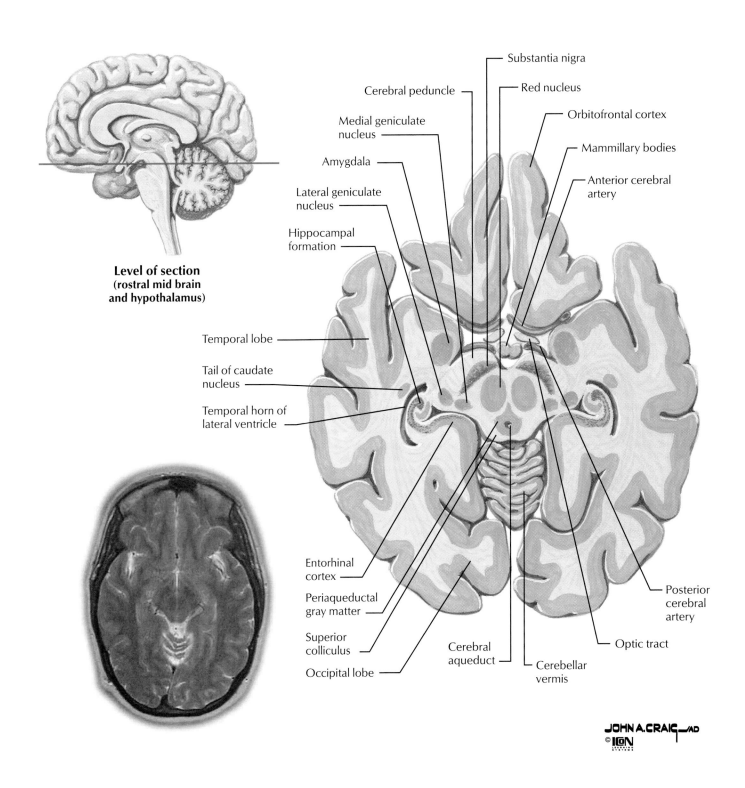

Level of section
(rostral mid brain
and hypothalamus)

Substantia nigra

Cerebral peduncle

Red nucleus

Medial geniculate
nucleus

Orbitofrontal cortex

Amygdala

Mammillary bodies

Lateral geniculate
nucleus

Anterior cerebral
artery

Hippocampal
formation

Temporal lobe

Tail of caudate
nucleus

Temporal horn of
lateral ventricle

Entorhinal
cortex

Periaqueductal
gray matter

Posterior
cerebral
artery

Superior
colliculus

Optic tract

Occipital lobe

Cerebral
aqueduct

Cerebellar
vermis

Rostral Midbrain and Hypothalamus

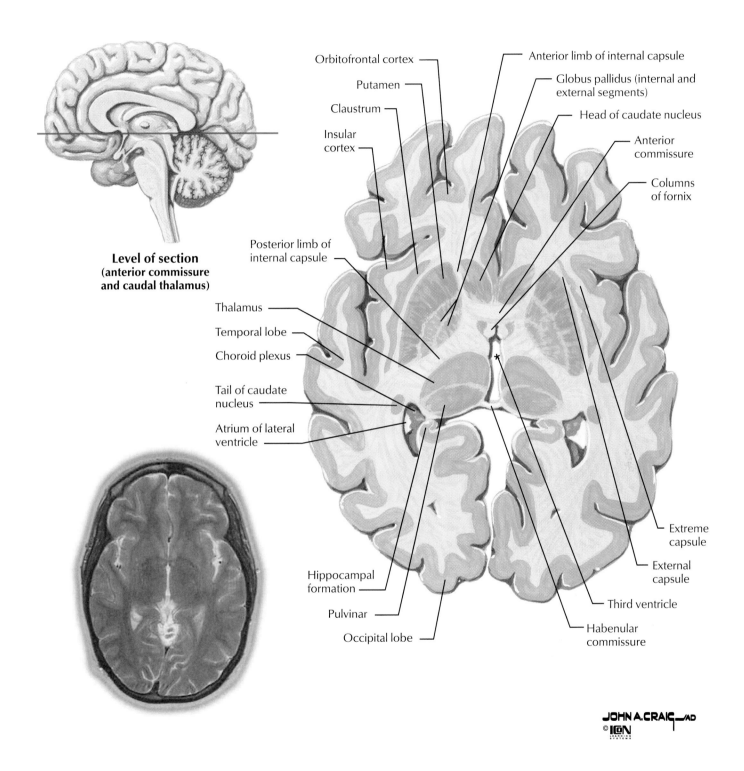

Level of section
(anterior commissure
and caudal thalamus)

Orbitofrontal cortex

Putamen

Claustrum

Insular cortex

Posterior limb of internal capsule

Thalamus

Temporal lobe

Choroid plexus

Tail of caudate nucleus

Atrium of lateral ventricle

Hippocampal formation

Pulvinar

Occipital lobe

Anterior limb of internal capsule

Globus pallidus (internal and external segments)

Head of caudate nucleus

Anterior commissure

Columns of fornix

Extreme capsule

External capsule

Third ventricle

Habenular commissure

JOHN A. CRAIG—AD
© ICN

Anterior Commissure and Caudal Thalamus

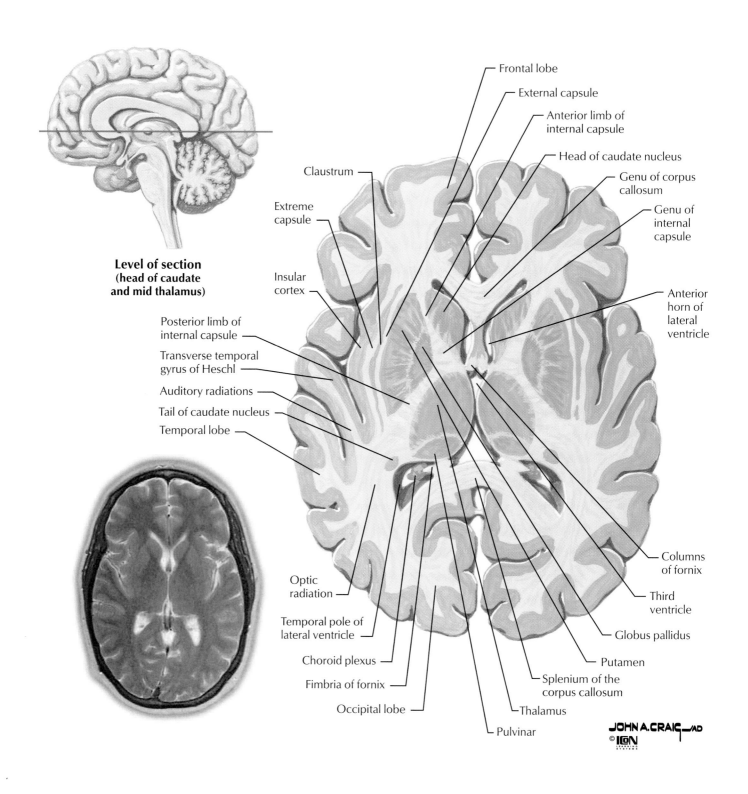

Level of section
(head of caudate
and mid thalamus)

Frontal lobe

External capsule

Anterior limb of
internal capsule

Head of caudate nucleus

Genu of corpus
callosum

Genu of
internal
capsule

Claustrum

Extreme
capsule

Insular
cortex

Anterior
horn of
lateral
ventricle

Posterior limb of
internal capsule

Transverse temporal
gyrus of Heschl

Auditory radiations

Tail of caudate nucleus

Temporal lobe

Columns
of fornix

Third
ventricle

Optic
radiation

Globus pallidus

Temporal pole of
lateral ventricle

Putamen

Choroid plexus

Splenium of the
corpus callosum

Fimbria of fornix

Occipital lobe

Thalamus

Pulvinar

JOHN A. CRAIG—AD
© ICN

Head of Caudate and Midthalamus

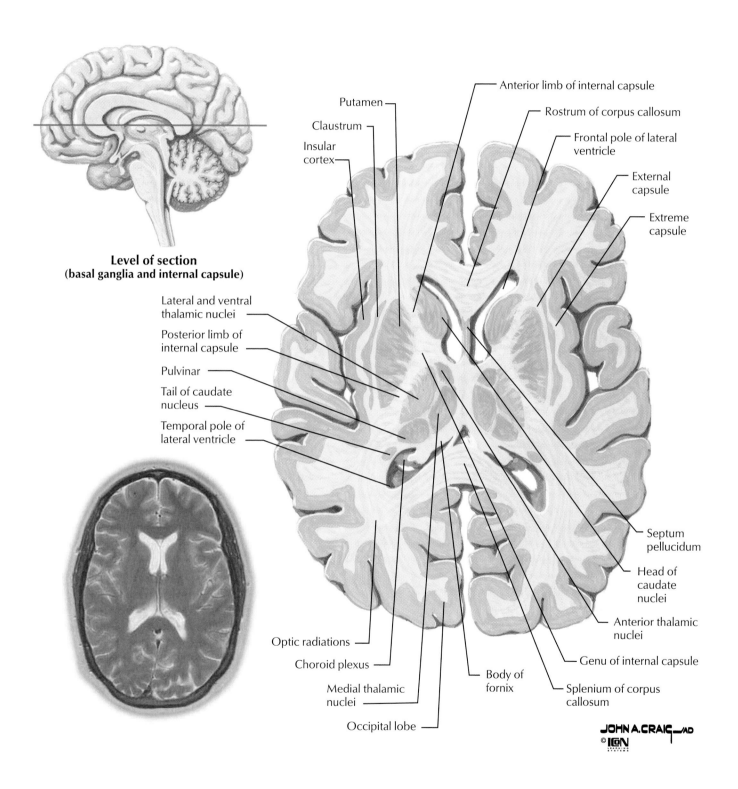

Level of section
(basal ganglia and internal capsule)

Putamen

Claustrum

Insular
cortex

Anterior limb of internal capsule

Rostrum of corpus callosum

Frontal pole of lateral
ventricle

External
capsule

Extreme
capsule

Lateral and ventral
thalamic nuclei

Posterior limb of
internal capsule

Pulvinar

Tail of caudate
nucleus

Temporal pole of
lateral ventricle

Septum
pellucidum

Head of
caudate
nuclei

Anterior thalamic
nuclei

Optic radiations

Choroid plexus

Medial thalamic
nuclei

Occipital lobe

Body of
fornix

Genu of internal capsule

Splenium of corpus
callosum

JOHN A. CRAIG—AD
© ICN

Basal Ganglia and Internal Capsule

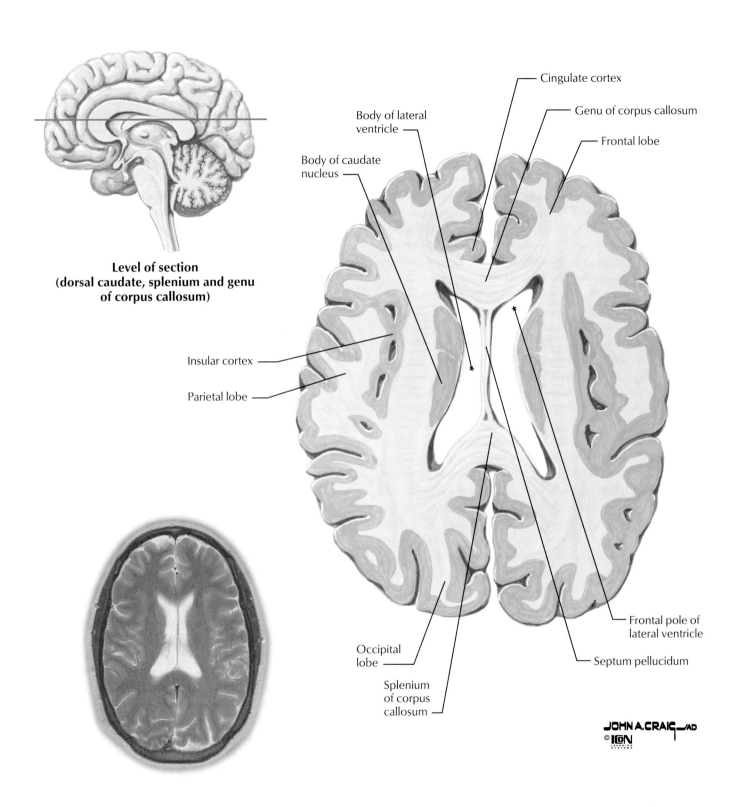

Level of section
(dorsal caudate, splenium and genu
of corpus callosum)

Cingulate cortex

Genu of corpus callosum

Frontal lobe

Body of lateral
ventricle

Body of caudate
nucleus

Insular cortex

Parietal lobe

Frontal pole of
lateral ventricle

Septum pellucidum

Occipital
lobe

Splenium
of corpus
callosum

JOHN A.CRAIG AD
© ICON
LEARNING SYSTEMS

Dorsal Caudate, Splenium, and Genu of Corpus Callosum

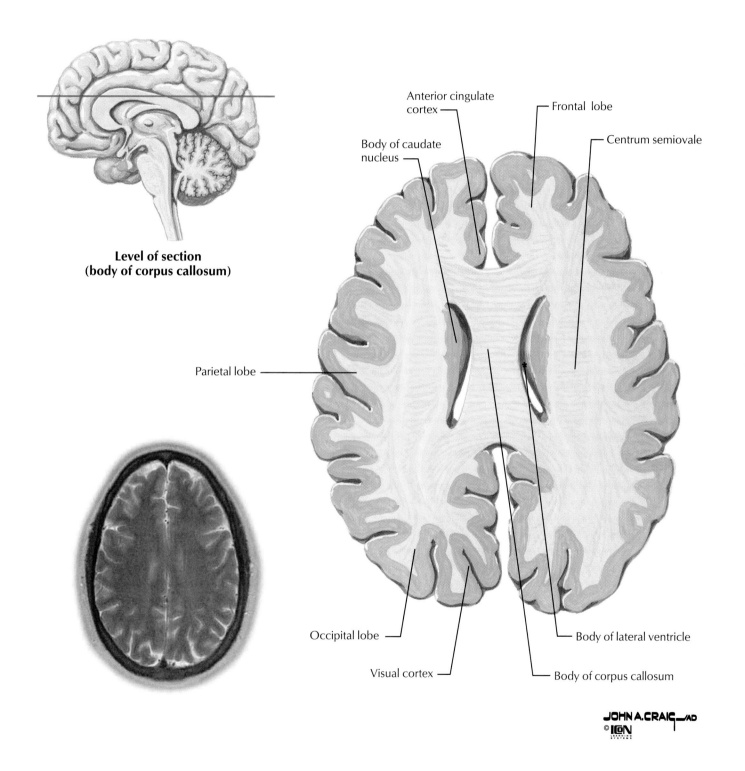

**Level of section
(body of corpus callosum)**

Anterior cingulate cortex

Frontal lobe

Body of caudate nucleus

Centrum semiovale

Parietal lobe

Occipital lobe

Body of lateral ventricle

Visual cortex

Body of corpus callosum

JOHN A. CRAIG—AD

©ICN

Body of Corpus Callosum

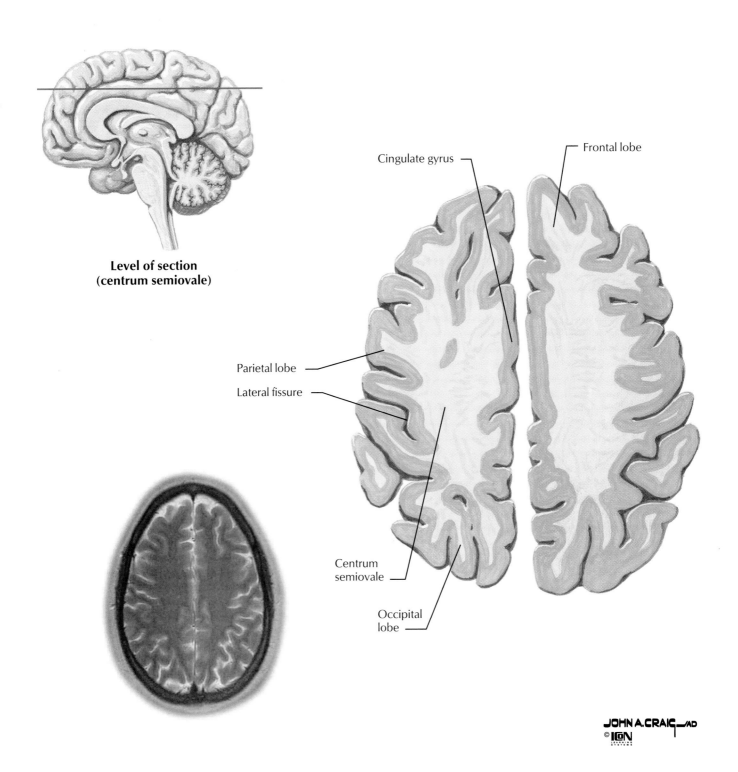

**Level of section
(centrum semiovale)**

Cingulate gyrus

Frontal lobe

Parietal lobe

Lateral fissure

Centrum
semiovale

Occipital
lobe

JOHN A.CRAIG—AD
©ICN

Centrum Semiovale

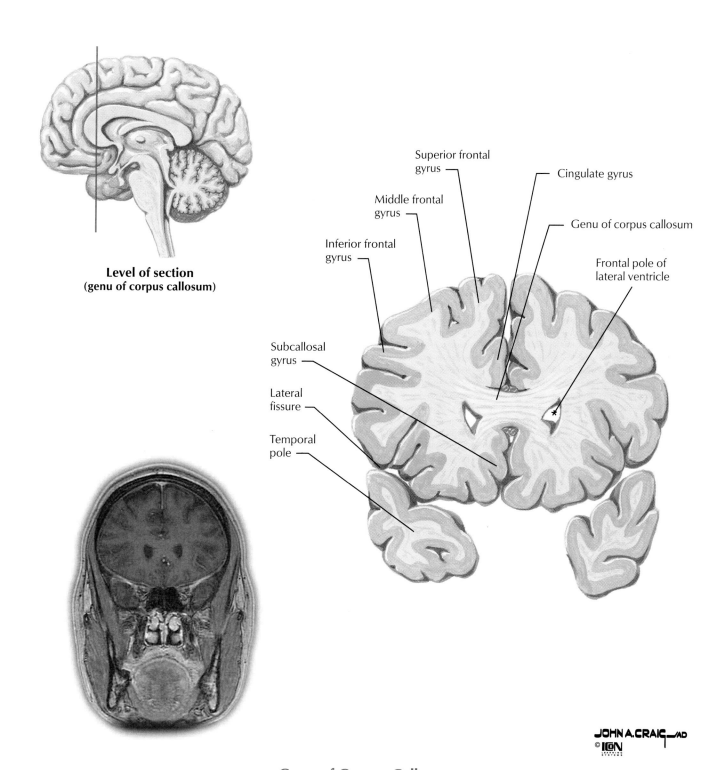

Level of section
(genu of corpus callosum)

Superior frontal gyrus

Cingulate gyrus

Middle frontal gyrus

Genu of corpus callosum

Inferior frontal gyrus

Frontal pole of lateral ventricle

Subcallosal gyrus

Lateral fissure

Temporal pole

JOHN A. CRAIG, AD
© ICN

Genu of Corpus Callosum

FIGURE II.88: CORONAL SECTIONS THROUGH THE FOREBRAIN

These plates compare coronal anatomical sections and MR images. They show important relationships of the IC, the basal ganglia, and the thalamus. Basal forebrain structures (such as the nucleus accumbens, the substantia innominata, and the nucleus basalis), thalamic nuclei, and the important temporal lobe structures (amygdaloid nuclei, hippocampal formation) and pathways (fornix, stria terminalis) are illustrated. The MR images for the coronal sections are T2-weighted, with a reversal technique (FLAIR) that results in the ventricles (cerebrospinal fluid) appearing dark.

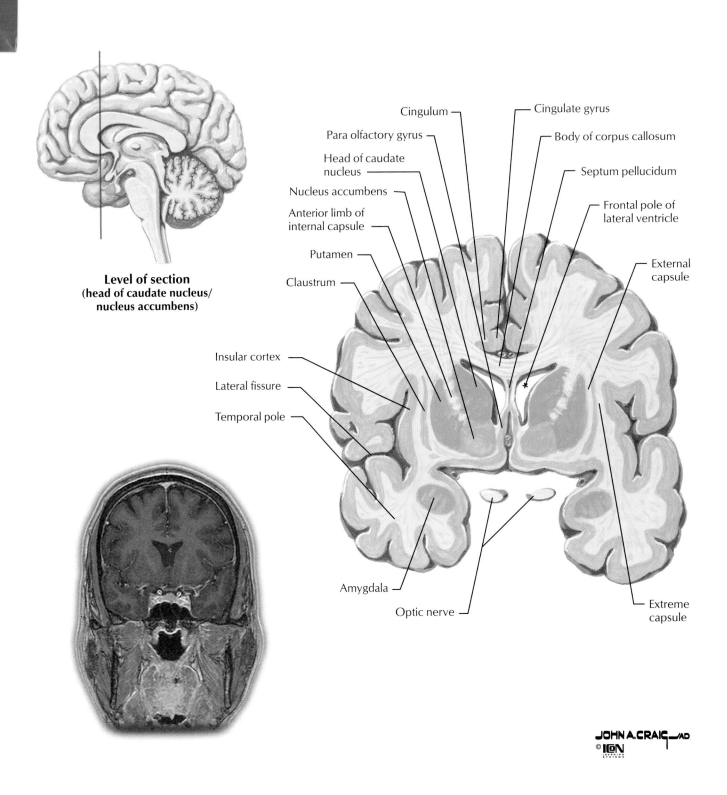

Level of section
(head of caudate nucleus/
nucleus accumbens)

Cingulum

Cingulate gyrus

Para olfactory gyrus

Body of corpus callosum

Head of caudate nucleus

Septum pellucidum

Nucleus accumbens

Frontal pole of lateral ventricle

Anterior limb of internal capsule

External capsule

Putamen

Claustrum

Insular cortex

Lateral fissure

Temporal pole

Amygdala

Optic nerve

Extreme capsule

JOHN A. CRAIG—AD
© ICN

Head of Caudate Nucleus/Nucleus Accumbens

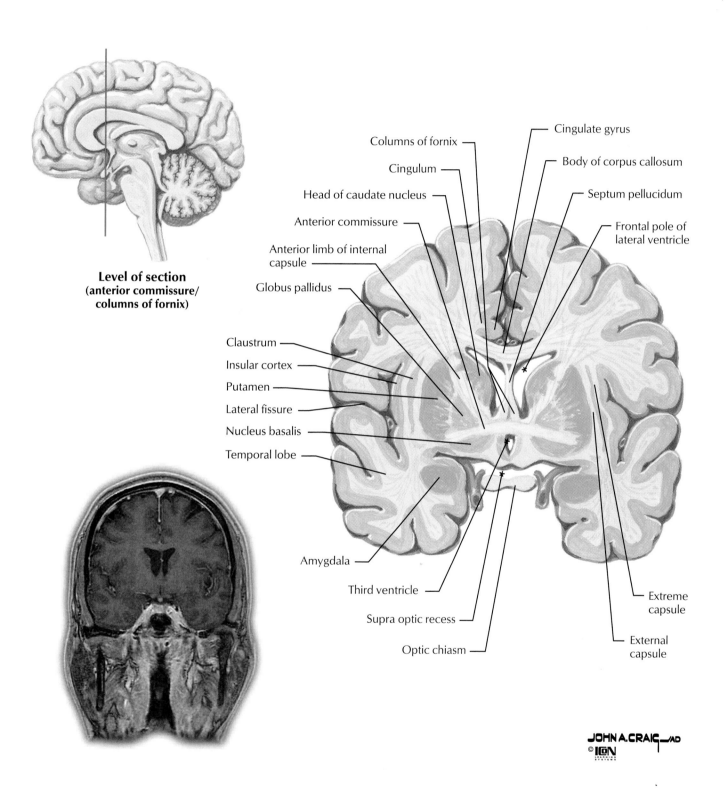

Level of section
(anterior commissure/
columns of fornix)

Columns of fornix

Cingulate gyrus

Cingulum

Body of corpus callosum

Head of caudate nucleus

Septum pellucidum

Anterior commissure

Frontal pole of
lateral ventricle

Anterior limb of internal
capsule

Globus pallidus

Claustrum

Insular cortex

Putamen

Lateral fissure

Nucleus basalis

Temporal lobe

Amygdala

Third ventricle

Supra optic recess

Optic chiasm

Extreme
capsule

External
capsule

JOHN A. CRAIG—AD
© ICN

Anterior Commissure/Columns of Fornix

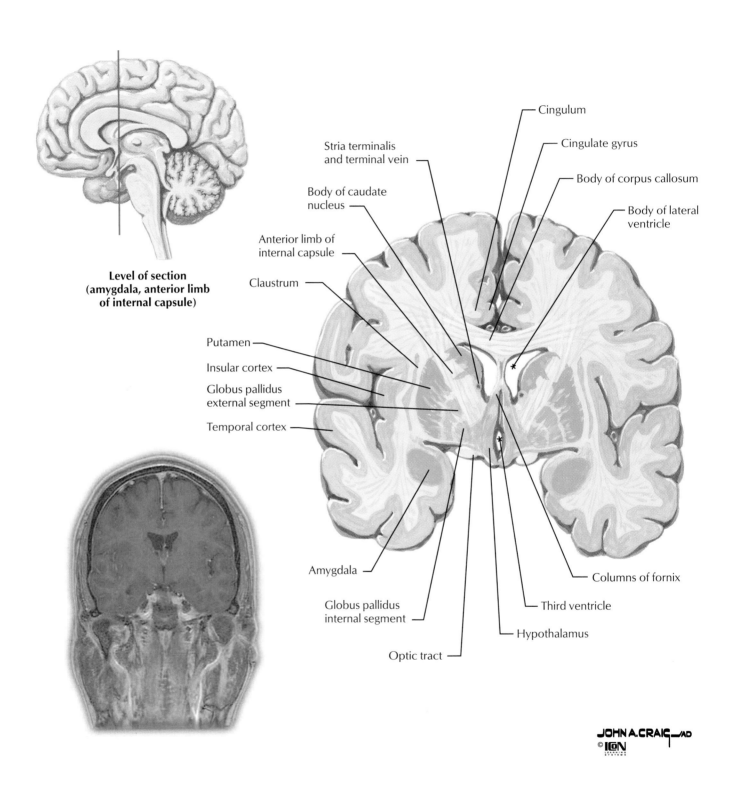

Level of section
(amygdala, anterior limb
of internal capsule)

Stria terminalis
and terminal vein

Body of caudate
nucleus

Anterior limb of
internal capsule

Claustrum

Putamen

Insular cortex

Globus pallidus
external segment

Temporal cortex

Amygdala

Globus pallidus
internal segment

Optic tract

Cingulum

Cingulate gyrus

Body of corpus callosum

Body of lateral
ventricle

Columns of fornix

Third ventricle

Hypothalamus

JOHN A. CRAIG MD
© ICN
LEARNING
SYSTEMS

Amygdala, Anterior Limb of Internal Capsule

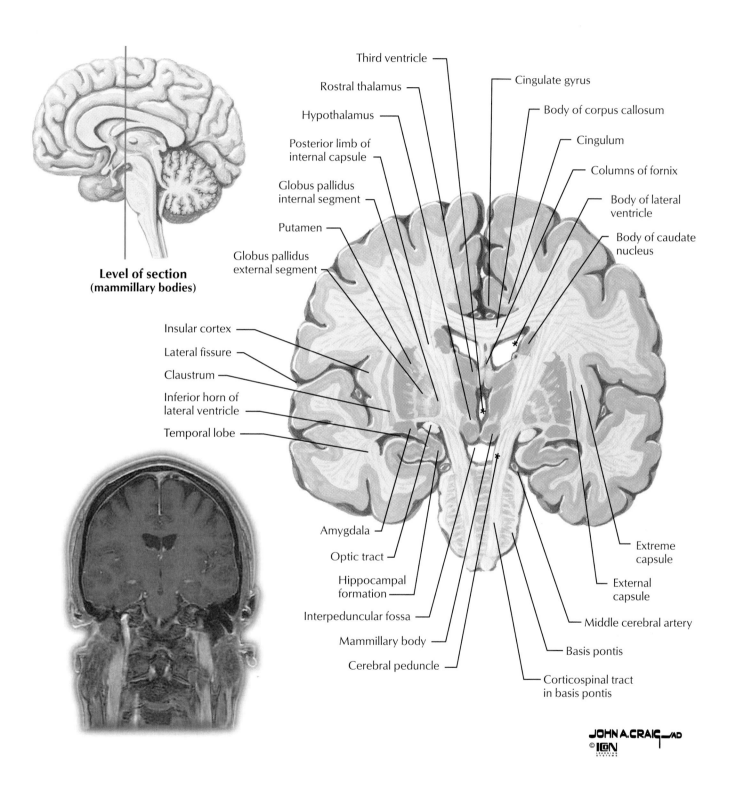

Level of section
(mammillary bodies)

Third ventricle

Rostral thalamus

Hypothalamus

Posterior limb of
internal capsule

Globus pallidus
internal segment

Putamen

Globus pallidus
external segment

Insular cortex

Lateral fissure

Claustrum

Inferior horn of
lateral ventricle

Temporal lobe

Amygdala

Optic tract

Hippocampal
formation

Interpeduncular fossa

Mammillary body

Cerebral peduncle

Cingulate gyrus

Body of corpus callosum

Cingulum

Columns of fornix

Body of lateral
ventricle

Body of caudate
nucleus

Extreme
capsule

External
capsule

Middle cerebral artery

Basis pontis

Corticospinal tract
in basis pontis

JOHN A.CRAIG AD
© ICN

Mammillary Bodies

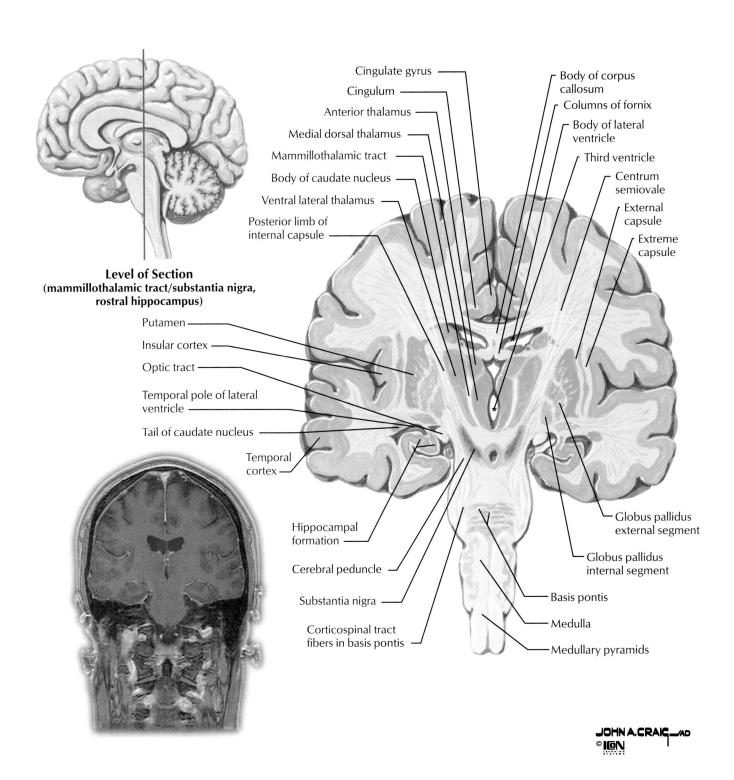

Level of Section
(mammillothalamic tract/substantia nigra,
rostral hippocampus)

Cingulate gyrus

Cingulum

Anterior thalamus

Medial dorsal thalamus

Mammillothalamic tract

Body of caudate nucleus

Ventral lateral thalamus

Posterior limb of
internal capsule

Body of corpus
callosum

Columns of fornix

Body of lateral
ventricle

Third ventricle

Centrum
semiovale

External
capsule

Extreme
capsule

Putamen

Insular cortex

Optic tract

Temporal pole of lateral
ventricle

Tail of caudate nucleus

Temporal
cortex

Hippocampal
formation

Cerebral peduncle

Substantia nigra

Corticospinal tract
fibers in basis pontis

Globus pallidus
external segment

Globus pallidus
internal segment

Basis pontis

Medulla

Medullary pyramids

JOHN A. CRAIG—MD
©ICON

Mammillothalamic Tract/Substantia Nigra, Rostral Hippocampus

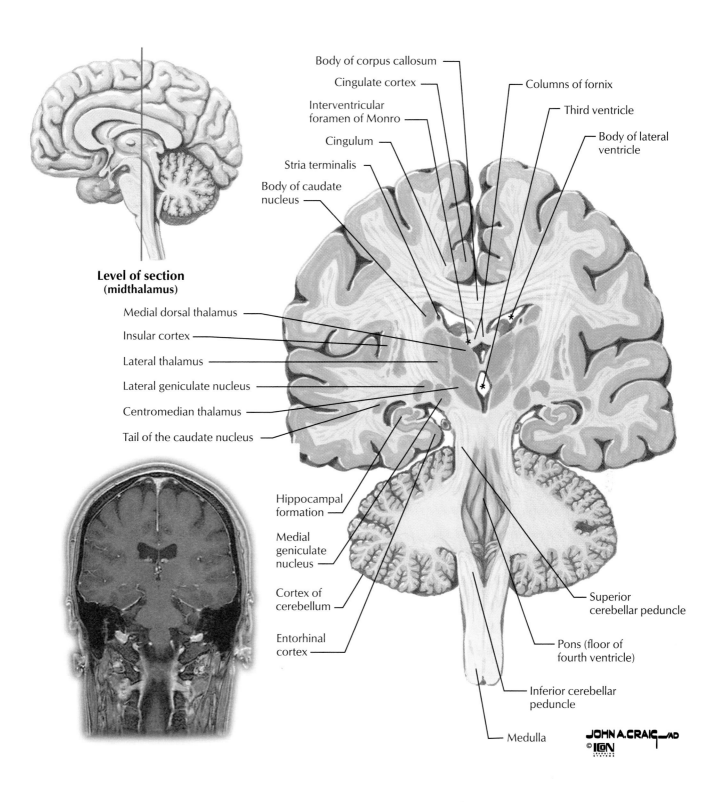

Level of section
(midthalamus)

Body of corpus callosum

Cingulate cortex

Columns of fornix

Interventricular foramen of Monro

Third ventricle

Cingulum

Body of lateral ventricle

Stria terminalis

Body of caudate nucleus

Medial dorsal thalamus

Insular cortex

Lateral thalamus

Lateral geniculate nucleus

Centromedian thalamus

Tail of the caudate nucleus

Hippocampal formation

Medial geniculate nucleus

Cortex of cerebellum

Entorhinal cortex

Superior cerebellar peduncle

Pons (floor of fourth ventricle)

Inferior cerebellar peduncle

Medulla

JOHN A.CRAIG—MD
©ICN

Midthalamus

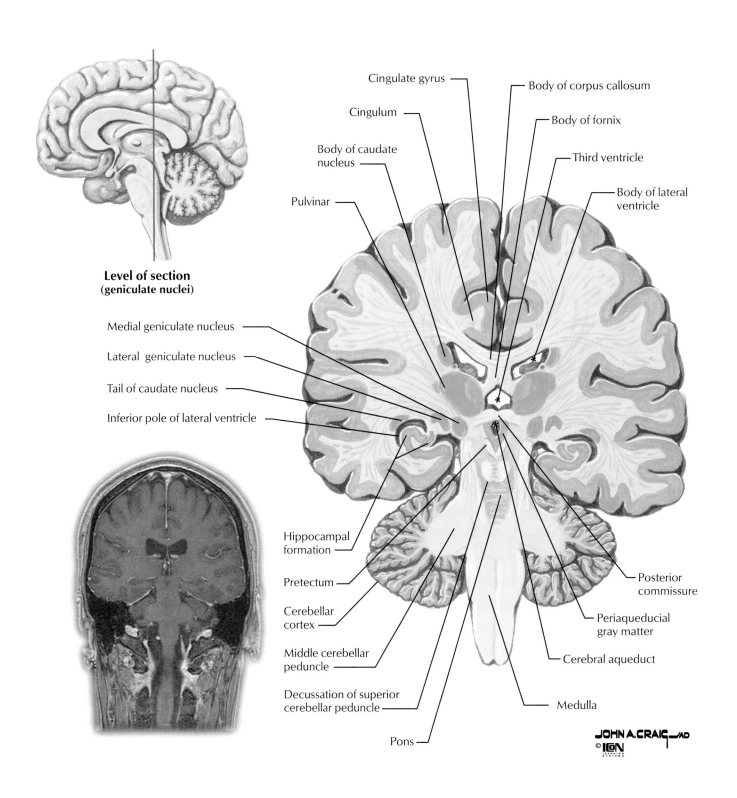

**Level of section
(geniculate nuclei)**

Cingulate gyrus

Body of corpus callosum

Cingulum

Body of fornix

Body of caudate nucleus

Third ventricle

Pulvinar

Body of lateral ventricle

Medial geniculate nucleus

Lateral geniculate nucleus

Tail of caudate nucleus

Inferior pole of lateral ventricle

Hippocampal formation

Pretectum

Posterior commissure

Cerebellar cortex

Periaqueducial gray matter

Middle cerebellar peduncle

Cerebral aqueduct

Decussation of superior cerebellar peduncle

Medulla

Pons

JOHN A. CRAIG AD
© ICON

Geniculate Nuclei

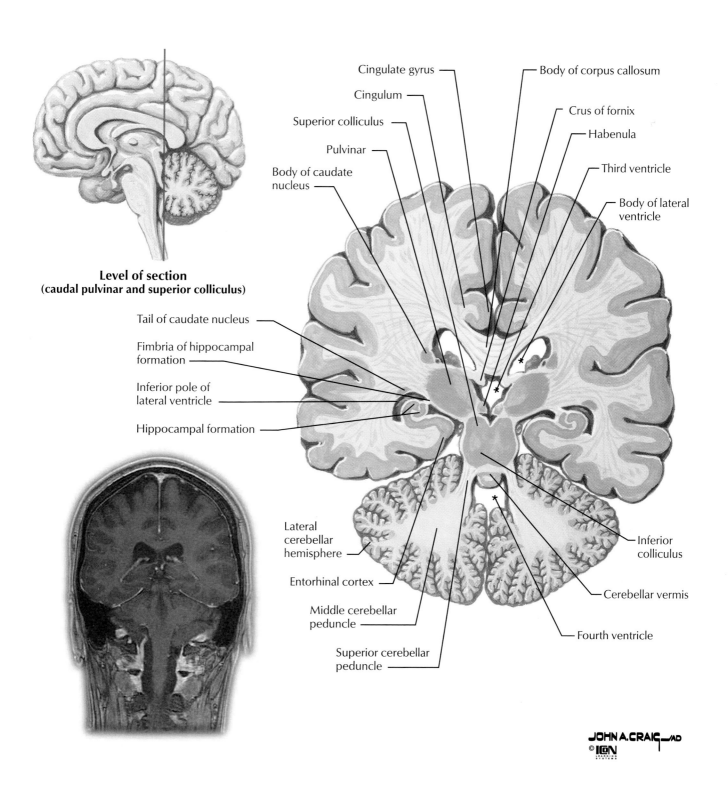

Level of section
(caudal pulvinar and superior colliculus)

Cingulate gyrus

Cingulum

Superior colliculus

Pulvinar

Body of caudate
nucleus

Body of corpus callosum

Crus of fornix

Habenula

Third ventricle

Body of lateral
ventricle

Tail of caudate nucleus

Fimbria of hippocampal
formation

Inferior pole of
lateral ventricle

Hippocampal formation

Lateral
cerebellar
hemisphere

Entorhinal cortex

Middle cerebellar
peduncle

Superior cerebellar
peduncle

Inferior
colliculus

Cerebellar vermis

Fourth ventricle

JOHN A. CRAIG MD
© ICN

Caudal Pulvinar and Superior Colliculus

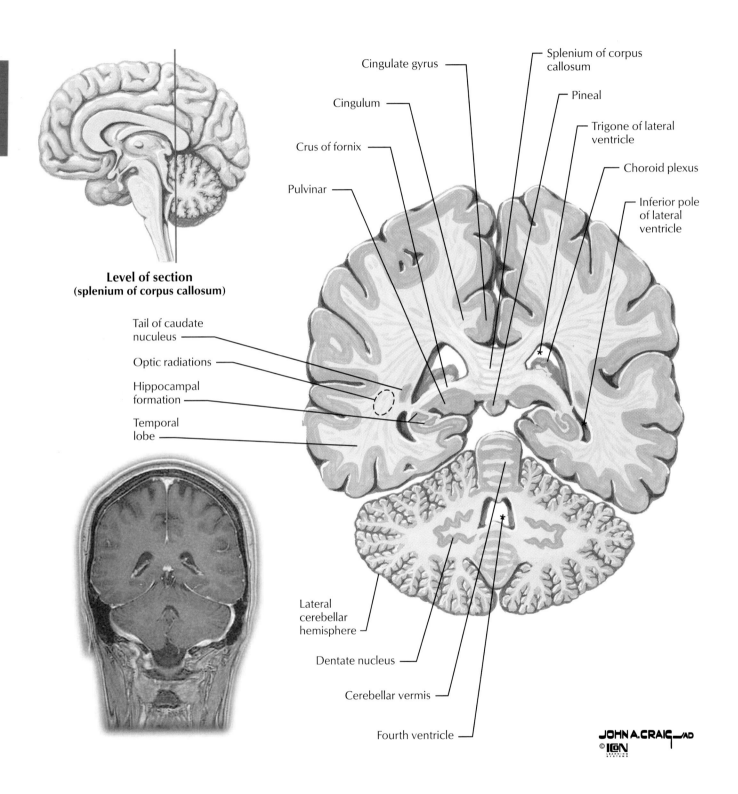

Level of section
(splenium of corpus callosum)

Cingulate gyrus

Cingulum

Crus of fornix

Pulvinar

Splenium of corpus callosum

Pineal

Trigone of lateral ventricle

Choroid plexus

Inferior pole of lateral ventricle

Tail of caudate nucleus

Optic radiations

Hippocampal formation

Temporal lobe

Lateral cerebellar hemisphere

Dentate nucleus

Cerebellar vermis

Fourth ventricle

JOHN A. CRAIG—AD
© ICON

Splenium of Corpus Callosum

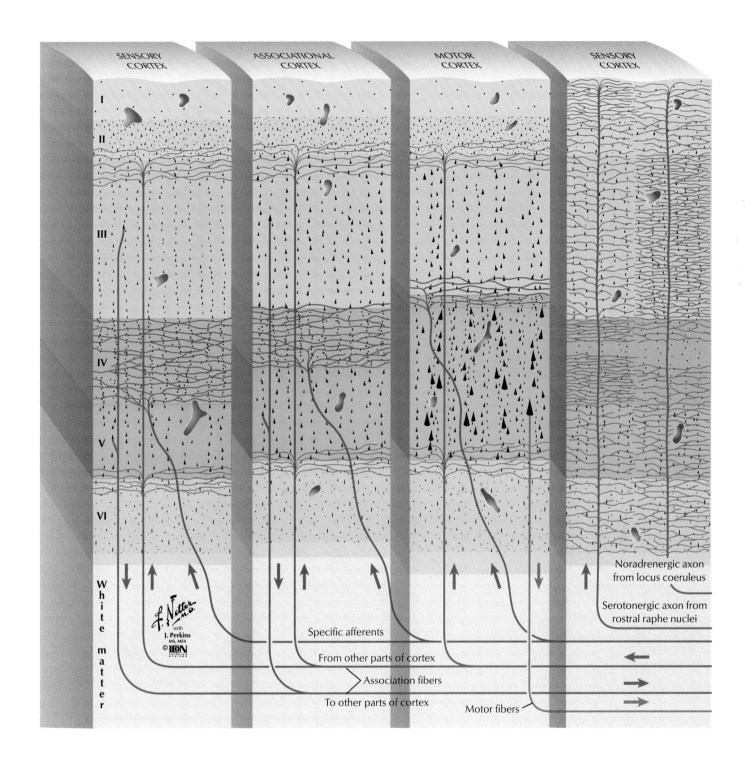

FIGURE II.89: LAYERS OF THE CEREBRAL CORTEX

Regions of the cerebral cortex with specific functional roles, such as the somatosensory cortex and the motor cortex, demonstrate histological characteristics that reflect their function. The sensory cortex has large granule cell layers (granular cortex) for receiving extensive input, whereas the motor cortex has sparse granule cell layers and extensive pyramidal cell layers, reflecting extensive output. Specific and nonspecific afferents terminate differentially in these structurally unique regions of the cortex. Monoamine inputs terminate more diffusely than do the specific inputs, reflecting the role of monoamines as modulators and enhancers of the activity of other neuronal systems.

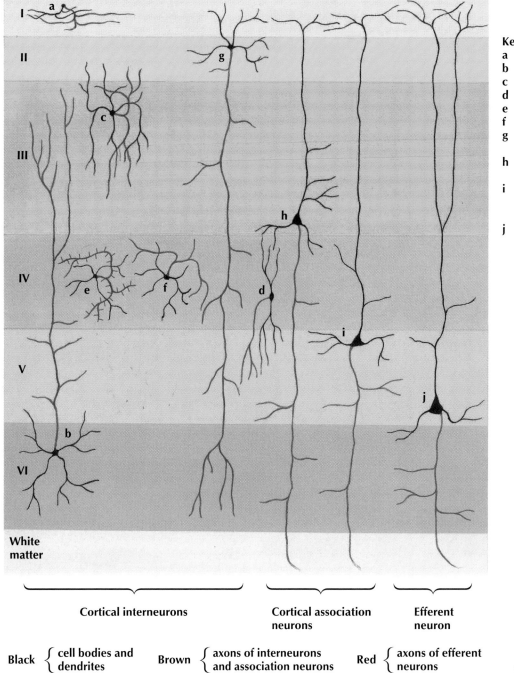

Key for Abbreviations
a Horizontal cell
b Cell of Martinotti
c Chandelier cell
d Aspiny granule cell
e Spiny granule cell
f Stellate (granule) cell
g Small pyramidal cell
   of layers II, III
h Small pyramidal
   association cell
i Small pyramidal
   association and projection
   cells of layer V
j Large pyramidal
   projection cell (Betz cell)

Cortical interneurons   Cortical association   Efferent
                               neurons   neuron

Black { cell bodies and   Brown { axons of interneurons   Red { axons of efferent
        dendrites   and association neurons   neurons

FIGURE II.90: CORTICAL NEURONAL CELL TYPES

The cerebral cortex has many anatomically unique cell types, with characteristic cell bodies, dendritic arborizations, and axonal distribution. Granule cells are local circuit neurons with small cell bodies, localized dendritic trees, and axons that distribute locally. Granule cells function as receiving neurons for thalamic and other input, and they modulate the excitability of other cortical neurons. Pyramidal cells possess more varied cell bodies, with large basolateral dendritic branching patterns and apical dendritic arborizations that run perpendicular to the cortical surface and arborize in upper layers. The axons of pyramidal cells, which function as projection neurons (e.g., corticospinal tract neurons), leave the cortex and may extend for up to a meter before synapsing on target neurons. These unique anatomical characteristics give rise to the concept that neuronal structure explains neuronal function.

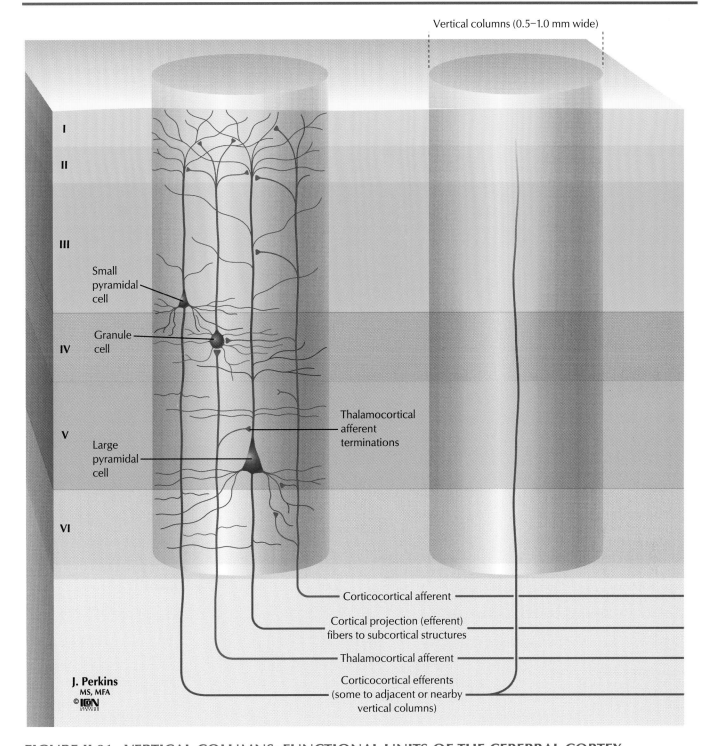

Vertical columns (0.5–1.0 mm wide)

I

II

III

Small pyramidal cell

Granule cell

IV

V

Large pyramidal cell

Thalamocortical afferent terminations

VI

Corticocortical afferent

Cortical projection (efferent) fibers to subcortical structures

Thalamocortical afferent

Corticocortical efferents (some to adjacent or nearby vertical columns)

J. Perkins
MS, MFA
©IGN

FIGURE II.91: VERTICAL COLUMNS: FUNCTIONAL UNITS OF THE CEREBRAL CORTEX

Experimental studies of sensory regions of the cerebral cortex provided anatomical and physiological evidence that discrete information from a specific region, or conveying specific functional characteristics, is processed in a cylindrical vertical zone of neurons in the cortex that spans all 6 layers of the neocortex. These vertical units vary from 0.5 to 1.0 mm in diameter. The diameter corresponds to the major horizontal expanse of a larger pyramidal cell in that unit. Both thalamic and cortical afferents arborize in the vertical column and synapse on both stellate (granule) cells and pyramidal neuron dendrites. Information from a vertical column can be sent to an adjacent or nearby column via corticocortical efferents, or it can be sent to distant structures by commissural fibers (cortex on the other side) or projection fibers (subcortical structures). The minimal elements of the vertical unit are shown.

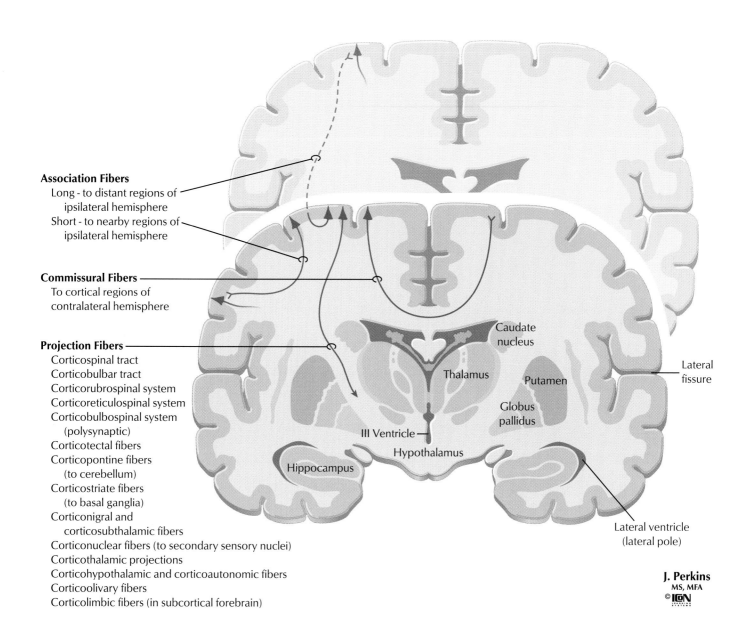

Association Fibers
  Long - to distant regions of
    ipsilateral hemisphere
  Short - to nearby regions of
    ipsilateral hemisphere

Commissural Fibers
  To cortical regions of
    contralateral hemisphere

Projection Fibers
  Corticospinal tract
  Corticobulbar tract
  Corticorubrospinal system
  Corticoreticulospinal system
  Corticobulbospinal system
    (polysynaptic)
  Corticotectal fibers
  Corticopontine fibers
    (to cerebellum)
  Corticostriate fibers
    (to basal ganglia)
  Corticonigral and
    corticosubthalamic fibers
  Corticonuclear fibers (to secondary sensory nuclei)
  Corticothalamic projections
  Corticohypothalamic and corticoautonomic fibers
  Corticoolivary fibers
  Corticolimbic fibers (in subcortical forebrain)

Caudate nucleus
Thalamus
Putamen
Globus pallidus
III Ventricle
Hypothalamus
Hippocampus
Lateral fissure
Lateral ventricle (lateral pole)

J. Perkins
MS, MFA
©ION

FIGURE II.92: EFFERENT CONNECTIONS OF THE CEREBRAL CORTEX

Neurons of the cerebral cortex send efferent connections to 3 major regions. Short or long association fibers are sent to other cortical regions of the same hemisphere by short association fibers (nearby) or long association fibers (at a distance). Commissural fibers are sent to cortical regions of the other hemisphere through the corpus callosum or the anterior commissure. Projection fibers are sent to numerous subcortical structures in the telencephalon, the diencephalon, the brain stem, and the spinal cord. The major sites of termination of these connections are listed in the diagram.

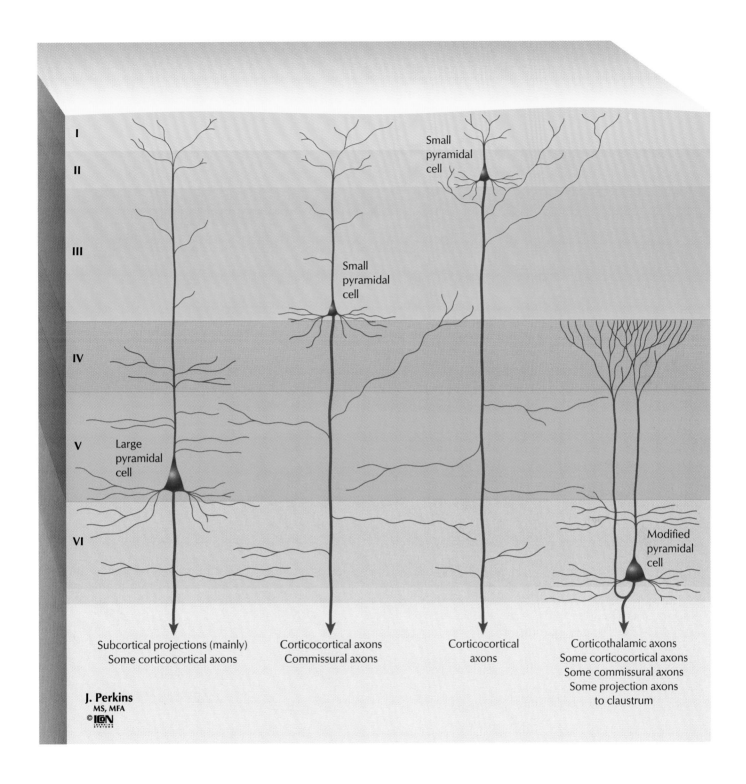

I

II

III

Small
pyramidal
cell

Small
pyramidal
cell

IV

V

Large
pyramidal
cell

VI

Modified
pyramidal
cell

Subcortical projections (mainly)
Some corticocortical axons

Corticocortical axons
Commissural axons

Corticocortical
axons

Corticothalamic axons
Some corticocortical axons
Some commissural axons
Some projection axons
to claustrum

J. Perkins
MS, MFA
©ICON

FIGURE II.93: NEURONAL ORIGINS OF EFFERENT CONNECTIONS OF THE CEREBRAL CORTEX

Association fibers destined for cortical regions of the same hemisphere arise mainly from smaller pyramidal cells in cortical layers II and III and from modified pyramidal cells in layer VI. Commissural fibers destined for cortical regions of the opposite hemisphere arise mainly from small pyramidal cells in cortical layer III and from some modified pyramidal cells in layer VI. Projection fibers arise from larger pyramidal cells in layer V and also from smaller pyramidal cells in layers V and VI. Only a small number of projection fibers arise from the giant Betz cells in layer V.

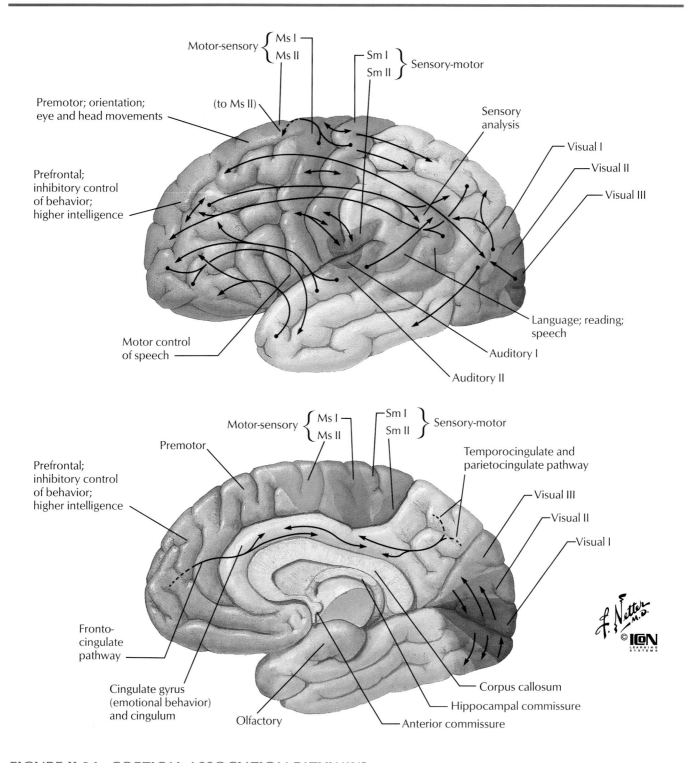

FIGURE II.94: CORTICAL ASSOCIATION PATHWAYS

Cerebral cortex neurons have extensive connections with other regions of the brain (projection neurons), with the opposite hemisphere (commissural neurons), and with other regions of the ipsilateral hemisphere (association fibers). The cortical association fibers may connect a primary sensory cortex with adjacent association areas (e.g., visual cortex, somatosensory cortex), or link multiple regions of cortex into complex association areas (e.g., polysensory analysis regions), or interlink important areas involved in language function, cognitive function, and emotional behavior and analysis. Damage to these pathways and associated cortical regions can result in loss of specific sensory and motor capabilities, aphasias (language disorders), agnosias (failure of recognition), and apraxias (performance deficits).

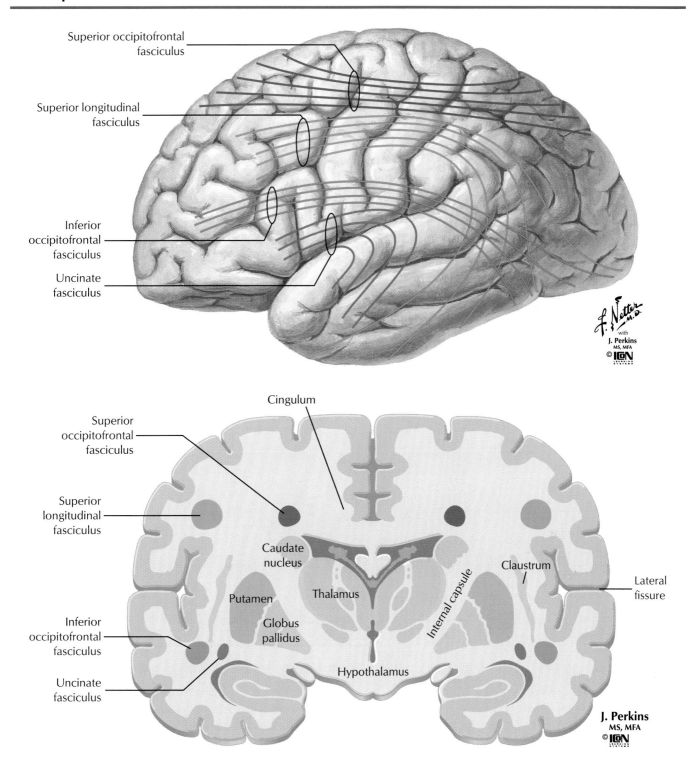

FIGURE II.95: MAJOR CORTICAL ASSOCIATION BUNDLES

Association fibers connecting cortical regions in one hemisphere with adjacent or distant regions of the same hemisphere are categorized as short association fibers (arcuate fibers) or long association fibers. The long association fibers often are recognized anatomically as specific association bundles and may have numerous fiber systems entering, exiting, and traversing them. Important named bundles include the uncinate fasciculus, the superior longitudinal fasciculus, the superior and inferior occipitofrontal fasciculi, and the cingulum. The cingulum is a bundle through which the major monoamines (dopamine, norepinephrine, serotonin) and part of the cholinergic projections travel to their widespread target sites.

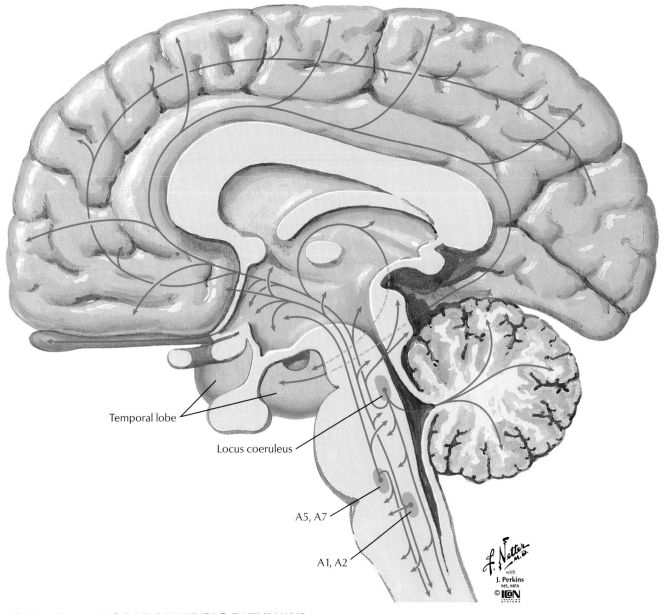

Temporal lobe

Locus coeruleus

A5, A7

A1, A2

FIGURE II.96: NORADRENERGIC PATHWAYS

Noradrenergic neurons in the brain stem project to widespread areas of the CNS. The neurons are found in the locus coeruleus (group A6) and in several cell groups in the RF (tegmentum) of the medulla and the pons (groups A1, A2, A5, A7). Axonal projections of the locus coeruleus branch to the cerebral cortex, the hippocampus, the hypothalamus, the cerebellum, brain stem nuclei, and the spinal cord. The locus coeruleus acts as a modulator of the excitability of other projection systems (including nociception), such as the glutamate system, and helps to regulate attention, alertness, and sleep-wake cycles. The RF groups are interconnected with spinal cord, brain stem, hypothalamic, and limbic regions involved in neuroendocrine control, visceral functions (temperature regulation, feeding and drinking behavior, reproductive behavior, autonomic regulation), and emotional behavior. A sparse set of epinephrine-containing neurons in the medullary RF are similarly interconnected with each other. The RF groups can work in concert with the locus coeruleus during challenge or in response to a stressor to coordinate alertness and appropriate neuroendocrine and autonomic responsiveness. The central noradrenergic and adrenergic neurons and their receptors are the targets of many pharmacological agents, including those for depression, analgesia, and hypertension.

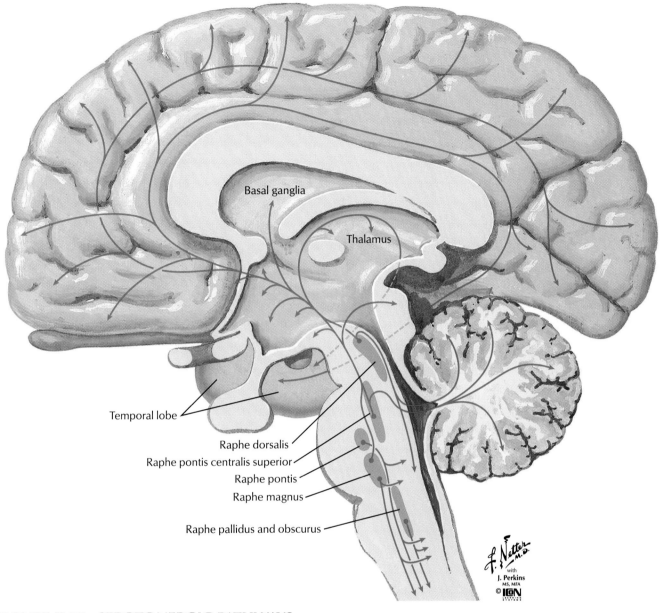

FIGURE II.97: SEROTONERGIC PATHWAYS

Serotonergic neurons (5-hydroxytryptamine [5-HT]), found in raphe nuclei of the brain stem and adjacent wings of cells, have widespread projections that innervate every major subdivision of the CNS. Neurons in the nucleus raphe dorsalis and the nucleus centralis superior project rostrally to innervate the cerebral cortex, many limbic forebrain structures (hippocampus, amygdala), the basal ganglia, many hypothalamic nuclei and areas, and some thalamic regions. Neurons in the raphe magnus, pontis, pallidus, and obscurus project more caudally to innervate many brain stem regions, the cerebellum, and the spinal cord. The projections of the nucleus raphe magnus to the dorsal horn of the spinal cord influence opiate analgesia and pain processing. The ascending serotonergic systems are involved in regulation of emotional behavior and a wide range of hypothalamic functions (neuroendocrine, visceral/autonomic). Serotonergic neurons are involved in sleep-wake cycles and stop firing during REM sleep. Projections to the cerebral cortex modulate the processing of afferent inputs (e.g., from the visual cortex). The descending serotonergic neurons enhance the effects of analgesia and are essential for opiate analgesia. They also modulate preganglionic autonomic neuronal excitability and enhance the excitability of LMNs. Many pharmacological agents (including drugs for treating depression, other cognitive and emotional behavioral states, headaches, and pain) target serotonergic neurons and their receptors.

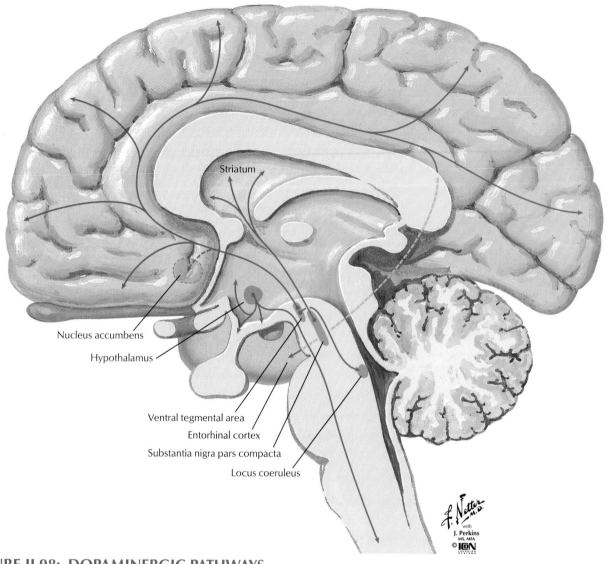

Striatum

Nucleus accumbens

Hypothalamus

Ventral tegmental area
Entorhinal cortex
Substantia nigra pars compacta
Locus coeruleus

FIGURE II.98: DOPAMINERGIC PATHWAYS

Dopaminergic (DA) neurons are found in the midbrain and the hypothalamus. In the midbrain, neurons in the substantia nigra pars compacta project axons mainly to the striatum (caudate nucleus, putamen) and to the globus pallidus and the subthalamus. The nigrostriatal projection is involved in basal ganglia circuitry that aids in the planning and execution of cortical activities, especially in the motor system. Damage to the nigrostriatal system results in Parkinson's disease. The antiparkinsonian drugs, such as L-dopa, target this system and its receptors. DA neurons in the ventral tegmental area and the mesencephalic RF send mesolimbic projections to the nucleus accumbens, the amygdala, and the hippocampus and mesocortical projections to the frontal cortex and some cortical association areas. The mesolimbic pathway to the nucleus accumbens is involved in motivation, reward, biological drives, and addictive behaviors,

particularly substance abuse. Projections to limbic structures can induce stereotyped, repetitive behaviors and activities. The mesocortical projections influence cognitive functions in the planning and carrying-out of frontal cortical activities and in attention mechanisms. The mesolimbic and mesocortical systems and their receptors are the targets of neuroleptic and antipsychotic agents that influence behaviors in schizophrenia, obsessive-compulsive disorder (OCD), attention deficit-hyperactivity disorder (ADHD), and other behavioral states. DA neurons in the hypothalamus form the tuberoinfundibular dopamine pathway, which projects from the arcuate nucleus to the contact zone of the median eminence, where dopamine acts as a prolactin inhibitory factor. Intrahypothalamic DA neurons also influence other neuroendocrine and visceral/autonomic hypothalamic functions.

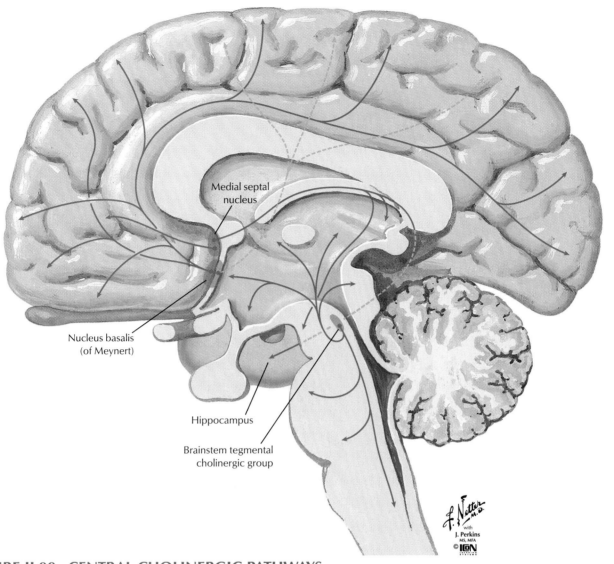

Medial septal nucleus

Nucleus basalis (of Meynert)

Hippocampus

Brainstem tegmental cholinergic group

FIGURE II.99: CENTRAL CHOLINERGIC PATHWAYS

Central cholinergic neurons are found mainly in the nucleus basalis (of Meynert) and in septal nuclei. Nucleus basalis neurons project cholinergic axons to the cerebral cortex, and septal cholinergic neurons project cholinergic axons to the hippocampal formation. These cholinergic projections are involved in cortical activation and memory function, particularly consolidation of short-term memory. They often appear to be damaged in Alzheimer's disease. Drugs that enhance cholinergic function are used for improvement of memory. Other cholinergic neurons, found in the brain stem tegmentum, project to structures in the thalamus, the brain stem, and the cerebellum. The projections to the thalamus modulate arousal and the sleep-wake cycle and appear to be important in the initiation of REM sleep. Cholinergic interneurons are present in the striatum and may participate in basal ganglia control of tone, posture, and initiation of movement or selection of wanted patterns of activity. Acetylcholine is the principal neurotransmitter in all preganglionic autonomic neurons and LMNs in the spinal cord and the brain stem.

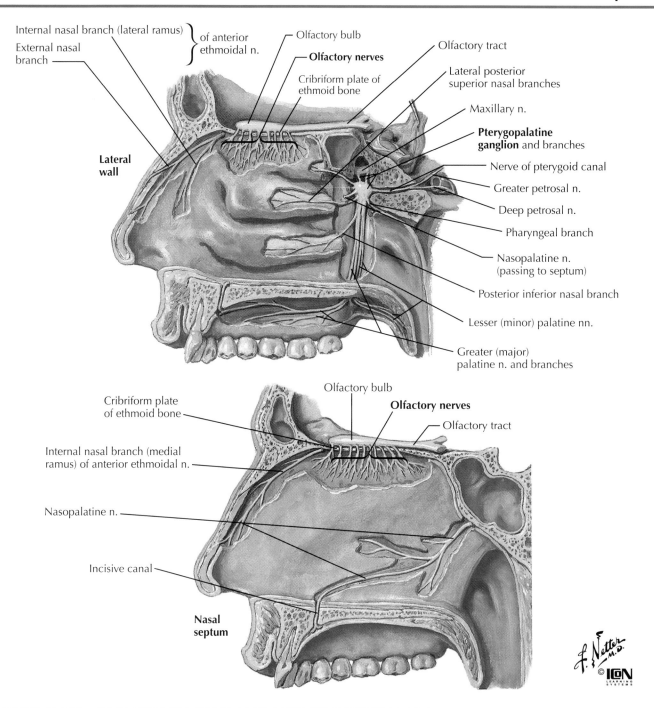

Internal nasal branch (lateral ramus)
External nasal branch
of anterior ethmoidal n.
Olfactory bulb
Olfactory nerves
Cribriform plate of ethmoid bone
Olfactory tract
Lateral posterior superior nasal branches
Maxillary n.
Pterygopalatine ganglion and branches
Nerve of pterygoid canal
Greater petrosal n.
Deep petrosal n.
Pharyngeal branch
Nasopalatine n. (passing to septum)
Posterior inferior nasal branch
Lesser (minor) palatine nn.
Greater (major) palatine n. and branches
Lateral wall

Cribriform plate of ethmoid bone
Olfactory bulb
Olfactory nerves
Olfactory tract
Internal nasal branch (medial ramus) of anterior ethmoidal n.
Nasopalatine n.
Incisive canal
Nasal septum

FIGURE II.100: OLFACTORY NERVE AND NERVES OF THE NOSE

The olfactory nerves and their projections into the CNS are an important component of forebrain function. Bipolar cells found in the olfactory epithelium are the primary sensory neurons. The peripheral axon, a chemosensory transducer, responds to the unique chemical stimuli of airborne molecules entering the nose. The central axons of bipolar neurons aggregate into approximately 20 olfactory nerves that traverse the cribriform plate and end in glomeruli of the ipsilateral olfactory bulb. These nerves are vulnerable to tearing, resulting in anosmia. Unlike neurons in other sensory systems, these bipolar neurons can proliferate and regenerate. After processing in the olfactory bulb, mitral neurons and tufted neurons project via the olfactory tract directly and indirectly to limbic forebrain structures, including septal nuclei and amygdaloid nuclei, and thereby influence the hypothalamus and its regulation of neuroendocrine and visceral/autonomic function. The olfactory system is involved in territorial recognition and defense, food and water acquisition, social behavior, reproductive behavior, and signaling of danger.

PART III. SYSTEMIC NEUROSCIENCE

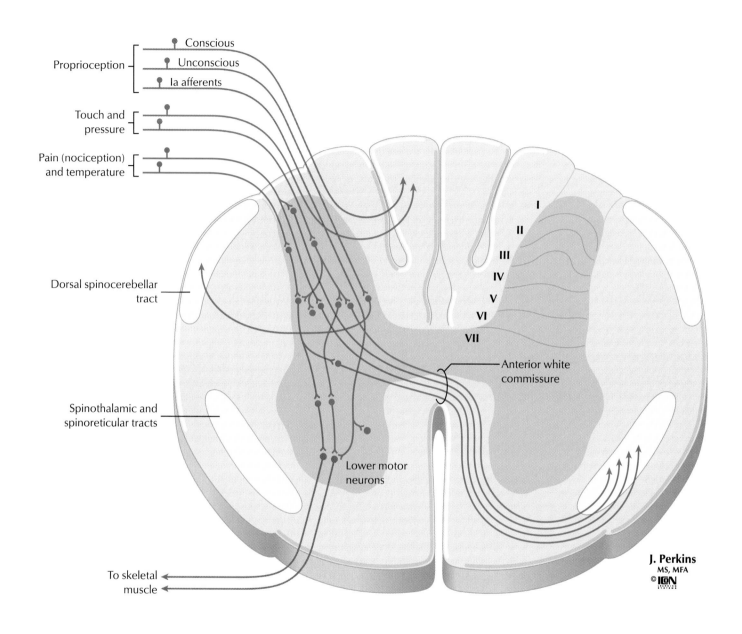

FIGURE III.1: SOMATOSENSORY AFFERENTS TO THE SPINAL CORD

Unmyelinated (UNM) and small myelinated (M) axons that convey nociception and temperature sensation terminate in laminae I and V (origin for spinothalamic tract). Other UNM axons terminate in the dorsal horn, from which neurons for polysynaptic reflexes and for the spinoreticular system originate. M axons for touch and pressure terminate in the dorsal horn, where additional reflex connections and spinothalamic projections originate. M axons also project into fasciculi gracilis and cuneatus for lemniscal pathways destined for conscious interpretation. M proprioceptive axons terminate directly on lower motor neurons (LMNs) (via Ia afferents) and the Ia interneuronal pool and also terminate on neurons of origin for the spinocerebellar tracts.

M = myelinated; UNM = unmyelinated.

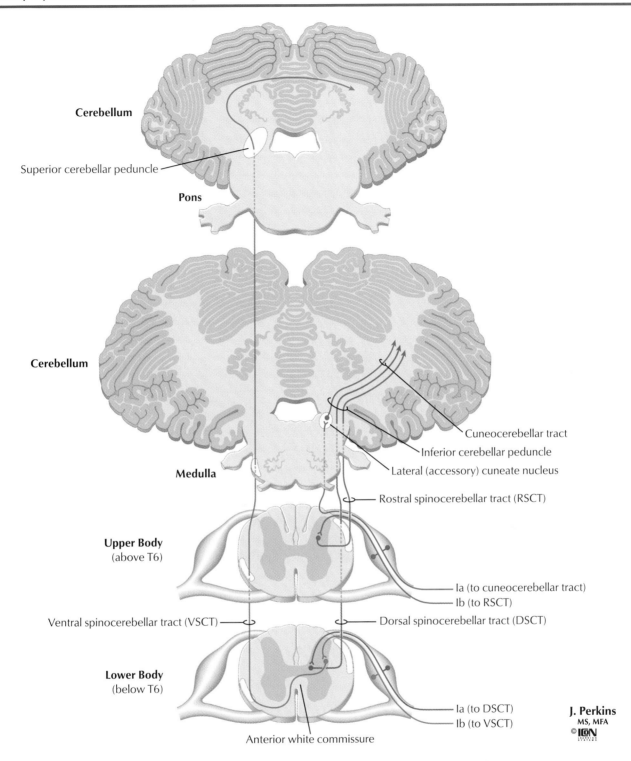

Cerebellum

Superior cerebellar peduncle

Pons

Cerebellum

Cuneocerebellar tract

Inferior cerebellar peduncle

Lateral (accessory) cuneate nucleus

Medulla

Rostral spinocerebellar tract (RSCT)

Upper Body
(above T6)

Ia (to cuneocerebellar tract)
Ib (to RSCT)

Ventral spinocerebellar tract (VSCT)   Dorsal spinocerebellar tract (DSCT)

Lower Body
(below T6)

Ia (to DSCT)
Ib (to VSCT)

J. Perkins
MS, MFA
©ICN

Anterior white commissure

FIGURE III.2: SOMATOSENSORY SYSTEM: SPINOCEREBELLAR PATHWAYS

Proprioceptive primary somatosensory axons from joints, tendons, and ligaments (represented by Ib afferents from Golgi tendon organs) terminate on neurons of origin (border cells, dorsal horn neurons) for the ventral spinocerebellar tract and the rostral spinocerebellar tract from the lower and upper body, respectively (T6 is cutoff). Proprioceptive primary somatosensory axons from muscle spindles (Ia afferents) terminate on neurons

of origin (Clarke's nucleus, lateral [external] cuneate nucleus of the medulla) for the dorsal spinocerebellar tract and the cuneocerebellar tract from the lower and upper body, respectively (T6 is cutoff). The dorsal spinocerebellar, rostral spinocerebellar, and cuneocerebellar tracts remain ipsilateral. The ventral spinocerebellar tract crosses twice, once in the anterior white commissure and again in the cerebellum.

215

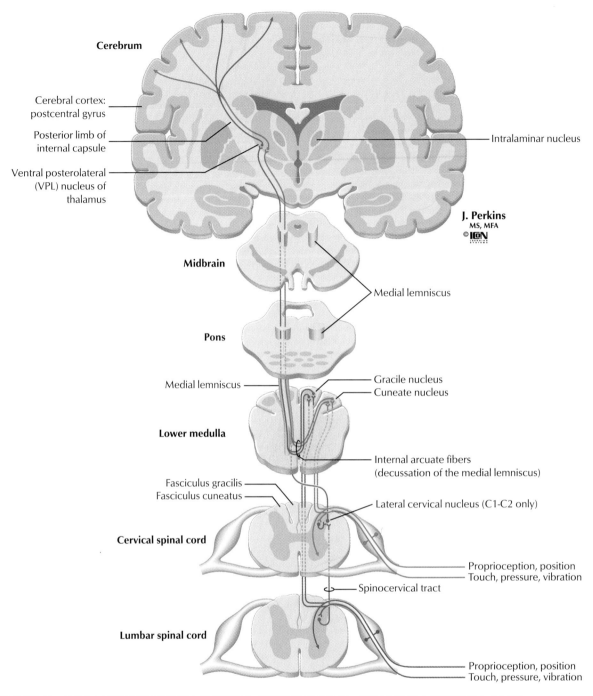

Cerebrum

Cerebral cortex: postcentral gyrus

Posterior limb of internal capsule

Ventral posterolateral (VPL) nucleus of thalamus

Intralaminar nucleus

J. Perkins
MS, MFA
© IGN

Midbrain

Medial lemniscus

Pons

Medial lemniscus

Gracile nucleus
Cuneate nucleus

Lower medulla

Internal arcuate fibers (decussation of the medial lemniscus)

Fasciculus gracilis
Fasciculus cuneatus

Lateral cervical nucleus (C1-C2 only)

Cervical spinal cord

Proprioception, position
Touch, pressure, vibration

Spinocervical tract

Lumbar spinal cord

Proprioception, position
Touch, pressure, vibration

FIGURE III.3: SOMATOSENSORY SYSTEM: THE DORSAL COLUMN SYSTEM AND EPICRITIC MODALITIES

Primary somatosensory M axons that convey fine discriminative touch, pressure, vibratory sensation, and conscious joint position sense project directly into the dorsal column system, where they are topographically organized (fasciculus gracilis for lower body [below T6], fasciculus cuneatus for upper body [T6 and above]). These axons terminate, respectively, in nucleus gracilis and nucleus cuneatus, from which the medial lemniscus origi-nates. This tract crosses in the medulla and projects to the ventral posterolateral (VPL) nucleus of the thalamus. The VPL nucleus terminates topographically in the primary sensory cortex. The spino-cervical system contributes polysynaptic mechanoreceptive information to supplement that in the dorsal column system.
M = myelinated.

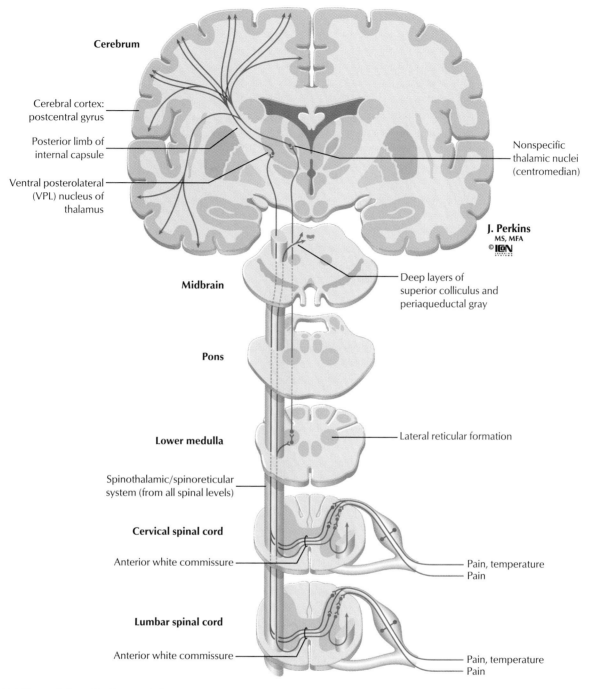

Cerebrum

Cerebral cortex:
postcentral gyrus

Posterior limb of
internal capsule

Ventral posterolateral
(VPL) nucleus of
thalamus

Nonspecific
thalamic nuclei
(centromedian)

J. Perkins
MS, MFA

Midbrain

Deep layers of
superior colliculus and
periaqueductal gray

Pons

Lower medulla

Lateral reticular formation

Spinothalamic/spinoreticular
system (from all spinal levels)

Cervical spinal cord

Anterior white commissure

Pain, temperature
Pain

Lumbar spinal cord

Anterior white commissure

Pain, temperature
Pain

FIGURE III.4: SOMATOSENSORY SYSTEM: THE SPINOTHALAMIC AND SPINORETICULAR SYSTEMS AND PROTOPATHIC MODALITIES

Primary somatosensory UNM (C fibers) and small M (Aδ fibers) axons that convey nociceptive information (fast, localized pain), temperature sensation, and light, moving touch terminate on neurons in laminae I and V. These neurons send crossed axons into the spinothalamic tract projecting to the VPL nucleus of the thalamus. These thalamic neurons project to the secondary somatosensory cortex (SII), as well as to the primary sensory cortex. Primary sensory C fibers contribute to a large, cascading network in the dorsal horn resulting in bilateral projections into the spinoreticular tract. This system ends mainly in the reticular formation (RF), from which polysynaptic projections lead to nonspecific, medial dorsal, and anterior thalamic nuclei. Some spinoreticular fibers terminate in the deeper layers of the superior colliculus (spinotectal pathway) and periaqueductal gray. Cortical regions such as the cingulate, insular, and prefrontal regions then process and interpret nociceptive information related to slow, excruciating pain. M = myelinated; UNM = unmyelinated.

Gating Mechanism

Spinal Mechanisms of Nociceptive Processing

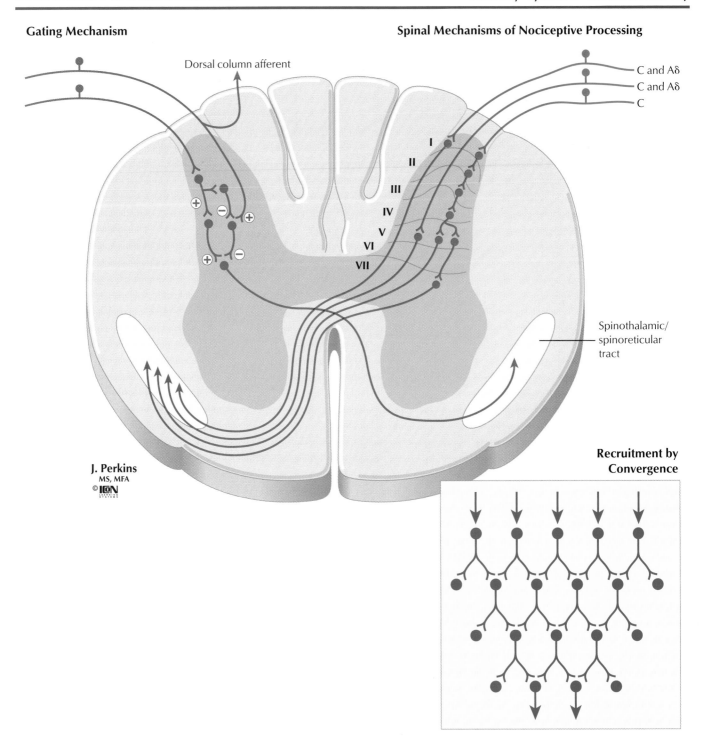

FIGURE III.5: SPINOTHALAMIC AND SPINORETICULAR NOCICEPTIVE PROCESSING IN THE SPINAL CORD

Unmyelinated primary afferents (C, Aδ fibers) that convey "fast, localized pain" and temperature sensation terminate in laminae I and V, from which the crossed spinothalamic axons originate. UNM primary afferents (C fibers) also terminate on neurons in the dorsal horn, from which a cascading system of recruitment, convergence, and polysynaptic interconnections originates. This system contributes to the spinoreticular tract (mainly crossed),

which projects into the RF and then projects polysynaptically to nonspecific, medial dorsal, and anterior thalamic nuclei. It contributes to perception of excruciating pain and its emotional connotation via cortical regions such as the cingulate, insular, and prefrontal cortices. The gating mechanism, shown on the left, allows primary dorsal column axon collaterals to dampen pain processing in the dorsal horn.

Mechanisms of Neuropathic Pain

1. Sprouting of sympathetic postganglionic nerve fibers on 1° afferent endings and 1° sensory cell bodies.
2. Lowered threshold for firing of C fibers (hyperesthesia) and Aδ fibers (allodynia).
3. Proliferation of α-adrenergic receptors on 1° sensory afferent endings and 1° sensory cell bodies.
4. Possible ephaptic afferent activation.
5. Permanent hyperactivation of wide dynamic range neurons.
6. Glutamate excitotoxic cell death of inhibitory neurons (glutamate storms).
7. Inadequacy of central descending serotonin, norepinephrine, opioid peptide pathways to control nociception.
8. Immobilization by pain decreases gating of nociceptive input, limiting physical therapy to initiate gating.
9. Sprouting of C fibers in spinal cord.
10. Extension of interneuron dendrites into additional spinal cord laminae.

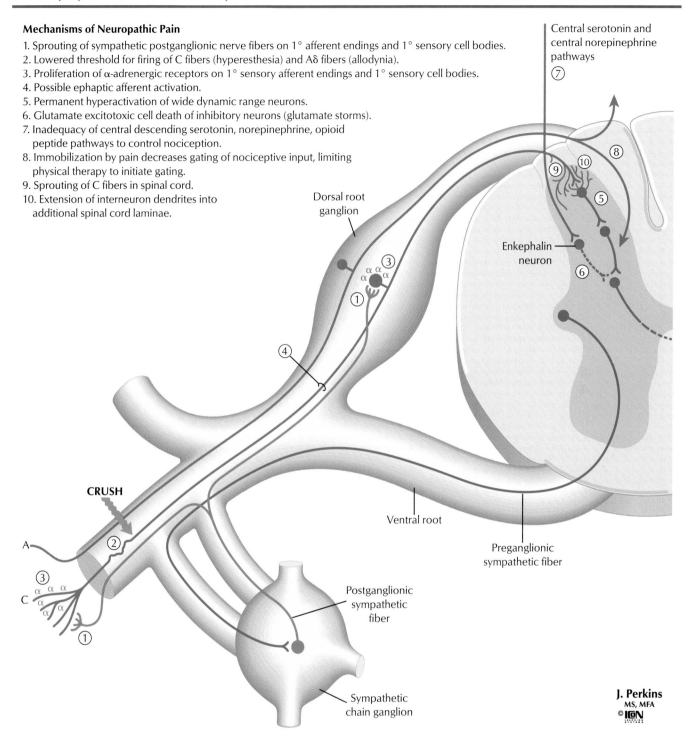

FIGURE III.6: MECHANISMS OF NEUROPATHIC PAIN AND SYMPATHETICALLY MAINTAINED PAIN

The cascading dorsal horn system—which receives primary afferent C fibers of nociceptive origin and projects into the spinoreticular system for the conscious interpretation of excruciating and neuropathic pain—is illustrated. The sympathetic connections, in addition to secreting norepinephrine into the blood and activating the secretion of epinephrine, can synapse with terminals and cell bodies of primary nociceptive neurons in neuropathic pain syndromes. Descending central noradrenergic and serotonergic projections are also shown. Specific mechanisms relevant to neuropathic pain, particularly complex regional pain syndrome (reflex sympathetic dystrophy), are described in the numbered sites.

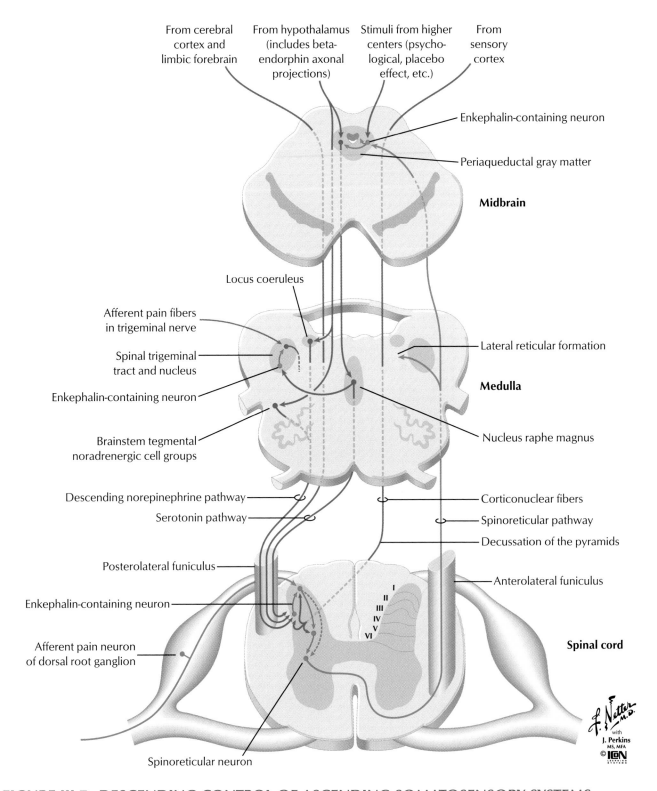

From cerebral cortex and limbic forebrain

From hypothalamus (includes beta-endorphin axonal projections)

Stimuli from higher centers (psychological, placebo effect, etc.)

From sensory cortex

Enkephalin-containing neuron

Periaqueductal gray matter

Midbrain

Locus coeruleus

Afferent pain fibers in trigeminal nerve

Spinal trigeminal tract and nucleus

Enkephalin-containing neuron

Lateral reticular formation

Medulla

Brainstem tegmental noradrenergic cell groups

Nucleus raphe magnus

Descending norepinephrine pathway

Serotonin pathway

Corticonuclear fibers

Spinoreticular pathway

Decussation of the pyramids

Posterolateral funiculus

Enkephalin-containing neuron

Anterolateral funiculus

Afferent pain neuron of dorsal root ganglion

I
II
III
IV
V
VI

Spinal cord

Spinoreticular neuron

FIGURE III.7: DESCENDING CONTROL OF ASCENDING SOMATOSENSORY SYSTEMS

Descending connections from the cerebral cortex, the limbic forebrain structures, the hypothalamus (the paraventricular nucleus and the periarcuate beta-endorphin neurons), the periaqueductal gray (PAG), the RF of the brain stem, central noradrenergic neurons (of the locus coeruleus and other brain stem tegmental groups), and serotonergic (5-HT) neurons (nucleus raphe magnus) modulate the processing of nociceptive information in the dorsal horn of the spinal cord. The central descending noradrenergic and serotonergic pathways, influenced by the PAG and other higher centers, are important for endogenous (and exogenous) modulation of pain.

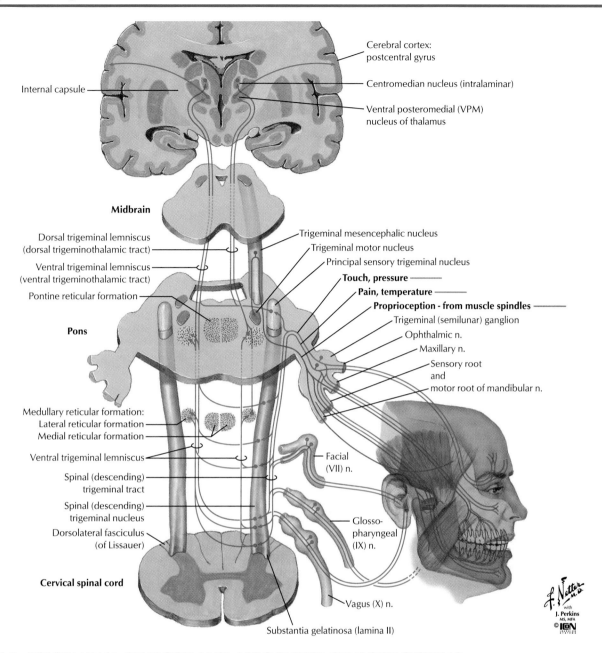

Cerebral cortex: postcentral gyrus

Internal capsule

Centromedian nucleus (intralaminar)

Ventral posteromedial (VPM) nucleus of thalamus

Midbrain

Dorsal trigeminal lemniscus (dorsal trigeminothalamic tract)

Ventral trigeminal lemniscus (ventral trigeminothalamic tract)

Pontine reticular formation

Pons

Trigeminal mesencephalic nucleus

Trigeminal motor nucleus

Principal sensory trigeminal nucleus

Touch, pressure

Pain, temperature

Proprioception - from muscle spindles

Trigeminal (semilunar) ganglion

Ophthalmic n.

Maxillary n.

Sensory root and motor root of mandibular n.

Medullary reticular formation: Lateral reticular formation Medial reticular formation

Ventral trigeminal lemniscus

Spinal (descending) trigeminal tract

Spinal (descending) trigeminal nucleus

Dorsolateral fasciculus (of Lissauer)

Cervical spinal cord

Facial (VII) n.

Glosso-pharyngeal (IX) n.

Vagus (X) n.

Substantia gelatinosa (lamina II)

FIGURE III.8: TRIGEMINAL SENSORY AND ASSOCIATED SENSORY SYSTEMS

Axons of primary sensory neurons enter the brain stem, travel in the descending (spinal) tract of V and terminate in the descending (spinal) nucleus of V. Axons of the trigeminal ganglion (V) supply the face, the anterior oral cavity, the teeth, and the gums; axons of the geniculate ganglion (VII) and the jugular ganglion (X) supply a small zone of the external ear; and axons of the petrosal ganglion (IX) supply general sensation to the posterior oral cavity and the pharynx. Axons from the descending nucleus of V project into the crossed trigeminal lemniscus (ventral trigeminothalamic tract [VTTT]), which terminates in the ventral posteromedial (VPM) nucleus of the thalamus. The VPM nucleus projects to the lateral primary sensory cortex (SI)

and to intralaminar thalamic nuclei, which are associated with nociceptive processing. The caudal descending nucleus of V also sends bilateral projections to the RF to process excruciating pain (similar to the spinoreticular system). Primary sensory axons that carry fine discriminative modalities from V (similar to the dorsal column) terminate in the rostral descending nucleus of V and the main sensory nucleus of V, which contribute to the VTTT. A portion of the main sensory nucleus also projects ipsilaterally to the VPM nucleus. The mesencephalic nucleus of V, a primary nucleus inside the CNS, mediates muscle spindle reflexes for masticatory and extraocular muscles.

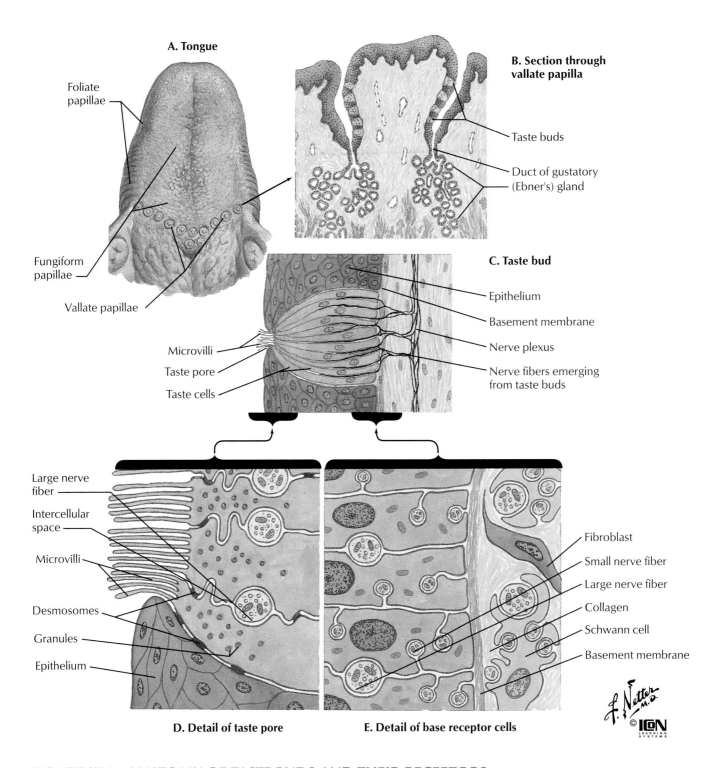

A. Tongue

Foliate papillae

Fungiform papillae

Vallate papillae

B. Section through vallate papilla

Taste buds

Duct of gustatory (Ebner's) gland

C. Taste bud

Microvilli

Taste pore

Taste cells

Epithelium

Basement membrane

Nerve plexus

Nerve fibers emerging from taste buds

Large nerve fiber

Intercellular space

Microvilli

Desmosomes

Granules

Epithelium

Fibroblast

Small nerve fiber

Large nerve fiber

Collagen

Schwann cell

Basement membrane

D. Detail of taste pore

E. Detail of base receptor cells

FIGURE III.9: ANATOMY OF TASTE BUDS AND THEIR RECEPTORS

Taste buds are chemosensory transducers that consist of bundles of columnar cells that lie within the epithelium. They translate individual molecular configurations or combinations of molecules for salty, sweet, sour, and bitter sensations into action potentials of both small and large primary sensory axons. The taste buds are found on the anterior and posterior regions of the tongue and, less frequently, on the palate and the epiglottis. Nerve fibers for taste show complex responses to electrical activity across populations of many nerve fibers. The integrative interpretation of taste takes place in the CNS.

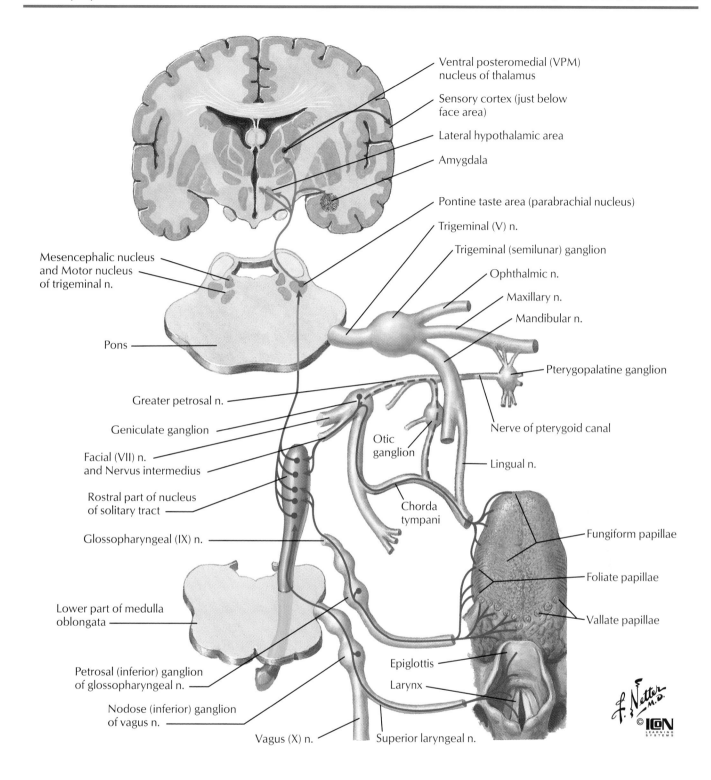

Ventral posteromedial (VPM) nucleus of thalamus

Sensory cortex (just below face area)

Lateral hypothalamic area

Amygdala

Pontine taste area (parabrachial nucleus)

Trigeminal (V) n.

Trigeminal (semilunar) ganglion

Ophthalmic n.

Maxillary n.

Mandibular n.

Mesencephalic nucleus and Motor nucleus of trigeminal n.

Pons

Pterygopalatine ganglion

Nerve of pterygoid canal

Greater petrosal n.

Geniculate ganglion

Otic ganglion

Lingual n.

Facial (VII) n. and Nervus intermedius

Chorda tympani

Rostral part of nucleus of solitary tract

Glossopharyngeal (IX) n.

Fungiform papillae

Foliate papillae

Vallate papillae

Lower part of medulla oblongata

Epiglottis

Petrosal (inferior) ganglion of glossopharyngeal n.

Larynx

Nodose (inferior) ganglion of vagus n.

Vagus (X) n.

Superior laryngeal n.

FIGURE III.10: TASTE PATHWAYS

Primary sensory axons of neurons of the geniculate ganglion (VII), the petrosal ganglion (IX), and the nodose (inferior) ganglion (X) supply taste buds in the anterior two-thirds of the tongue, the posterior third of the tongue, and the epiglottis and palate, respectively. These axons terminate in the rostral part of the nucleus solitarius (nucleus of the solitary tract), which sends ipsilateral projections mainly to the parabrachial nucleus in the pons. The parabrachial nucleus projects to the VPM nucleus of the thalamus, the hypothalamus (lateral hypothalamic area, paraventricular nucleus), and the amygdaloid nuclei. These nonthalamic projections are associated with the emotional, motivational, and behavioral aspects of taste and food intake.

Frontal section

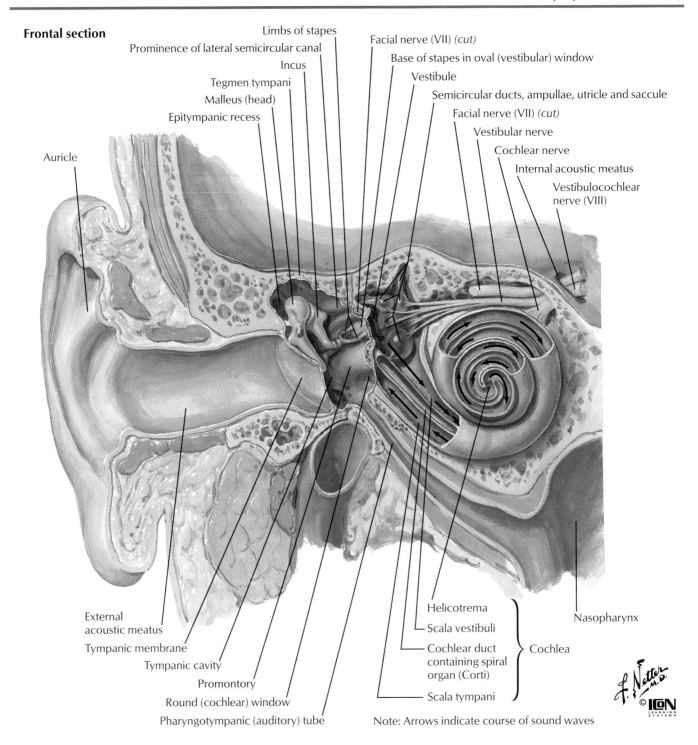

Limbs of stapes
Prominence of lateral semicircular canal
Incus
Tegmen tympani
Malleus (head)
Epitympanic recess
Facial nerve (VII) *(cut)*
Base of stapes in oval (vestibular) window
Vestibule
Semicircular ducts, ampullae, utricle and saccule
Facial nerve (VII) *(cut)*
Vestibular nerve
Cochlear nerve
Internal acoustic meatus
Vestibulocochlear nerve (VIII)
Auricle
External acoustic meatus
Tympanic membrane
Tympanic cavity
Promontory
Round (cochlear) window
Pharyngotympanic (auditory) tube
Helicotrema
Scala vestibuli
Cochlear duct containing spiral organ (Corti)
Scala tympani
Cochlea
Nasopharynx

Note: Arrows indicate course of sound waves

FIGURE III.11: PERIPHERAL PATHWAYS FOR SOUND RECEPTION

The sound transduction process involves movement of mechanical sound through the external ear and the external acoustic meatus, across the tympanic membrane, leveraged as a mechanical force by the bones of the middle ear (ossicles) via the oval window to produce a fluid wave in the cochlear duct. This fluid wave causes differential movement of the basilar membrane, stimulating hairs on the apical portion of hair cells to release neurotransmitters that stimulate primary sensory axons of neurons of the cochlear (spiral) ganglion. The basilar membrane in the cochlea shows maximal displacement spatially according to the frequency of impinging tones, with low frequencies stimulating the apex (helicotrema) and high frequencies stimulating the base. The eustachian (pharyngotympanic) tube permits pressure equilibration between the middle ear and the outside world.

Bony and membranous labyrinths: schema

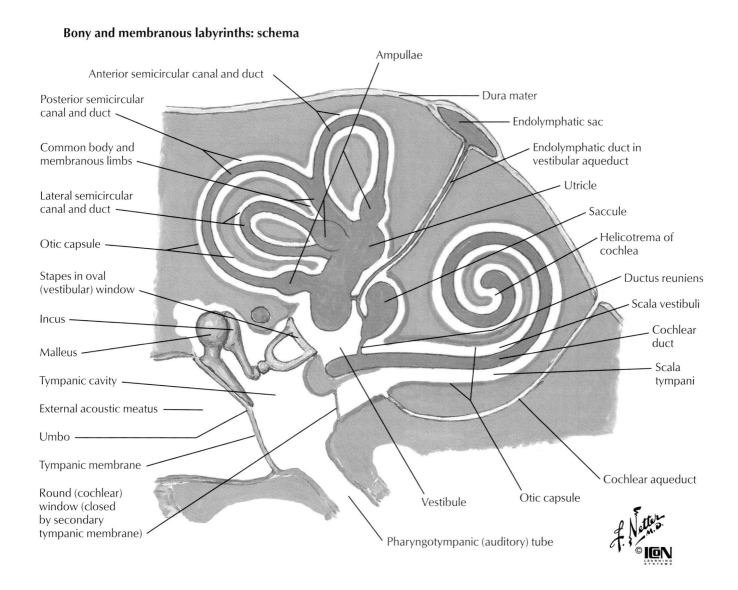

Ampullae

Anterior semicircular canal and duct

Dura mater

Posterior semicircular canal and duct

Endolymphatic sac

Common body and membranous limbs

Endolymphatic duct in vestibular aqueduct

Lateral semicircular canal and duct

Utricle

Otic capsule

Saccule

Helicotrema of cochlea

Stapes in oval (vestibular) window

Ductus reuniens

Incus

Scala vestibuli

Malleus

Cochlear duct

Tympanic cavity

Scala tympani

External acoustic meatus

Umbo

Tympanic membrane

Round (cochlear) window (closed by secondary tympanic membrane)

Cochlear aqueduct

Vestibule

Otic capsule

Pharyngotympanic (auditory) tube

FIGURE III.12: BONY AND MEMBRANOUS LABYRINTHS

The relationship between the cochlea and the vestibular apparatus (utricle, saccule, semicircular canals and ducts) and the bony labyrinth that surrounds them is illustrated. The ossicles (malleus, incus, stapes) leverage movement of the tympanic membrane to produce movement of the oval window. Movement of the oval window causes the fluid wave to move through the scala vestibuli and the scala tympani of the cochlea and ricochet onto the round window. The 3 semicircular canals are located at 90° angles to each other, representing tilted X, Y, and Z axes.

Section through turn of cochlea

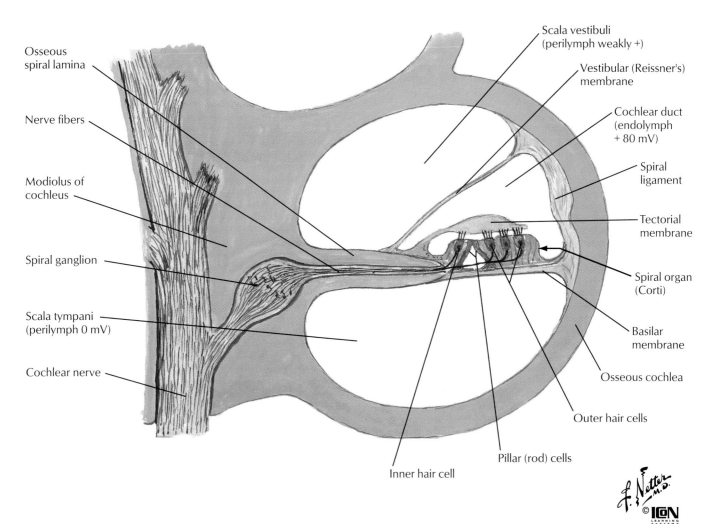

Osseous
spiral lamina

Nerve fibers

Modiolus of
cochleus

Spiral ganglion

Scala tympani
(perilymph 0 mV)

Cochlear nerve

Scala vestibuli
(perilymph weakly +)

Vestibular (Reissner's)
membrane

Cochlear duct
(endolymph
+ 80 mV)

Spiral
ligament

Tectorial
membrane

Spiral organ
(Corti)

Basilar
membrane

Osseous cochlea

Outer hair cells

Pillar (rod) cells

Inner hair cell

FIGURE III.13: VIII NERVE INNERVATION OF HAIR CELLS OF THE ORGAN OF CORTI

Primary sensory axons of the spiral (cochlear) ganglion innervate inner and outer hair cells of the organ of Corti, located on the basilar membrane. The axons are activated by release of neurotransmitters from the hair cells, which occurs when the hairs on the apical surface are moved by shearing forces from movement of the fluid basilar membrane in relation to the rigid tectorial membrane. This represents the complex transduction process of the converting external sound waves to action potentials in spiral ganglion axons.

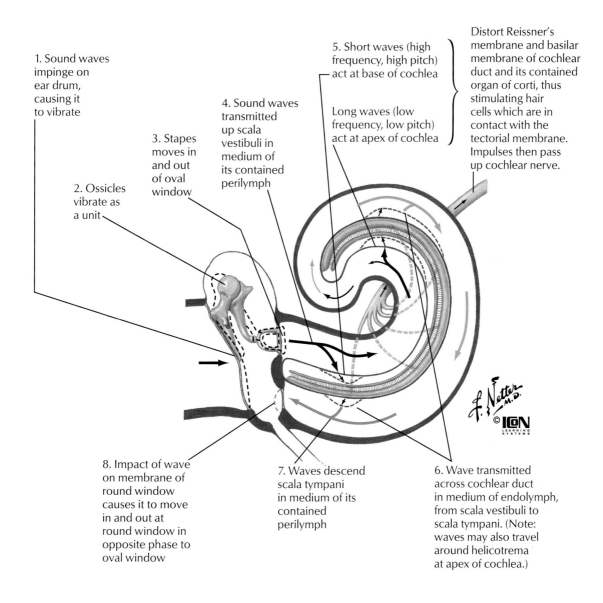

1. Sound waves impinge on ear drum, causing it to vibrate

2. Ossicles vibrate as a unit

3. Stapes moves in and out of oval window

4. Sound waves transmitted up scala vestibuli in medium of its contained perilymph

5. Short waves (high frequency, high pitch) act at base of cochlea

Long waves (low frequency, low pitch) act at apex of cochlea

Distort Reissner's membrane and basilar membrane of cochlear duct and its contained organ of corti, thus stimulating hair cells which are in contact with the tectorial membrane. Impulses then pass up cochlear nerve.

8. Impact of wave on membrane of round window causes it to move in and out at round window in opposite phase to oval window

7. Waves descend scala tympani in medium of its contained perilymph

6. Wave transmitted across cochlear duct in medium of endolymph, from scala vestibuli to scala tympani. (Note: waves may also travel around helicotrema at apex of cochlea.)

FIGURE III.14: COCHLEAR RECEPTORS

Fluid movement through the scala vestibuli, around the helicotrema, and back through the scala tympani moves the basilar membrane on which the organ of Corti and its hair cells reside differentially. Movement of hairs by shearing forces of the tectorial membrane on the apical portion of the hair cells results in their depolarization and in the release of neurotransmitters. This release stimulates action potentials in the primary afferent axons of spiral ganglion cells. Efferent axons from the olivocochlear bundle that can modulate the sensory transduction process and the excitability of hair cells are controlled by descending central auditory pathways.

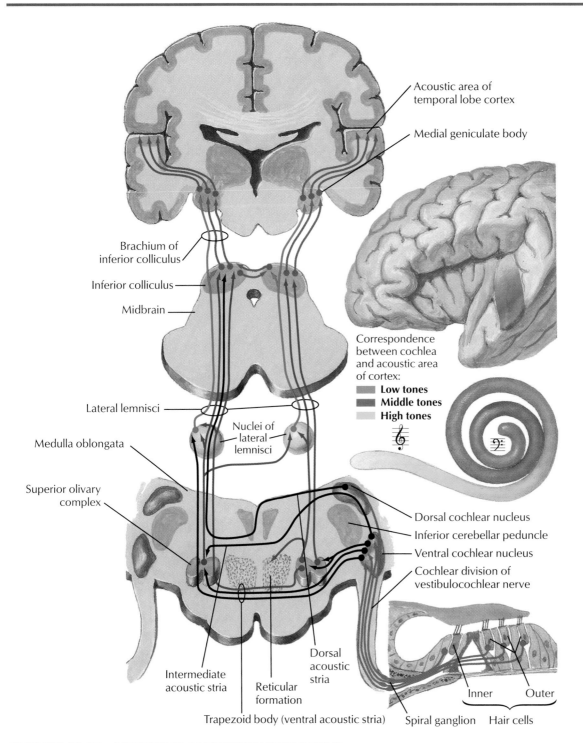

FIGURE III.15: AFFERENT AUDITORY PATHWAYS

Central axon projections of the spiral ganglion neurons terminate in dorsal and ventral cochlear nuclei in several tonotopic maps (shown in the cochlea in colors). These cochlear nuclei project into the lateral lemniscus (LL), via acoustic stria, but many projections remain ipsilateral. The LL terminates in the nucleus of the inferior colliculus. The inferior colliculus, in turn, projects via its brachium to the medial geniculate body (MGB) of the thalamus. The thalamus sends tonotopic projections to the primary auditory cortex on the transverse gyrus of Heschl. The accessory auditory brain stem nuclei (superior olivary nucleus for lateral sound localization, nuclei of the trapezoid body [not shown] and the LL) send crossed and uncrossed projections through the LL. Because sound is represented bilaterally, a unilateral lesion in the LL, the auditory thalamus, auditory radiations, or auditory cortex results in diminution in hearing and auditory neglect contralateral to simultaneous stimulation.

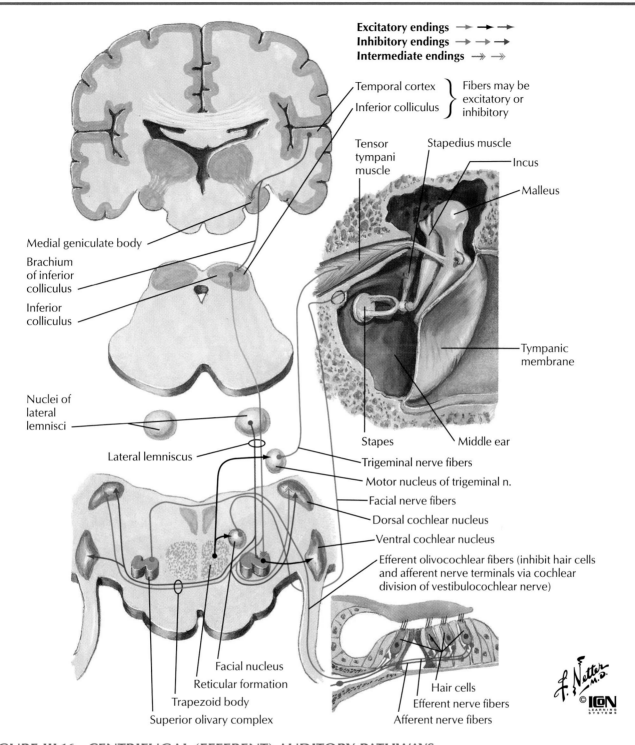

Excitatory endings
Inhibitory endings
Intermediate endings

Temporal cortex
Inferior colliculus
} Fibers may be
excitatory or
inhibitory

Tensor tympani muscle
Stapedius muscle
Incus
Malleus
Medial geniculate body
Brachium of inferior colliculus
Inferior colliculus
Tympanic membrane
Nuclei of lateral lemnisci
Lateral lemniscus
Stapes
Middle ear
Trigeminal nerve fibers
Motor nucleus of trigeminal n.
Facial nerve fibers
Dorsal cochlear nucleus
Ventral cochlear nucleus
Efferent olivocochlear fibers (inhibit hair cells and afferent nerve terminals via cochlear division of vestibulocochlear nerve)
Facial nucleus
Reticular formation
Trapezoid body
Superior olivary complex
Hair cells
Efferent nerve fibers
Afferent nerve fibers

FIGURE III.16: CENTRIFUGAL (EFFERENT) AUDITORY PATHWAYS

Descending pathways travel from the auditory cortex, the MGB of the thalamus, the inferior colliculus, and accessory auditory nuclei of the brain stem to caudal structures in the pathway to terminate in the cochlear nuclei and the superior olivary nucleus. These centrifugal connections permit descending control of incoming auditory information. The olivocochlear bundle from the superior olivary nuclei projects back to the hair cells in the organ of Corti to modulate the transduction process between the hair cells and the primary afferent axons. The motor nuclei of V and VII send LMN axonal projections to the tensor tympani and stapedius muscles, respectively, to dampen reflexes of the ossicles in response to sustained loud noise.

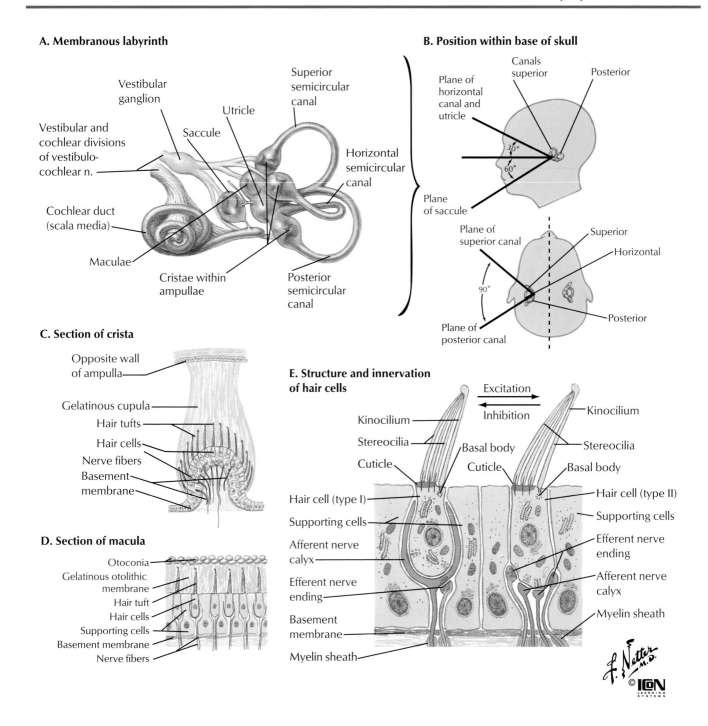

A. Membranous labyrinth

B. Position within base of skull

C. Section of crista

D. Section of macula

E. Structure and innervation of hair cells

FIGURE III.17: VESTIBULAR RECEPTORS

The vestibular receptors include hair cells in the cristae ampullaris of the utricle (linear acceleration or gravity) and saccule (low-frequency vibration) and in the maculae of the orthogonally oriented semicircular canals (angular acceleration or movement of the head). Hair tufts from the cristae ampullaris and the maculae are embedded in a gelatinous substance, which is moved by gravity (utricle) exerting force on the calcium carbonate crystals (otoliths) resting on top of the hairs, or by fluid in a semicircular canal (head movement). Bending of the kinocilium in the hair tufts depolarizes the hair cell, causing the release of neurotransmitters that stimulate action potentials of primary sensory axons of the vestibular (Scarpa's) ganglion. Additional efferent projections from the CNS modulate this transduction process.

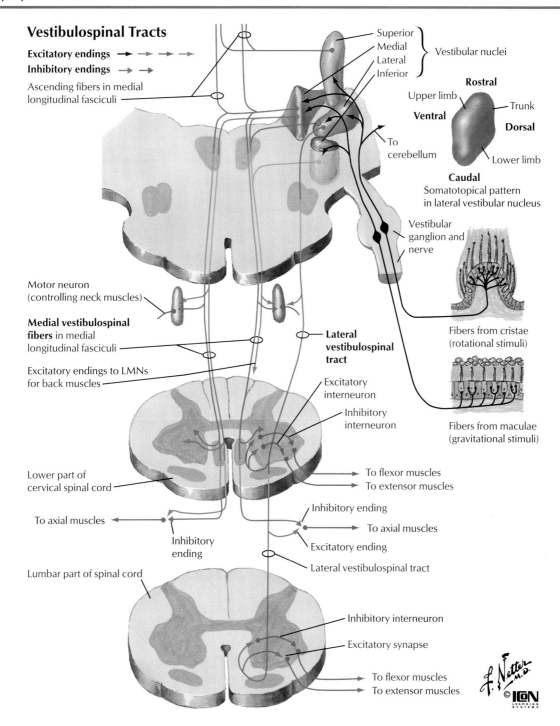

Vestibulospinal Tracts

Excitatory endings → → → →
Inhibitory endings → →

Ascending fibers in medial longitudinal fasciculi

Superior
Medial
Lateral
Inferior } Vestibular nuclei

Rostral
Upper limb
Ventral   **Dorsal**

Lower limb

Caudal
Somatotopical pattern in lateral vestibular nucleus

To cerebellum

Vestibular ganglion and nerve

Fibers from cristae (rotational stimuli)

Fibers from maculae (gravitational stimuli)

Motor neuron (controlling neck muscles)

Medial vestibulospinal fibers in medial longitudinal fasciculi

Excitatory endings to LMNs for back muscles

Lateral vestibulospinal tract

Excitatory interneuron

Inhibitory interneuron

Lower part of cervical spinal cord

To flexor muscles
To extensor muscles

To axial muscles

Inhibitory ending

Inhibitory ending

To axial muscles

Excitatory ending

Lateral vestibulospinal tract

Lumbar part of spinal cord

Inhibitory interneuron

Excitatory synapse

To flexor muscles
To extensor muscles

FIGURE III.18: VESTIBULAR PATHWAYS

Primary afferent vestibular axons from the vestibular ganglion terminate in the superior, inferior, medial, and lateral vestibular nuclei and directly in the cerebellum (deep nuclei and cortex). Descending axons are sent from the medial vestibulospinal tract (medial nucleus) to spinal cord LMNs to regulate head and neck movements. Descending axons are sent from the lateral vestibulospinal tract (lateral nucleus) to all levels of spinal cord LMNs to activate extensor movements. Multiple vestibular nuclei project to the cerebellum to modulate and coordinate muscle activity for basic tone and posture (shown in figure III.45) and to extraocular LMNs via the medial longitudinal fasciculus to coordinate eye movements with head and neck movements. Some ascending axons from the vestibular nuclei may reach the thalamus (near VPM and posterior nuclei), with projections to the lateral postcentral gyrus (area 2, motion perception and spatial orientation) and the insular and temporoparietal cortices.

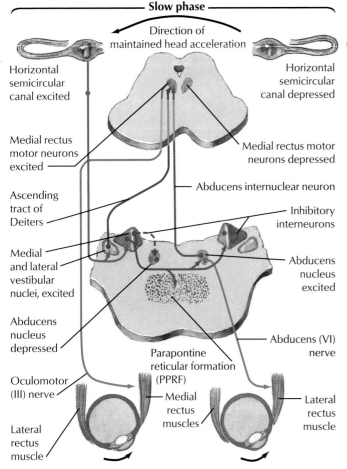

Eyes move in opposite direction to head; tend to preserve visual fixation: rate determined by degree of horizontal canal excitation

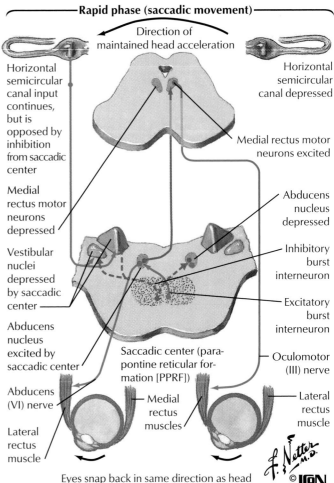

Eyes snap back in same direction as head

FIGURE III.19: NYSTAGMUS

Nystagmus, the alternating back-and-forth movements of the eye, requires central coordination of extraocular LMNs and eye movements. Optokinetic nystagmus, the visually activated movement of the eyes via tracking mechanisms, allows the eyes to return to a forward position by visual association cortex projections through the superior colliculus to extraocular LMNs. Vestibular nystagmus involves vestibular projections via the medial longitudinal fasciculus to extraocular nuclei (LMNs). The slow phase (or drift) of vestibular nystagmus results in the provocation of eye movements as if the head were turning. It is caused by asymmetrical input from receptors of the semicircular canals or from damage to vestibular nuclei or the vestibular cerebellum. The fast phase (saccadic movement) is the provoked return to a forward position.

Horizontal section

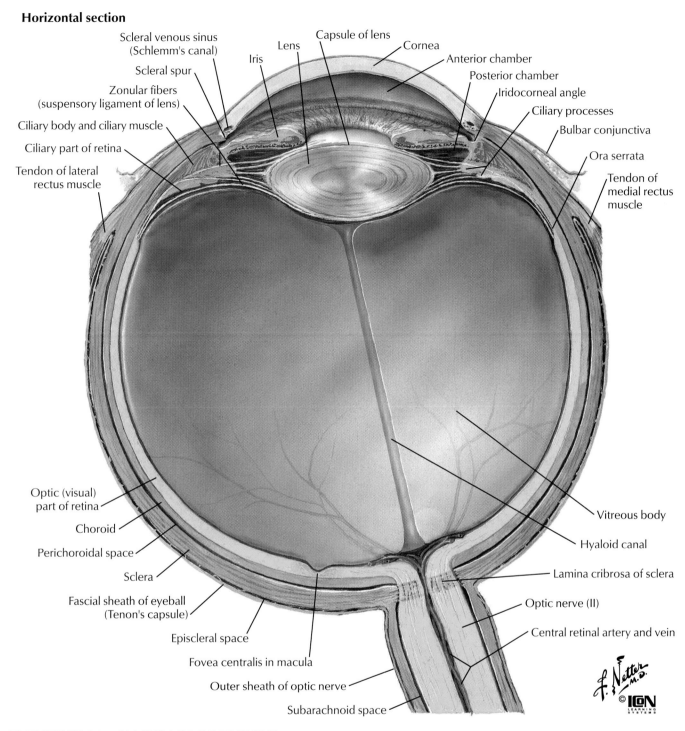

Scleral venous sinus (Schlemm's canal)
Scleral spur
Zonular fibers (suspensory ligament of lens)
Ciliary body and ciliary muscle
Ciliary part of retina
Tendon of lateral rectus muscle
Iris
Lens
Capsule of lens
Cornea
Anterior chamber
Posterior chamber
Iridocorneal angle
Ciliary processes
Bulbar conjunctiva
Ora serrata
Tendon of medial rectus muscle
Optic (visual) part of retina
Choroid
Perichoroidal space
Sclera
Fascial sheath of eyeball (Tenon's capsule)
Episcleral space
Fovea centralis in macula
Outer sheath of optic nerve
Subarachnoid space
Vitreous body
Hyaloid canal
Lamina cribrosa of sclera
Optic nerve (II)
Central retinal artery and vein

FIGURE III.20: ANATOMY OF THE EYE

There are 3 major layers of the eye. The outer layer, the fibrous tunic, consists of the protective cornea (transparent) and sclera (opaque). The middle layer, the vascular tunic (uveal tract), consists of the choroid, the ciliary body, and the iris. The transparent biconvex lens surrounded by a capsule of zonular fibers is suspended from the ciliary process of the ciliary body. The inner layer, the internal tunic, consists of the neuroretina, the nonpigment epithelium of the ciliary body, and the pigment epithelium of the posterior iris. The retina contains the photoreceptors for transduction of photon energy into neuronal activity. Aqueous humor is secreted from blood vessels of the iris into the posterior chamber and flows through the pupil into the anterior chamber, where it is absorbed into the trabecular meshwork into Schlemm's canal at the iridocorneal angle. Glaucoma results when absorption of aqueous humor is blocked. Vitreous humor fills the interior of the eyeball.

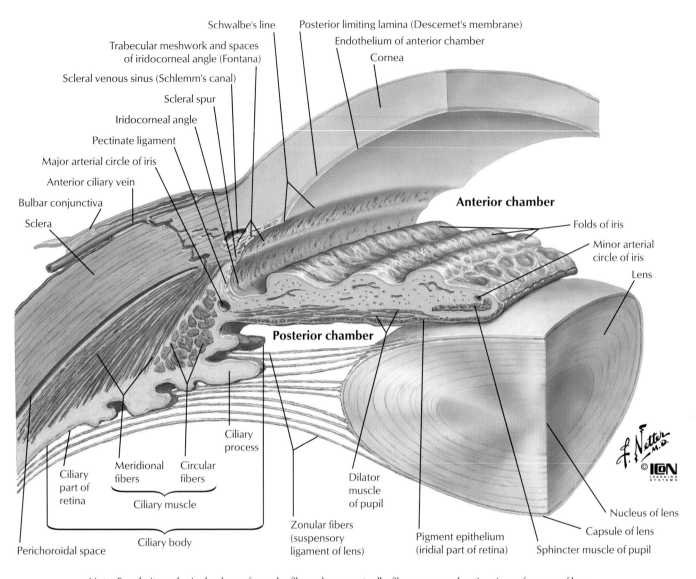

Schwalbe's line
Trabecular meshwork and spaces of iridocorneal angle (Fontana)
Scleral venous sinus (Schlemm's canal)
Scleral spur
Iridocorneal angle
Pectinate ligament
Major arterial circle of iris
Anterior ciliary vein
Bulbar conjunctiva
Sclera

Posterior limiting lamina (Descemet's membrane)
Endothelium of anterior chamber
Cornea

Anterior chamber

Folds of iris
Minor arterial circle of iris
Lens

Posterior chamber

Ciliary process

Ciliary part of retina
Meridional fibers
Circular fibers
Ciliary muscle
Perichoroidal space
Ciliary body

Dilator muscle of pupil
Zonular fibers (suspensory ligament of lens)
Pigment epithelium (iridial part of retina)

Nucleus of lens
Capsule of lens
Sphincter muscle of pupil

Note: For clarity, only single plane of zonular fibers shown; actually, fibers surround entire circumference of lens

FIGURE III.21: ANTERIOR AND POSTERIOR CHAMBERS OF THE EYE

The ciliary muscle and the pupillary constrictor muscle are supplied by parasympathetic postganglionic M nerve fibers from the ciliary ganglion (preganglionics in the Edinger-Westphal nucleus, axons in CN III). Ciliary muscle contraction reduces the tension on zonular fibers and causes the lens to curve, which induces accommodation for near vision. In the pupillary light reflex, light shone in one eye enters the CNS via the optic nerve (CN II) (afferent limb) and terminates in the pretectum. Neurons of the pretectum project bilaterally (crossed axons through the posterior commissure) to the Edinger-Westphal nucleus. This nucleus projects to the ciliary ganglion via CN III (efferent limb), which results in both direct (ipsilateral) and consensual (contralateral) pupillary constriction. The pupillary dilator muscle is supplied by sympathetic postganglionic UNM nerve fibers from the superior cervical ganglion (preganglionics in T1 and T2).

M = myelinated; UNM = unmyelinated.

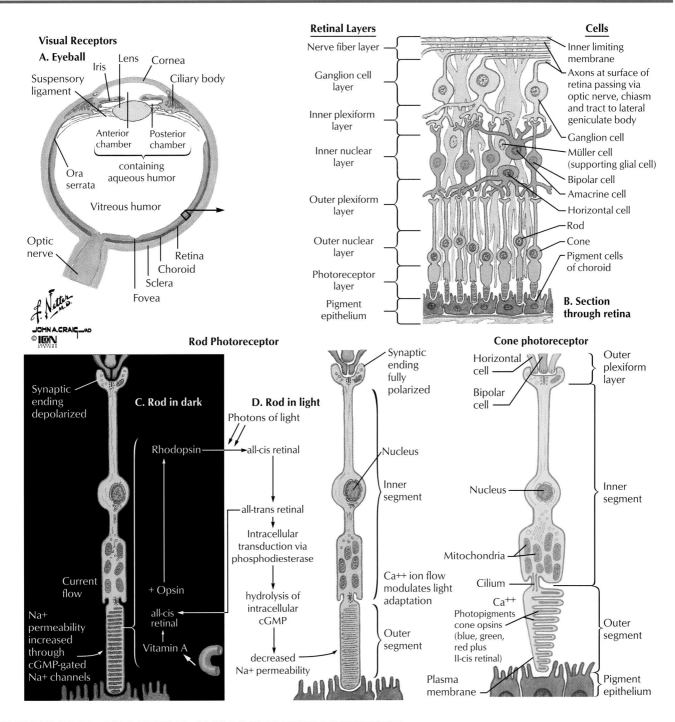

FIGURE III.22: THE RETINA AND THE PHOTORECEPTORS

The retina, a tissue-thin piece of CNS containing the photoreceptors, is attached to the vascular tunic at the ora serrata. The outer segments (rods and cones) of the photoreceptors are embedded in a pigment epithelium to prevent backscatter in the outer part of the retina. The rods and cones connect synaptically with bipolar cells, which in turn connect with the ganglion cells of the retina (equivalent of secondary sensory nuclei). Horizontal and amacrine cells provide horizontal interconnections in the retina. In the macula (3 mm in diameter), the fovea centralis (0.4 mm in diameter), the central point for visual focusing, consists of cones for color vision (photopic), which project, with very little convergence, to ganglion cells. The peripheral retinal photoreceptors, mainly rods for night vision (scotopic), project, with great convergence, to ganglion cells. Rod light transduction involves conversion of ll-cis-retinal (from rhodopsin) to an all-trans form, provoking calcium influx with hyperpolarization and a decrease in sodium conductance.

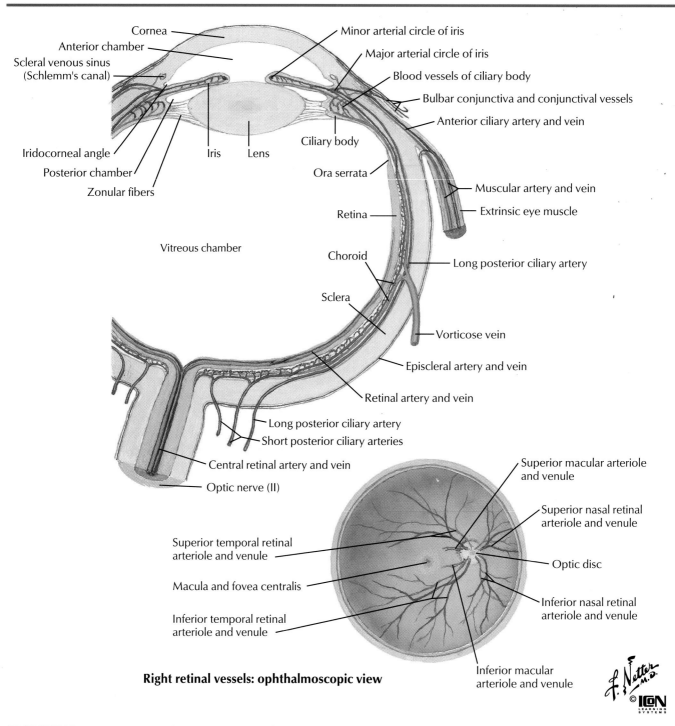

Cornea
Anterior chamber
Scleral venous sinus (Schlemm's canal)
Iridocorneal angle
Posterior chamber
Zonular fibers
Iris
Lens
Vitreous chamber
Minor arterial circle of iris
Major arterial circle of iris
Blood vessels of ciliary body
Bulbar conjunctiva and conjunctival vessels
Anterior ciliary artery and vein
Ciliary body
Ora serrata
Muscular artery and vein
Extrinsic eye muscle
Retina
Choroid
Long posterior ciliary artery
Sclera
Vorticose vein
Episcleral artery and vein
Retinal artery and vein
Long posterior ciliary artery
Short posterior ciliary arteries
Central retinal artery and vein
Optic nerve (II)

Superior temporal retinal arteriole and venule
Macula and fovea centralis
Inferior temporal retinal arteriole and venule
Superior macular arteriole and venule
Superior nasal retinal arteriole and venule
Optic disc
Inferior nasal retinal arteriole and venule
Inferior macular arteriole and venule

Right retinal vessels: ophthalmoscopic view

FIGURE III.23: ARTERIES AND VEINS OF THE EYE

The central retinal artery and its branches supply blood to the retina. This arterial system, derived from the ophthalmic artery (the first branch off the internal carotid artery), is often the site where ischemic or embolic events (transient ischemic attacks) herald the presence of serious vascular disease. Ciliary arteries supply the middle vascular tunic, which also contributes blood to the retina. Blood supply to the retina can be disrupted if the retina becomes detached. Vessels enter and exit the retina at the optic disk (nerve head), located nasally and slightly inferiorly from the geometric midpoint of the eyeball. The macula is located temporally and slightly inferiorly from this midpoint.

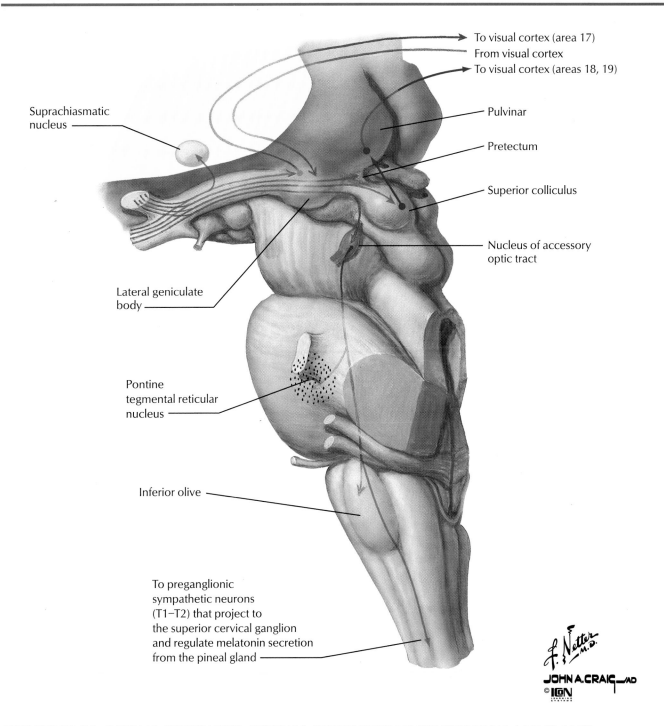

To visual cortex (area 17)
From visual cortex
To visual cortex (areas 18, 19)

Suprachiasmatic nucleus

Pulvinar

Pretectum

Superior colliculus

Nucleus of accessory optic tract

Lateral geniculate body

Pontine tegmental reticular nucleus

Inferior olive

To preganglionic sympathetic neurons (T1–T2) that project to the superior cervical ganglion and regulate melatonin secretion from the pineal gland

JOHN A. CRAIG—AD
© ICN

FIGURE III.24: VISUAL PATHWAYS: RETINAL PROJECTIONS TO THE THALAMUS AND THE BRAIN STEM

Retinal projections travel through the optic nerve, chiasm, and tract and terminate in several regions. The lateral geniculate body mediates conscious interpretation of visual input. The superior colliculus, a second pathway through the pulvinar to the associative visual cortex, provides localizing information for visual stimuli. It also provides descending contralateral connections (tectospinal tract) to cervical LMNs to mediate reflex visual effects on head and neck movements. The pretectum mediates the pupillary light reflex. The suprachiasmatic nucleus of the hypothalamus integrates light flux and regulates circadian rhythms and diurnal cycles. The nucleus of the inferior accessory optic tract may help to mediate brain stem responses for visual tracking and may interconnect with sympathetic preganglionic neurons in T1 and T2 (regulating the superior cervical ganglion).

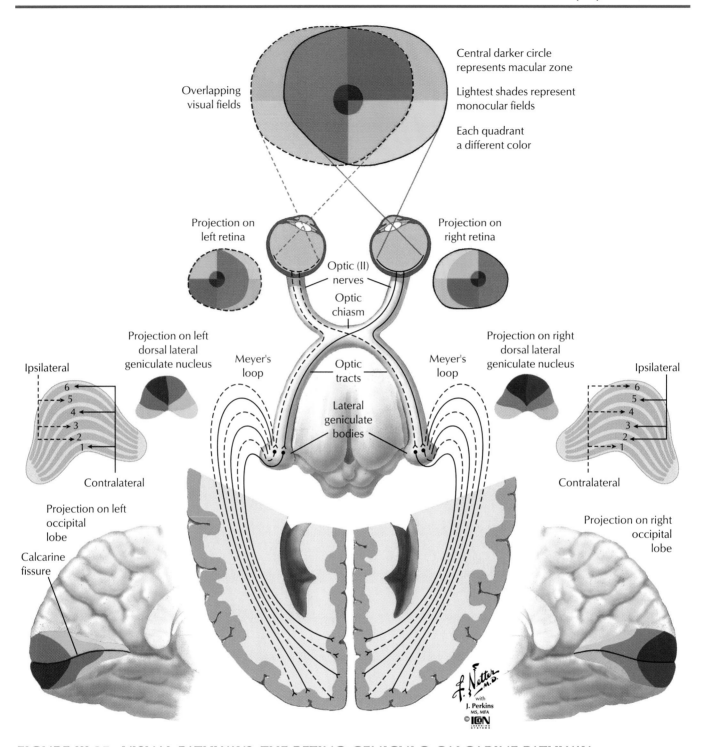

Overlapping visual fields

Central darker circle represents macular zone

Lightest shades represent monocular fields

Each quadrant a different color

Projection on left retina

Projection on right retina

Optic (II) nerves

Optic chiasm

Projection on left dorsal lateral geniculate nucleus

Projection on right dorsal lateral geniculate nucleus

Ipsilateral

Ipsilateral

Meyer's loop

Meyer's loop

Optic tracts

Lateral geniculate bodies

Contralateral

Contralateral

Projection on left occipital lobe

Projection on right occipital lobe

Calcarine fissure

FIGURE III.25: VISUAL PATHWAYS: THE RETINO-GENICULO-CALCARINE PATHWAY

This visual pathway conveys information for fine-grained conscious visual analysis of the outside world. It is organized topographically (retinotopic) through its course to the calcarine cortex in the occipital lobe. The nasal hemiretinal ganglion cell axons cross the midline in the optic chiasm, whereas the temporal hemiretinal ganglion cell axons remain ipsilateral. Thus, each optic tract conveys information from the contralateral visual field, and damage produces a contralateral hemianopia.

The optic tracts terminate in the lateral geniculate body or nucleus, which is organized in 6 layers. The optic radiations project to the calcarine (striate) cortex (area 17). The portion of the optic radiations that loops through the temporal lobe (Meyer's loop) can be damaged by a tumor or mass; such damage results in a contralateral upper quadrantanopia (quadrant deficit). Bilateral convergence from the right and left retinas takes place first in the primary visual cortex, area 17.

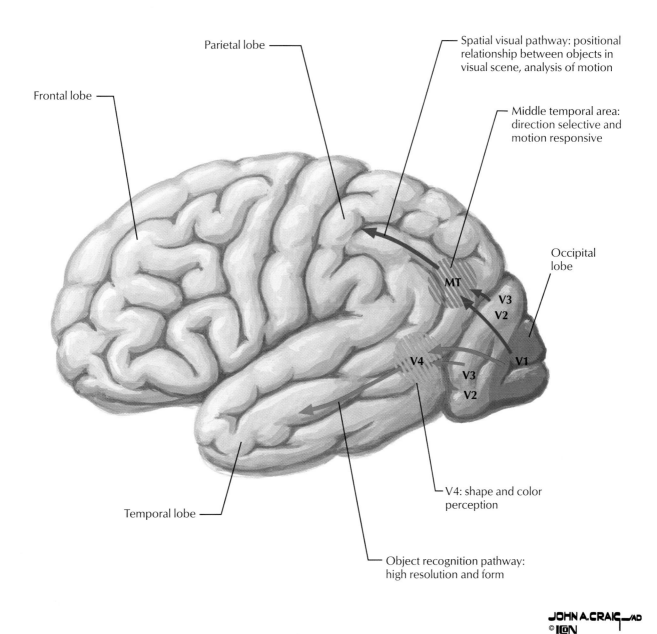

Parietal lobe

Spatial visual pathway: positional relationship between objects in visual scene, analysis of motion

Frontal lobe

Middle temporal area: direction selective and motion responsive

Occipital lobe

MT

V3
V2

V4

V3
V2

V1

V4: shape and color perception

Temporal lobe

Object recognition pathway: high resolution and form

JOHN A. CRAIG—AD
© IGN

FIGURE III.26: VISUAL PATHWAYS IN THE PARIETAL AND TEMPORAL LOBES

Neurons in the primary visual cortex (V1, area 17) send axons to the association visual cortex (V2 and V3, areas 18 and 19). V2 and V3 also receive input from the superior colliculus via the pulvinar. V1, V2, and V3 project to the middle temporal area and V4. Middle temporal neurons are direction selective and motion responsive and further project into the parietal lobe for spatial visual processing.

The parietal neurons provide analysis of motion and of positional relationships between objects in the visual field. V4 neurons are involved in shape and color perception. V4 projects into the temporal lobe, in which neurons provide high-resolution object recognition, including faces, animate objects, and classification and orientation of objects.

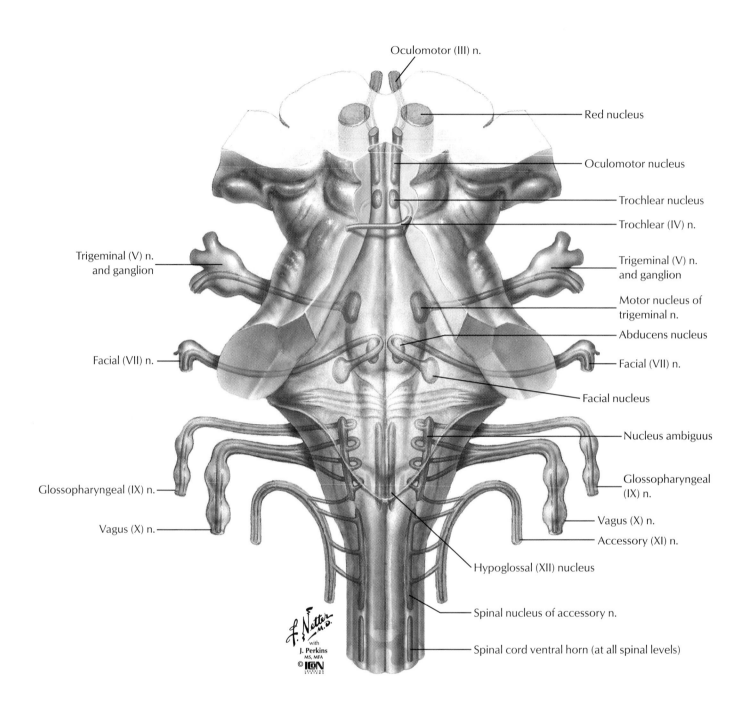

Oculomotor (III) n.

Red nucleus

Oculomotor nucleus

Trochlear nucleus

Trochlear (IV) n.

Trigeminal (V) n. and ganglion

Trigeminal (V) n. and ganglion

Motor nucleus of trigeminal n.

Abducens nucleus

Facial (VII) n.

Facial (VII) n.

Facial nucleus

Nucleus ambiguus

Glossopharyngeal (IX) n.

Glossopharyngeal (IX) n.

Vagus (X) n.

Vagus (X) n.

Accessory (XI) n.

Hypoglossal (XII) nucleus

Spinal nucleus of accessory n.

Spinal cord ventral horn (at all spinal levels)

FIGURE III.27: LOWER MOTOR NEURON DISTRIBUTION IN THE SPINAL CORD AND THE BRAIN STEM

Lower motor neurons (LMNs) are found in the ventral (anterior) horn at all levels of the spinal cord and in motor cranial nerve nuclei in the medulla, pons, and the midbrain. These LMNs send axons into the ventral root and then into spinal nerves from the spinal cord ventral horn, and into cranial nerves from the brain stem. The LMN axons terminate as neuromuscular junctions on skeletal muscle fibers.

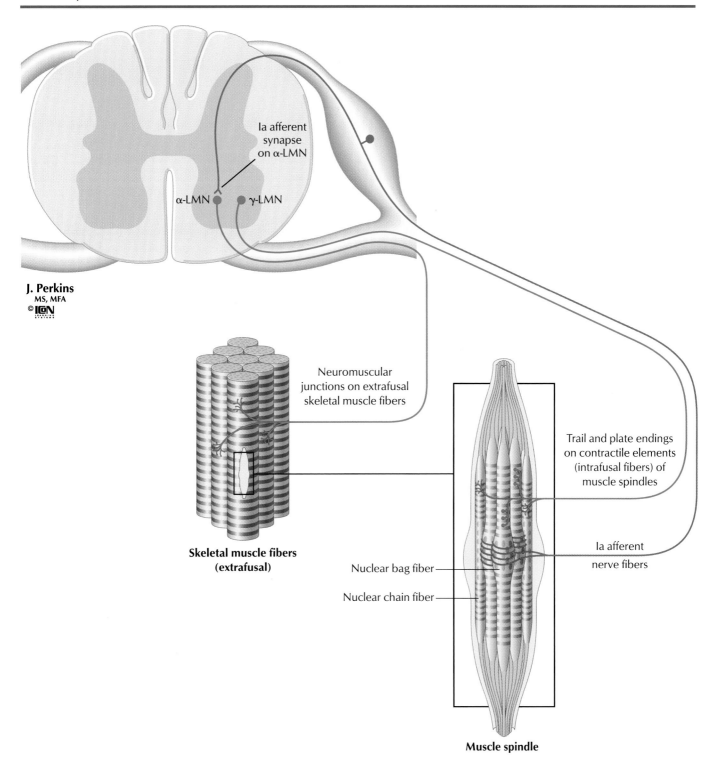

J. Perkins
MS, MFA
©ICN

Ia afferent
synapse
on α-LMN

α-LMN   γ-LMN

Neuromuscular
junctions on extrafusal
skeletal muscle fibers

Skeletal muscle fibers
(extrafusal)

Trail and plate endings
on contractile elements
(intrafusal fibers) of
muscle spindles

Ia afferent
nerve fibers

Nuclear bag fiber

Nuclear chain fiber

Muscle spindle

FIGURE III.28: ALPHA AND GAMMA LOWER MOTOR NEURONS

All LMN groups, except the facial nerve nucleus that supplies the muscles of facial expression, contain both alpha motor neurons (α-LMNs) that supply the skeletal muscle fibers (extrafusal fibers) and gamma motor neurons (γ-LMNs) that supply the small contractile elements of muscle spindles (intrafusal fibers). The muscles of facial expression do not have muscle spindles and are not supplied by γ-LMNs. The α-LMNs regulate contraction of the skeletal muscles to produce movement. The γ-LMNs regulate the sensitivity of the muscle spindles for Ia and group II afferent modulation of α-LMN excitability.

Cerebral Cortex: Efferent Pathways

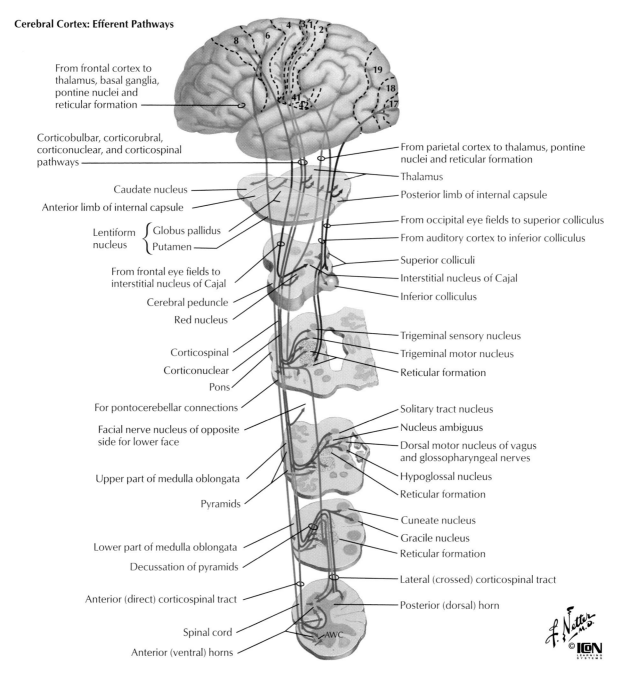

From frontal cortex to thalamus, basal ganglia, pontine nuclei and reticular formation

Corticobulbar, corticorubral, corticonuclear, and corticospinal pathways

Caudate nucleus

Anterior limb of internal capsule

Lentiform nucleus { Globus pallidus / Putamen }

From frontal eye fields to interstitial nucleus of Cajal

Cerebral peduncle

Red nucleus

Corticospinal

Corticonuclear

Pons

For pontocerebellar connections

Facial nerve nucleus of opposite side for lower face

Upper part of medulla oblongata

Pyramids

Lower part of medulla oblongata

Decussation of pyramids

Anterior (direct) corticospinal tract

Spinal cord

Anterior (ventral) horns

From parietal cortex to thalamus, pontine nuclei and reticular formation

Thalamus

Posterior limb of internal capsule

From occipital eye fields to superior colliculus

From auditory cortex to inferior colliculus

Superior colliculi

Interstitial nucleus of Cajal

Inferior colliculus

Trigeminal sensory nucleus

Trigeminal motor nucleus

Reticular formation

Solitary tract nucleus

Nucleus ambiguus

Dorsal motor nucleus of vagus and glossopharyngeal nerves

Hypoglossal nucleus

Reticular formation

Cuneate nucleus

Gracile nucleus

Reticular formation

Lateral (crossed) corticospinal tract

Posterior (dorsal) horn

AWC

FIGURE III.29: CORTICAL EFFERENT PATHWAYS

Neurons in the motor cortex (area 4) and the supplemental and premotor cortices (area 6) send axons to the basal ganglia (caudate nucleus and putamen), the thalamus (ventroanterior [VA] and ventrolateral [VL] nuclei), the red nucleus, pontine nuclei, motor cranial nerve nuclei on both sides, and the spinal cord ventral horn mainly on the contralateral side. These axons form the corticospinal tract, the corticobulbar tract, corticostriate projections, corticopontine projections, corticothalamic projections, and cortical connections to upper motor neurons (UMNs) of the brain stem (reticular formation [RF], red nucleus, superior colliculus).

Neurons of the sensory cortex (areas 3, 1, 2) send axons mainly to secondary sensory nuclei to regulate incoming lemniscal sensory projections destined for conscious interpretation. Neurons in the frontal eye fields (area 8) project to the superior colliculus, the horizontal and vertical gaze centers of the brain stem, and the interstitial nucleus of Cajal to coordinate voluntary eye movements and associated head movements. Other regions of the sensory cortex project axons to thalamic and brain stem structures that regulate incoming lemniscal sensory information.

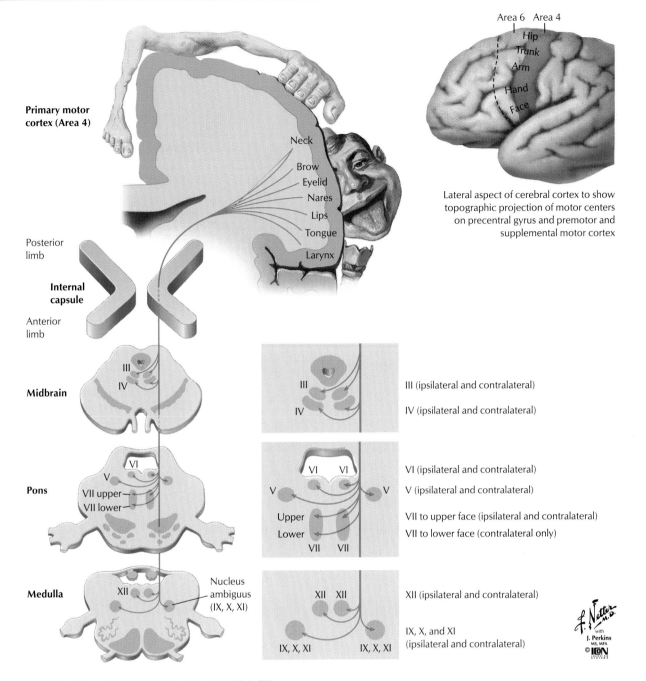

Area 6 Area 4
Hip
Trunk
Arm
Hand
Face

Lateral aspect of cerebral cortex to show topographic projection of motor centers on precentral gyrus and premotor and supplemental motor cortex

Primary motor cortex (Area 4)

Neck
Brow
Eyelid
Nares
Lips
Tongue
Larynx

Posterior limb
Internal capsule
Anterior limb

Midbrain
III
IV

III (ipsilateral and contralateral)
IV (ipsilateral and contralateral)

Pons
VI
V
VII upper
VII lower

VI (ipsilateral and contralateral)
V (ipsilateral and contralateral)
VII to upper face (ipsilateral and contralateral)
VII to lower face (contralateral only)

Upper
Lower

Medulla
XII
Nucleus ambiguus (IX, X, XI)

XII (ipsilateral and contralateral)
IX, X, and XI (ipsilateral and contralateral)

FIGURE III.30: CORTICOBULBAR TRACT

The corticobulbar tract (CBT) arises mainly from the lateral portion of the primary motor cortex (area 4). CBT axons project through the genu of the internal capsule into the cerebral peduncle, the basis pontis, and the medullary pyramids on the ipsilateral side. The axons distribute to motor cranial nerve nuclei on the ipsilateral and contralateral sides, except for the portion of the facial nerve (CN VII) nucleus that supplies the muscles of facial expression for the lower face, which receive contralateral projections exclusively. CBT projections to the hypoglossal nucleus are mainly contralateral; projections to the spinal accessory nucleus are mainly ipsilateral. In contrast to Bell's palsy (CN VII palsy), in which the entire ipsilateral face is paralyzed, CBT lesions result mainly in a contralateral drooping lower face that is paretic to voluntary commands (central facial palsy).

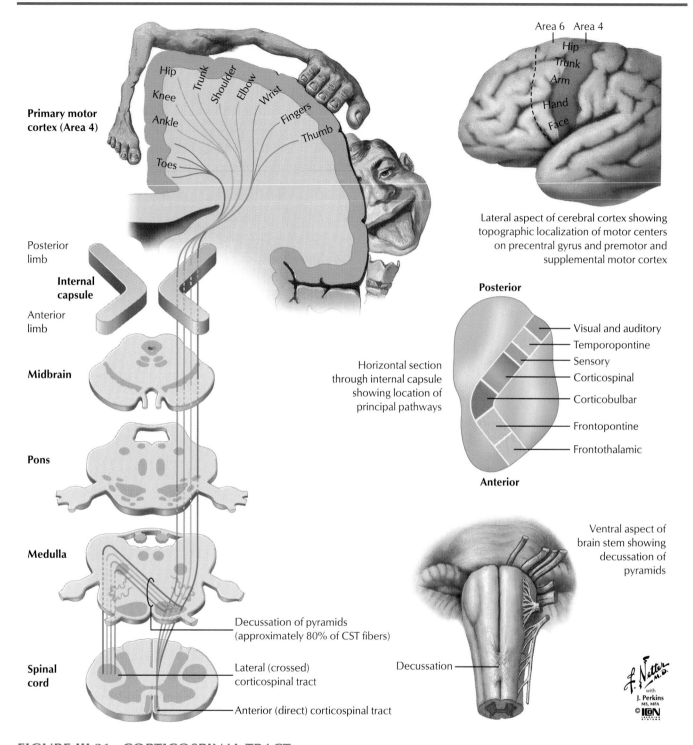

Lateral aspect of cerebral cortex showing
topographic localization of motor centers
on precentral gyrus and premotor and
supplemental motor cortex

Horizontal section
through internal capsule
showing location of
principal pathways

Ventral aspect of
brain stem showing
decussation of
pyramids

FIGURE III.31: CORTICOSPINAL TRACT

The motor portion of the corticospinal tract (CST) originates from neurons of many sizes mainly from the primary motor cortex (area 4) and the supplemental and premotor cortices (area 6). The primary sensory cortex (areas 3, 1, 2) contributes axons to the CST that terminate mainly in secondary sensory nuclei to regulate incoming lemniscal sensory information processing. The CST travels through the posterior limb of the internal capsule, the cerebral peduncle, the basis pontis, and the medullary

pyramid on the ipsilateral side. Most CST axons decussate in the decussation of the pyramids at the medullary–spinal cord junction and descend in the lateral CST to synapse on α-LMNs and γ-LMNs both directly and indirectly through interneurons. CST axons that do not decussate continue as the anterior CST and then decussate at the appropriate level to terminate directly and indirectly on LMNs contralateral to the cells of origin.

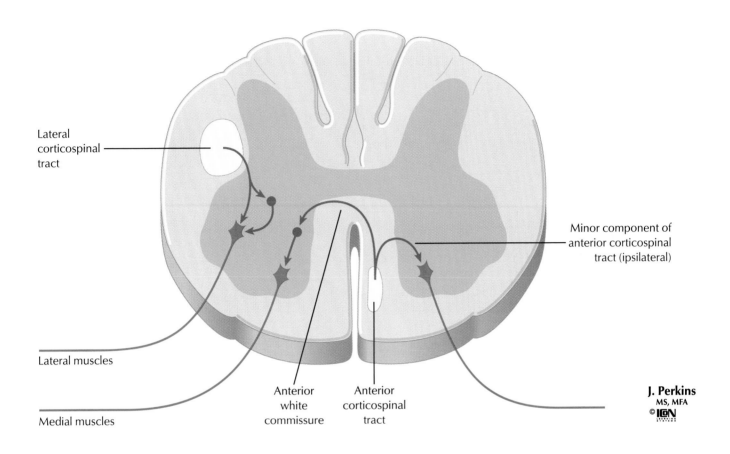

Lateral corticospinal tract

Minor component of anterior corticospinal tract (ipsilateral)

Lateral muscles

Medial muscles

Anterior white commissure

Anterior corticospinal tract

J. Perkins
MS, MFA
©ICN

FIGURE III.32: CORTICOSPINAL TRACT TERMINATIONS IN THE SPINAL CORD

Crossed CST axons in the lateral CST, intermixed with axons of the rubrospinal tract, travel in the lateral funiculus. Most of these CST axons terminate directly and indirectly on LMNs associated with distal musculature, especially for skilled hand and finger movements. The uncrossed anterior CST axons decussate predominantly in the anterior white commissure and terminate directly and indirectly mainly on LMNs that supply medial musculature. A small number of anterior CST axons terminate ipsilateral to the cortical cells of origin. An isolated lesion of the CST in the medullary pyramids results in weakness of contralateral fine hand and finger movements. All lesions involving the CST intermixed with other descending motor systems (internal capsule, cerebral peduncle, pons) produce contralateral spastic hemiplegia with hypertonia, hyperreflexia, and a plantar extensor response. Lesions of the lateral CST produce similar symptoms ipsilaterally below the level of the lesion.

245

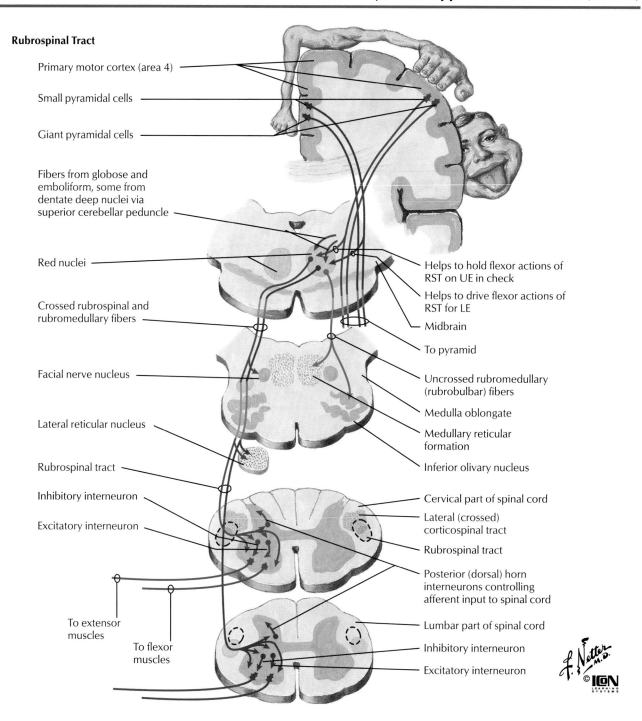

Rubrospinal Tract

- Primary motor cortex (area 4)
- Small pyramidal cells
- Giant pyramidal cells
- Fibers from globose and emboliform, some from dentate deep nuclei via superior cerebellar peduncle
- Red nuclei
- Crossed rubrospinal and rubromedullary fibers
- Facial nerve nucleus
- Lateral reticular nucleus
- Rubrospinal tract
- Inhibitory interneuron
- Excitatory interneuron
- To extensor muscles
- To flexor muscles

- Helps to hold flexor actions of RST on UE in check
- Helps to drive flexor actions of RST for LE
- Midbrain
- To pyramid
- Uncrossed rubromedullary (rubrobulbar) fibers
- Medulla oblongate
- Medullary reticular formation
- Inferior olivary nucleus
- Cervical part of spinal cord
- Lateral (crossed) corticospinal tract
- Rubrospinal tract
- Posterior (dorsal) horn interneurons controlling afferent input to spinal cord
- Lumbar part of spinal cord
- Inhibitory interneuron
- Excitatory interneuron

FIGURE III.33: RUBROSPINAL TRACT

The red nucleus receives ipsilateral topographical input from the motor cortex and functions as an indirect corticospinal system. Axons of the rubrospinal tract (RST) decussate in the ventral tegmental decussation and descend in the lateral brain stem and the lateral funiculus of the spinal cord, where they are intermixed extensively with axons of the lateral CST. The RST terminates directly and indirectly on α-LMNs and γ-LMNs in the spinal cord, particularly those associated with flexor movements of the extremities. The RST helps to drive flexor movements for the lower extremity but helps to hold flexor movements in check for the upper extremity. RST lesions usually occur in conjunction with the CST in the spinal cord; corticorubral lesions also occur in conjunction with the CST in the internal capsule and the cerebral peduncle. These lesions result in contralateral spastic hemiplegia. Brain stem lesions caudal to the red nucleus result in decerebration (extensor spasticity).

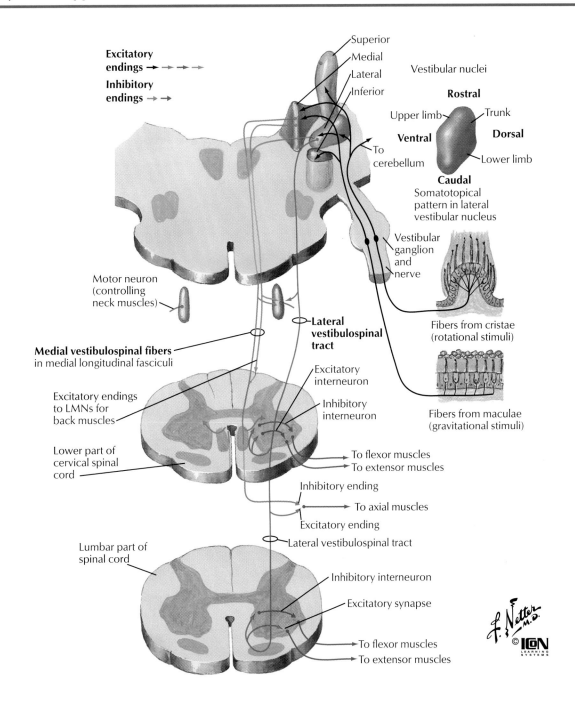

Excitatory endings → ⇢ ⇢ ⇢
Inhibitory endings ⇢ →

Superior
Medial
Lateral
Inferior
Vestibular nuclei

Rostral
Upper limb — Trunk
Ventral — **Dorsal**
Lower limb
Caudal
Somatotopical pattern in lateral vestibular nucleus

To cerebellum

Vestibular ganglion and nerve

Fibers from cristae (rotational stimuli)

Fibers from maculae (gravitational stimuli)

Motor neuron (controlling neck muscles)

Lateral vestibulospinal tract

Medial vestibulospinal fibers in medial longitudinal fasciculi

Excitatory interneuron

Inhibitory interneuron

Excitatory endings to LMNs for back muscles

Lower part of cervical spinal cord

To flexor muscles
To extensor muscles

Inhibitory ending

To axial muscles

Excitatory ending

Lateral vestibulospinal tract

Lumbar part of spinal cord

Inhibitory interneuron

Excitatory synapse

To flexor muscles
To extensor muscles

FIGURE III.34: VESTIBULOSPINAL TRACTS

The lateral vestibulospinal tract (LVST) arises from the lateral vestibular nucleus (LVN) and terminates directly and indirectly on ipsilateral α-LMNs and γ-LMNs associated with extensor musculature, especially proximal musculature. If this powerful antigravity extensor system were not kept in check by descending connections from the red nucleus and the cerebellum, it would produce a constant state of extensor hypertonia. The medial vestibulospinal tract (MVST) arises from the medial vestibular nucleus (MVN) to provide inhibition of the α-LMNs and the γ-LMNs that control neck and axial musculature. The MVST terminates mainly on interneurons in the cervical spinal cord ventral horn. These 2 vestibulospinal tracts stabilize and coordinate the position of the head, the neck, and the body and provide important reflex and brain stem control over tone and posture. The vestibulospinal tracts work with the reticulospinal tracts to control tone and posture.

Reticulospinal and Corticoreticular Pathways

Thickness of blue line indicates density of cortical projection

Parietal
Frontal
Orbito-frontal

6 4 3,1,2

Excitatory endings → → →

Inhibitory endings → →

Occipital

Temporal

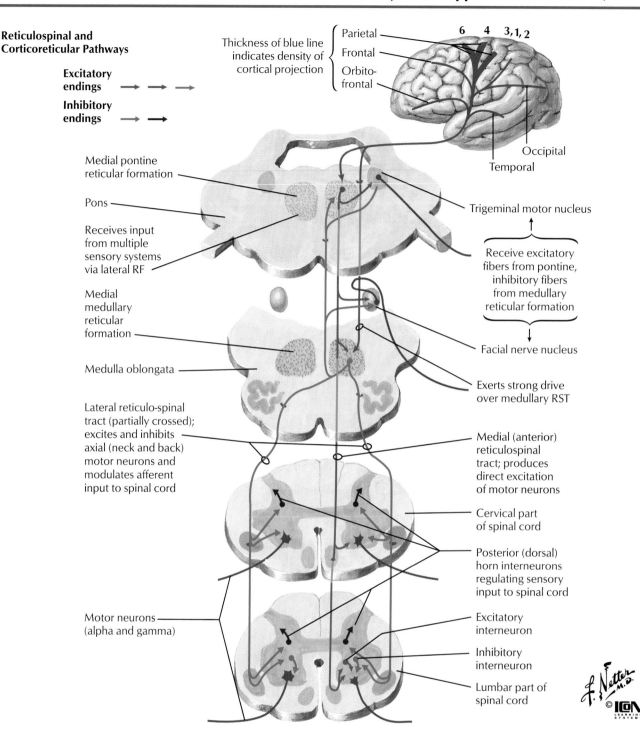

Medial pontine reticular formation

Pons

Receives input from multiple sensory systems via lateral RF

Medial medullary reticular formation

Medulla oblongata

Lateral reticulo-spinal tract (partially crossed); excites and inhibits axial (neck and back) motor neurons and modulates afferent input to spinal cord

Motor neurons (alpha and gamma)

Trigeminal motor nucleus

Receive excitatory fibers from pontine, inhibitory fibers from medullary reticular formation

Facial nerve nucleus

Exerts strong drive over medullary RST

Medial (anterior) reticulospinal tract; produces direct excitation of motor neurons

Cervical part of spinal cord

Posterior (dorsal) horn interneurons regulating sensory input to spinal cord

Excitatory interneuron

Inhibitory interneuron

Lumbar part of spinal cord

FIGURE III.35: RETICULOSPINAL AND CORTICORETICULAR PATHWAYS

The pontine reticulospinal tract (RetST) arises from neurons of the medial pontine RF (nuclei pontis caudalis and oralis). Axons descend as the pontine (medial) RetST mainly ipsilaterally and terminate directly and indirectly on α-LMNs and γ-LMNs at all levels. This tract has a distinct extensor bias with axial musculature, and it reinforces the action of the LVST. The cerebral cortex exerts minimal influence on the pontine RetST; it is driven by poly-sensory input from trigeminal and somatosensory sources. The medullary RetST originates from the medial RF (nucleus gigantocellularis) and is heavily driven by cortical input, especially from the motor and premotor/supplemental motor cortices. Axons of the medullary (lateral) RetST terminate bilaterally, directly and indirectly, on α-LMNs and γ-LMNs at all levels. The medullary RetST exerts a flexor bias, reinforcing the CST and the RST. The reticulospinal tracts are important regulators of basic tone and posture. They are not organized somatotopically.

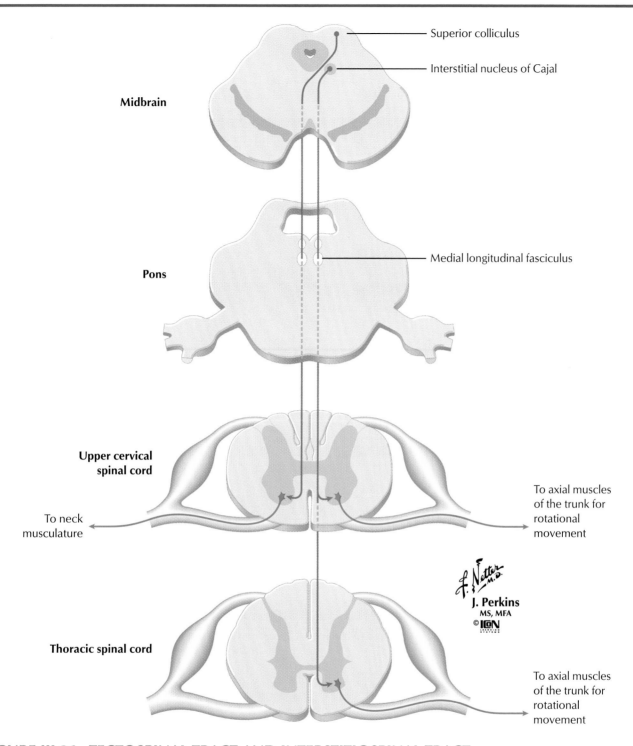

Superior colliculus

Interstitial nucleus of Cajal

Midbrain

Medial longitudinal fasciculus

Pons

Upper cervical
spinal cord

To neck
musculature

To axial muscles
of the trunk for
rotational
movement

J. Perkins
MS, MFA

Thoracic spinal cord

To axial muscles
of the trunk for
rotational
movement

FIGURE III.36: TECTOSPINAL TRACT AND INTERSTITIOSPINAL TRACT

The tectospinal tract (TST) arises from neurons in deep layers of the superior colliculus, decussates in the dorsal tegmental decussation, descends contralaterally near the midline, and terminates directly and indirectly on α-LMNs and γ-LMNs in the cervical spinal cord associated with head and neck movements. This pathway mediates reflex and visual tracking influences for positioning the head with regard to visual input. The interstitiospinal tract (IST) arises from the interstitial nucleus of Cajal, a region that helps to coordinate eye movements and gaze centers. The IST descends ipsilaterally in the medial longitudinal fasciculus (MLF) and terminates directly and indirectly on α-LMNs and γ-LMNs associated with axial musculature of the trunk involved in rotational movement.

A. Corticospinal tracts

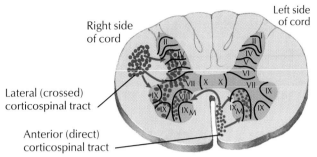

Right side of cord

Left side of cord

Lateral (crossed) corticospinal tract

Anterior (direct) corticospinal tract

Fibers from left motor cortex
Fibers from left sensory cortex

B. Rubrospinal tracts

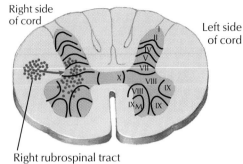

Right side of cord

Left side of cord

Right rubrospinal tract

Fibers from left red nucleus

C. Reticulospinal tracts

Lateral reticulospinal tract

Medial reticulospinal tract

Fibers from left pontine reticular formation
Fibers from left medullary reticular formation

D. Vestibulospinal tracts

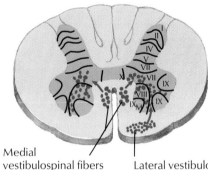

Medial vestibulospinal fibers

Lateral vestibulospinal tract

Fibers from left lateral (Deiters') nucleus
Fibers from left medial and inferior nuclei (only to cervical and thoracic levels)

FIGURE III.37: SPINAL CORD TERMINATIONS OF MAJOR DESCENDING UPPER MOTOR NEURON TRACTS

The lateral CST and RST terminations are directed mainly toward LMNs associated with distal limb musculature. The anterior CST, the reticulospinal tracts, and the vestibulospinal tracts are directed mainly toward LMNs associated with more proximal and axial musculature.

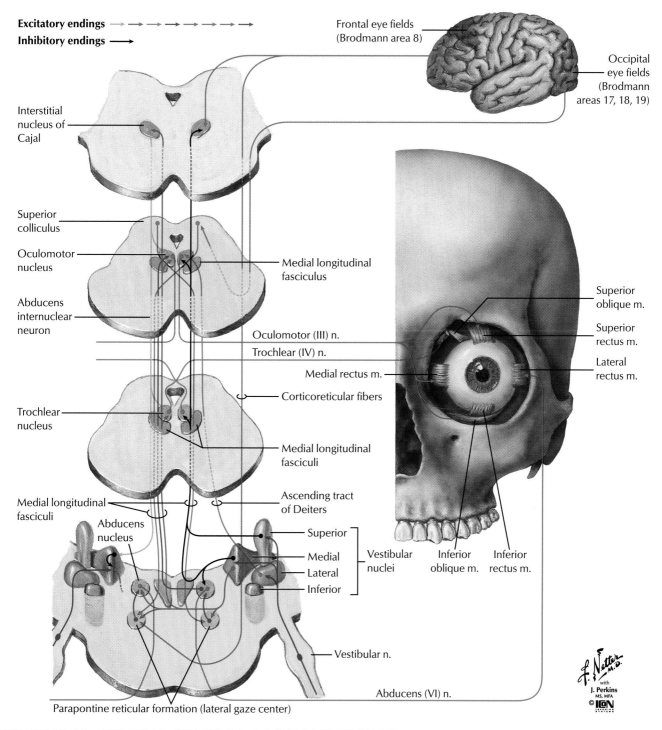

Excitatory endings → → → → → → → →
Inhibitory endings ⟶

Frontal eye fields (Brodmann area 8)

Occipital eye fields (Brodmann areas 17, 18, 19)

Interstitial nucleus of Cajal

Superior colliculus

Oculomotor nucleus

Medial longitudinal fasciculus

Abducens internuclear neuron

Oculomotor (III) n.

Trochlear (IV) n.

Medial rectus m.

Superior oblique m.

Superior rectus m.

Lateral rectus m.

Trochlear nucleus

Corticoreticular fibers

Medial longitudinal fasciculi

Medial longitudinal fasciculi

Ascending tract of Deiters

Abducens nucleus

Superior
Medial
Lateral
Inferior

Vestibular nuclei

Inferior oblique m.

Inferior rectus m.

Vestibular n.

Parapontine reticular formation (lateral gaze center)

Abducens (VI) n.

with J. Perkins MS, MFA

FIGURE III.38: CENTRAL CONTROL OF EYE MOVEMENTS

Central control of eye movements is achieved through the coordination of extraocular motor nuclei for cranial nerve CN III (oculomotor), CN IV (trochlear), and CN VI (abducens). The parapontine reticular formation (PPRF) (horizontal gaze center) receives input from the vestibular nuclei, the deep layers of the superior colliculus (input from V1, V2, V3), the cerebral cortex (frontal eye fields), and the interstitial nucleus of Cajal (input from the vestibular nuclei and the frontal eye fields). The PPRF supplies the ipsilateral CN VI nucleus and the contralateral CN III nucleus (via interneurons in the CN VI nucleus) for the medial rectus, thus coordinating horizontal eye movements. The interstitial nucleus of Cajal helps to coordinate vertical and oblique eye movements. Secondary sensory vestibular projections also terminate in the extraocular motor cranial nerve nuclei. Axons interconnecting the extraocular motor cranial nerve nuclei travel through the MLF.

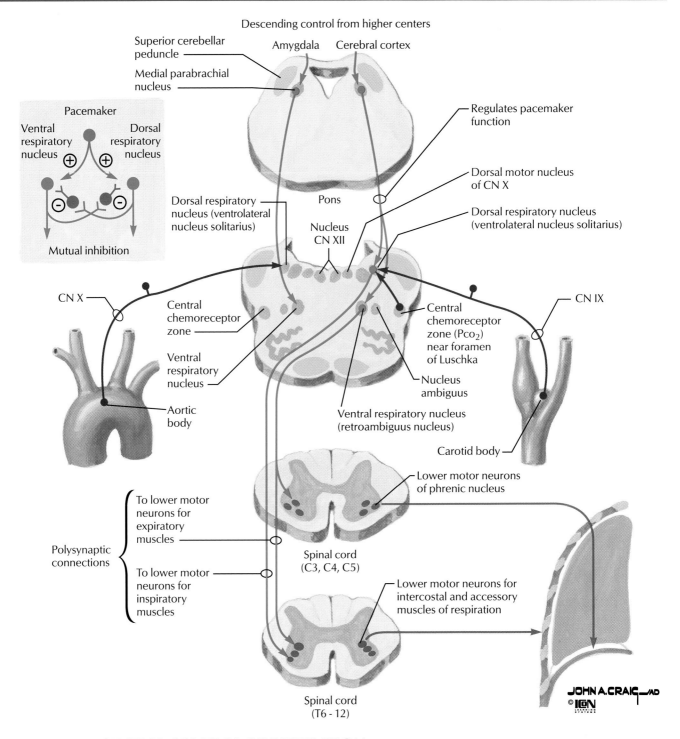

Descending control from higher centers

Superior cerebellar peduncle
Amygdala
Cerebral cortex
Medial parabrachial nucleus

Pacemaker

Ventral respiratory nucleus ⊕ ⊕ Dorsal respiratory nucleus
⊖ ⊖

Mutual inhibition

Regulates pacemaker function

Dorsal motor nucleus of CN X

Dorsal respiratory nucleus (ventrolateral nucleus solitarius)

Dorsal respiratory nucleus (ventrolateral nucleus solitarius)

Pons

Nucleus CN XII

CN X

Central chemoreceptor zone

Ventral respiratory nucleus

Aortic body

Central chemoreceptor zone (Pco_2) near foramen of Luschka

Nucleus ambiguus

Ventral respiratory nucleus (retroambiguus nucleus)

CN IX

Carotid body

Lower motor neurons of phrenic nucleus

To lower motor neurons for expiratory muscles

Polysynaptic connections

To lower motor neurons for inspiratory muscles

Spinal cord (C3, C4, C5)

Lower motor neurons for intercostal and accessory muscles of respiration

Spinal cord (T6 - 12)

JOHN A. CRAIG—AD
© IICN

FIGURE III.39: CENTRAL CONTROL OF RESPIRATION

Inspiration and expiration are regulated by nuclei of the RF. The dorsal respiratory nucleus (DRN) (lateral nucleus solitarius) sends crossed axons to terminate on cervical spinal cord LMNs of the phrenic nucleus and on thoracic spinal cord LMNs that supply intercostals and accessory respiratory musculature associated with inspiration. The ventral respiratory nucleus (VRN) (nucleus retro-ambiguus) sends crossed axons to terminate on thoracic spinal cord LMNs that supply accessory musculature associated with expiration. The DRN receives input from the carotid body chemosensors (via CN IX) and the aortic body chemosensors (via CN X) and from the central chemoreceptive zones of the lateral medulla. The DRN and the VRN mutually inhibit each other. The medial parabrachial nucleus (PBN) acts as a respiratory pacemaker to regulate the DRN and the VRN. The medial PBN receives input from higher centers such as the amygdala and the cerebral cortex.

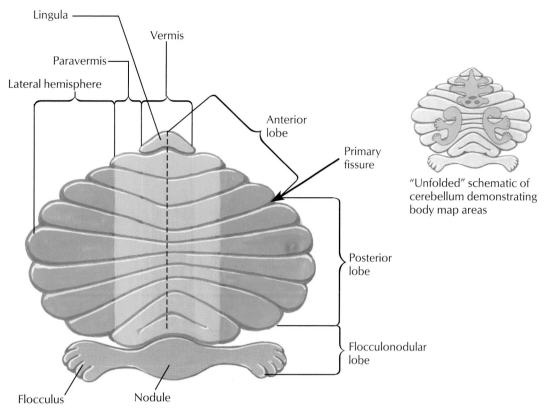

Lingula

Vermis

Paravermis

Lateral hemisphere

Anterior lobe

Primary fissure

Posterior lobe

Flocculonodular lobe

Flocculus

Nodule

"Unfolded" schematic of cerebellum demonstrating body map areas

"Unfolded" schematic of cerebellum demonstrating regions and lobes

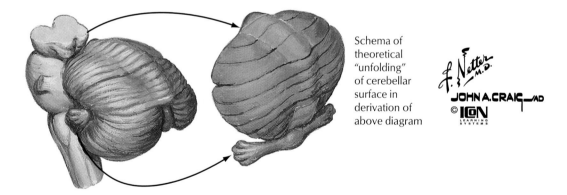

Schema of theoretical "unfolding" of cerebellar surface in derivation of above diagram

FIGURE III.40: FUNCTIONAL SUBDIVISIONS OF THE CEREBELLUM

The cerebellum is classically subdivided into anterior, middle (posterior), and flocculonodular (FN) lobes. Damage to each lobe is associated with ipsilateral syndromes such as stiff legged gate (anterior lobe), loss of coordination with dysmetria, action tremor, hypotonia, ataxia, decomposition of movement (middle lobe), and truncal ataxia (FN lobe). The cerebellum is also classified according to a longitudinal scheme, based on cerebellar cortical regions that project to deep cerebellar nuclei, which in turn project to and coordinate the activity of UMN cell groups. This scheme includes the vermis and the FN lobe (projecting to the fastigial nucleus and the LVN), the paravermis (projecting to globose and emboliform nuclei), and the lateral hemispheres (projecting to the dentate nucleus). Each cerebellar subdivision is interlinked with circuitry related to specific UMN systems.

Cerebellar Cortex

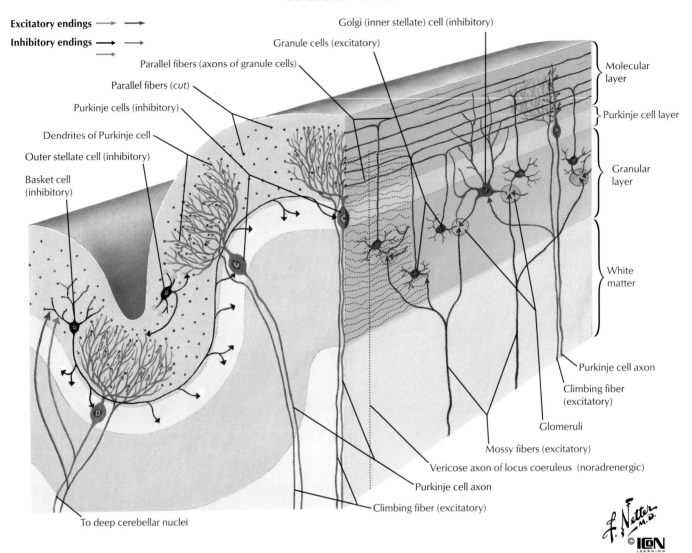

Excitatory endings →
Inhibitory endings ▸

Golgi (inner stellate) cell (inhibitory)
Granule cells (excitatory)
Parallel fibers (axons of granule cells)
Parallel fibers (*cut*)
Purkinje cells (inhibitory)
Dendrites of Purkinje cell
Outer stellate cell (inhibitory)
Basket cell (inhibitory)

Molecular layer
Purkinje cell layer
Granular layer
White matter
Purkinje cell axon
Climbing fiber (excitatory)
Glomeruli
Mossy fibers (excitatory)
Vericose axon of locus coeruleus (noradrenergic)
Purkinje cell axon
Climbing fiber (excitatory)
To deep cerebellar nuclei

FIGURE III.41: CEREBELLAR NEURONAL CIRCUITRY

The cerebellum is organized into an outer 3-layered cortex, white matter, deep cerebellar nuclei, and cerebellar peduncles that connect with the spinal cord, the brain stem, and the thalamus. In the cortex, the Purkinje cells (the major output neurons) have their dendritic trees in the molecular layer (arranged in parallel "plates"), their cell bodies in the Purkinje cell layer, and their axons in the granular layer and the deeper white matter. Inputs to the cerebellar cortex arrive as climbing fibers (from the inferior olivary nucleus) or mossy fibers (all other inputs). The mossy fibers synapse on granule cells, whose axons form an array of parallel fibers that extend through the dendritic trees of several hundred Purkinje cells. Additional interneurons modulate interconnections in the molecular layer (outer stellate cells), at the Purkinje cell body (basket cells), and at granule cell and molecular layer associations (Golgi cells). Noradrenergic axons of the locus coeruleus neurons terminate in all 3 layers and modulate the excitability of other cerebellar connectivity.

A. General Scheme

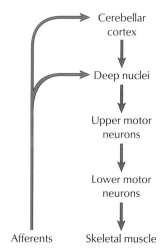

B. Deep Nuclei Relationship With Afferents

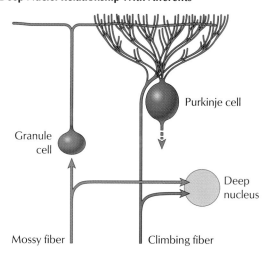

C. Circuitry of Cerebellar Neurons - Mossy Fibers

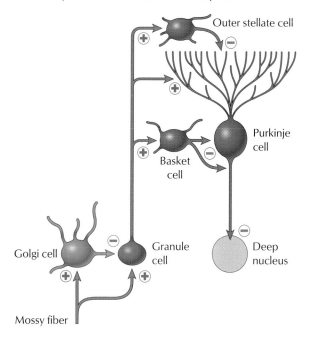

D. Circuitry of Cerebellar Neurons - Climbing Fibers

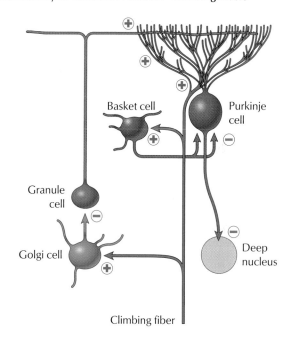

J. Perkins
MS, MFA
©ION

FIGURE III.42: CIRCUIT DIAGRAMS OF AFFERENT CONNECTIONS IN THE CEREBELLUM

Afferents to the cerebellum include mossy fibers, climbing fibers, and locus coeruleus noradrenergic fibers. The mossy fibers synapse in the deep nuclei and on granule cells. The climbing fibers intertwine around the Purkinje cell dendritic tree. The noradrenergic locus coeruleus axons terminate with all cell types in the cerebellar cortex. The loops and circuits in C and D show interneuronal modulation of afferent connections and Purkinje cell outflow. The entire circuitry of the cerebellar cortex provides fine-tuning of the original processing in the deep cerebellar nuclei. The entire Purkinje cell output to the deep nuclei is mediated by inhibition, using GABA as the neurotransmitter.

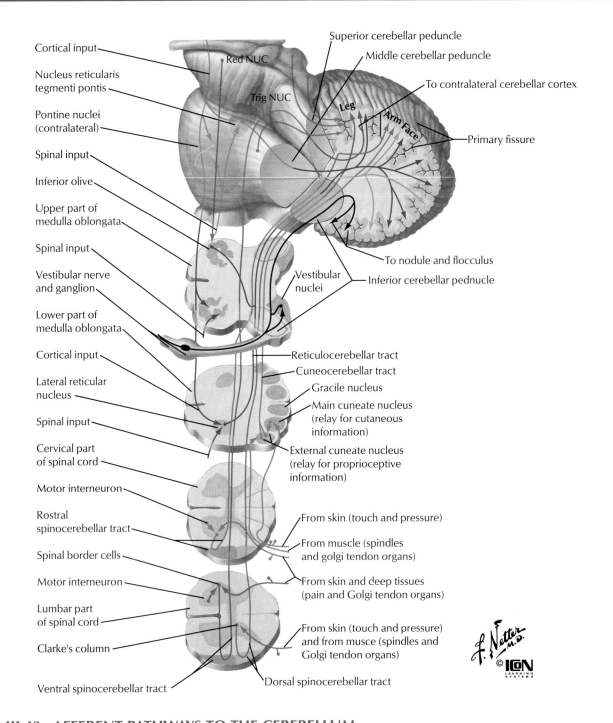

Cortical input

Nucleus reticularis
tegmenti pontis

Pontine nuclei
(contralateral)

Spinal input

Inferior olive

Upper part of
medulla oblongata

Spinal input

Vestibular nerve
and ganglion

Lower part of
medulla oblongata

Cortical input

Lateral reticular
nucleus

Spinal input

Cervical part
of spinal cord

Motor interneuron

Rostral
spinocerebellar tract

Spinal border cells

Motor interneuron

Lumbar part
of spinal cord

Clarke's column

Ventral spinocerebellar tract

Red NUC

Trig NUC

Leg

Arm Face

Superior cerebellar peduncle

Middle cerebellar peduncle

To contralateral cerebellar cortex

Primary fissure

To nodule and flocculus

Inferior cerebellar pednucle

Vestibular
nuclei

Reticulocerebellar tract

Cuneocerebellar tract

Gracile nucleus

Main cuneate nucleus
(relay for cutaneous
information)

External cuneate nucleus
(relay for proprioceptive
information)

From skin (touch and pressure)

From muscle (spindles
and golgi tendon organs)

From skin and deep tissues
(pain and Golgi tendon organs)

From skin (touch and pressure)
and from musce (spindles and
Golgi tendon organs)

Dorsal spinocerebellar tract

FIGURE III.43: AFFERENT PATHWAYS TO THE CEREBELLUM

Afferents to the cerebellum terminate in topo-graphically organized zones in both the deep nuclei and the cerebellar cortex. The body is repre-sented in the cerebellar cortex in at least 3 separate regions. Afferents traveling through the inferior cerebellar peduncle include spinocerebellar path-ways (dorsal and rostral spinocerebellar tracts, cuneocerebellar tract), the inferior olivary input, RF input from the lateral reticular nucleus and other regions, vestibular input from the ganglion and vestibular nuclei, and some trigeminal input. The

dorsal spinocerebellar tract and cuneocerebellar tract derive mainly from muscle spindle output, whereas the ventral and rostral spinocerebellar tracts derive mainly from golgi tendon organ out-put. The middle cerebellar peduncle conveys mainly pontocerebellar axons that carry crossed corticopontocerebellar inputs. Afferents traveling through the superior cerebellar peduncle include the ventral spinocerebellar tract, visual and audi-tory tectocerebellar input, some trigeminal input, and noradrenergic locus coeruleus input.

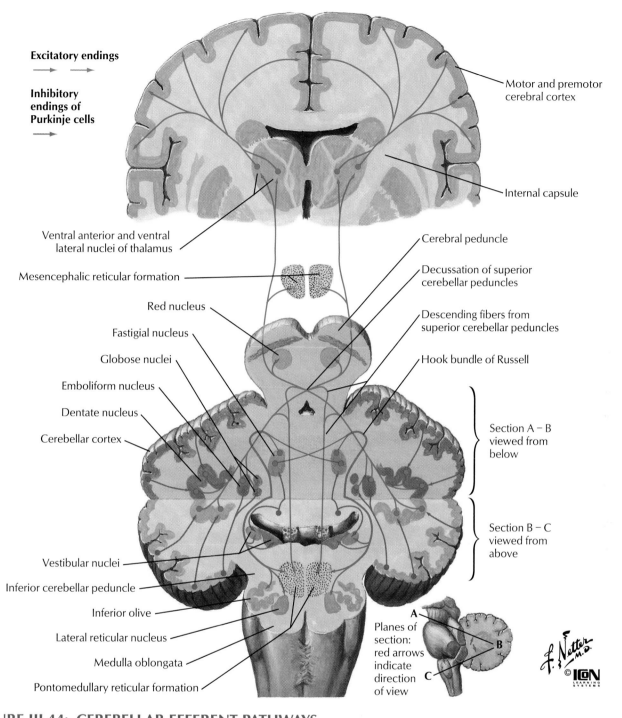

Excitatory endings

→   →

Inhibitory
endings of
Purkinje cells

→

Motor and premotor
cerebral cortex

Internal capsule

Ventral anterior and ventral
lateral nuclei of thalamus

Cerebral peduncle

Mesencephalic reticular formation

Decussation of superior
cerebellar peduncles

Red nucleus

Descending fibers from
superior cerebellar peduncles

Fastigial nucleus

Hook bundle of Russell

Globose nuclei

Emboliform nucleus

Dentate nucleus

Cerebellar cortex

Section A – B
viewed from
below

Section B – C
viewed from
above

Vestibular nuclei

Inferior cerebellar peduncle

Inferior olive

A

Lateral reticular nucleus

B

Medulla oblongata

Planes of
section:
red arrows
indicate
direction
of view

C

Pontomedullary reticular formation

FIGURE III.44: CEREBELLAR EFFERENT PATHWAYS

Efferents from the cerebellum derive from the deep nuclei. Projections from the fastigial nucleus exit mainly through the inferior cerebellar peduncle and terminate mainly ipsilaterally in the LVN and other vestibular nuclei, and in pontine and medullary reticular nuclei, regulating the vestibulospinal and reticulospinal tracts. Projections from the globose and emboliform nuclei project mainly contralaterally through the decussation of the superior cerebellar peduncle to the red nucleus, with a smaller contribution to the VL nucleus of the thalamus, and mainly modulate activity of the RST. Projections from the dentate nucleus project mainly contralaterally through the decussation of the superior cerebellar peduncle to the VL nucleus and, to a lesser extent, the VA nucleus of the thalamus, and mainly modulate activity of the CST. A small projection from the dentate nucleus also projects to the contralateral red nucleus and to brain stem reticular formation.

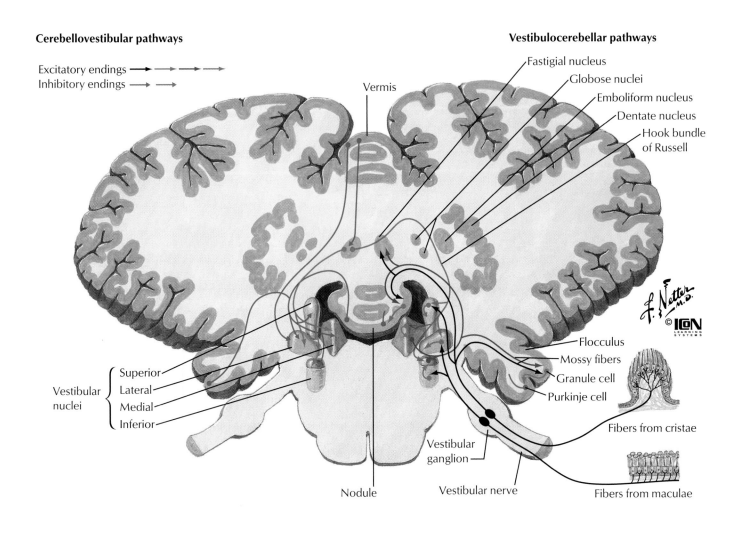

Cerebellovestibular pathways

Excitatory endings ⟶
Inhibitory endings ⟶

Vermis

Vestibulocerebellar pathways

Fastigial nucleus
Globose nuclei
Emboliform nucleus
Dentate nucleus
Hook bundle of Russell

Flocculus
Mossy fibers
Granule cell
Purkinje cell

Fibers from cristae

Vestibular nuclei
Superior
Lateral
Medial
Inferior

Vestibular ganglion

Vestibular nerve

Fibers from maculae

Nodule

FIGURE III.45: VESTIBULOCEREBELLAR AND CEREBELLOVESTIBULAR PATHWAYS

Primary sensory vestibular inputs terminate in the 4 vestibular nuclei and in the fastigial nucleus and the cerebellar cortex of the vermis and the FN lobe. The vestibular nuclei also project to the cerebellar cortex of the vermis and the FN lobe. Purkinje cells in the vermis and the FN lobe, in turn, project back to the vestibular nuclei and the fastigial nucleus. The fastigial nucleus projects to the vestibular nuclei and to the pontine and medullary medial RF. Thus, primary and secondary vestibular neurons project to the fastigial nucleus and the cerebellar cortex, and both the cerebellar cortex and the deep nuclei project back to the vestibular nuclei. This extensive reciprocal vestibulocerebellar circuitry regulates basic spatial position and body tone and posture.

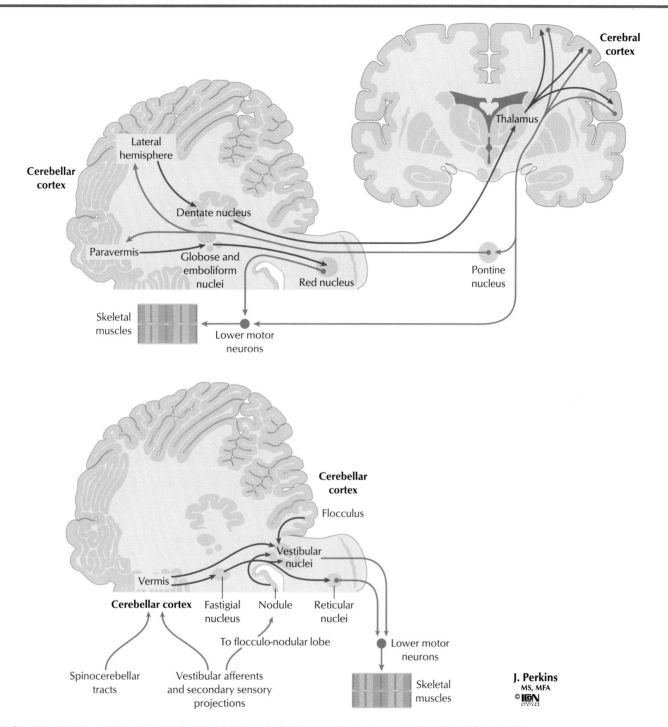

FIGURE III.46: SCHEMATIC DIAGRAMS OF EFFERENT PATHWAYS FROM THE CEREBELLUM TO UPPER MOTOR NEURONAL SYSTEMS

The lateral cerebellar hemisphere connects through the dentate nucleus with VA and VL nuclei of the thalamus, the major thalamic inputs to the cells of origin of the CST in the motor and premotor/supplemental motor cortices. The paravermal cerebellar cortex connects through the globose and emboliform nuclei with the red nucleus, cells of origin for the RST. The cerebellar connections to the cells of origin for the CST and the RST are mainly crossed, and these UMN systems cross

again before terminating on LMNs. Thus, the cerebellum is associated with the ipsilateral LMNs through 2 crossings. The vermis and the FN lobe connect with the fastigial nucleus and lateral vestibular nuclei. The fastigial nucleus projects mainly ipsilaterally to cells of origin for the vestibulospinal and reticulospinal tracts, exerting mainly an ipsilateral influence on spinal cord LMNs through these UMN systems.

Connections of Basal Ganglia

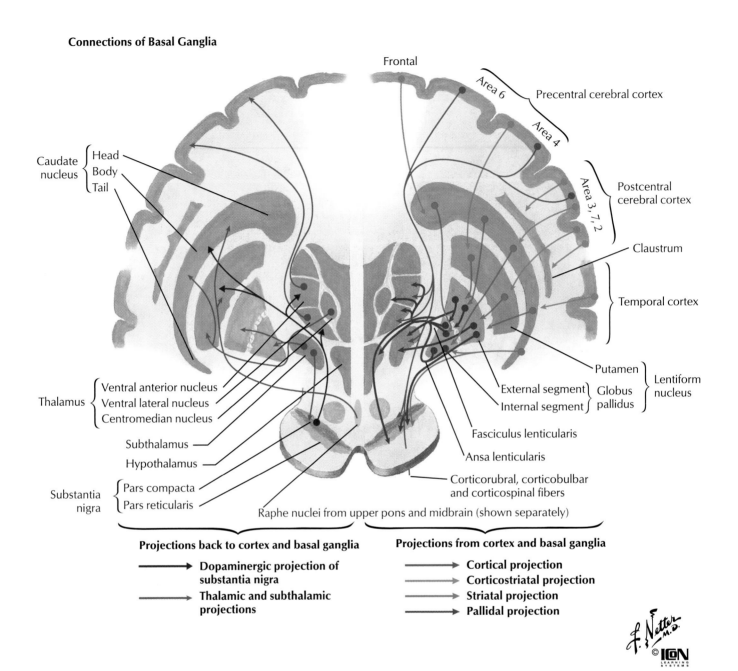

FIGURE III.47: CONNECTIONS OF THE BASAL GANGLIA

The basal ganglia consist of the striatum (caudate nucleus and putamen) and the globus pallidus (GP). The substantia nigra (SN) and the subthalamic nucleus (STN), which are reciprocally connected with the basal ganglia, are often included as part of the basal ganglia. Inputs to the basal ganglia from the cerebral cortex, the thalamus (intralaminar nuclei), the SN pars compacta (dopaminergic input), and the rostral raphe nuclei (serotonergic input) are directed mainly toward the striatum, and

the STN projects mainly to the globus pallidus. The striatum projects to the GP. The GP internal segment projects to the thalamus (VA, VL, and centromedian nuclei), and the external segment projects to the STN. Thalamic VA and VL nuclei provide input to the cells of origin for the CST. Damage to basal ganglia components often results in movement disorders. Damage to the dopamine neurons in the SN pars compacta results in Parkinson's disease.

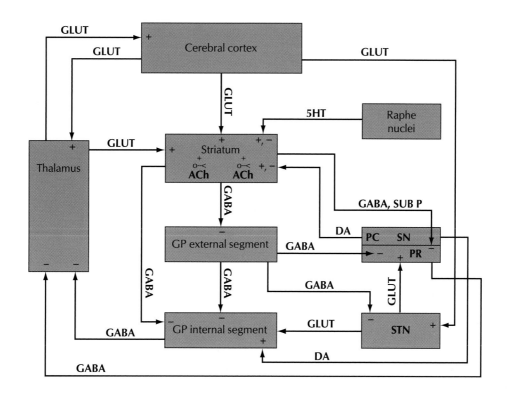

SN = Substantia nigra
STN = Subthalamic nucleus
GLUT = Glutamate
GABA = Gamma aminobutyric acid
DA = Dopamine

5HT = 5-Hydroxytryptamine (serotonin)
PC = Pars compacta
PR = Pars reticularis
ACh = Acetylcholine
GP = Globus pallidus
SUB P = Substance P

FIGURE III.48: BASIC BASAL GANGLIA CIRCUITRY AND NEUROTRANSMITTERS

Inputs from the cerebral cortex and the thalamus to the striatum are excitatory (glutamate). The striatopallidal and pallidothalamic connections are inhibitory (GABA). The combination of these excitatory and inhibitory influences results in a net drive over the thalamocortical (and resultant corticospinal) output. Extensive inhibitory and excitatory circuitry that produce complex modulation of basal ganglia output also derive from the internal segment of the GP, the SN, and the STN. The dopaminergic nigrostriatal connections can exert both inhibitory and excitatory effects on the striatum. In Parkinson's disease, the loss of nigrostriatal dopamine axons allows both negative symptoms (bradykinesia) and positive symptoms (resting tremor, muscular rigidity, postural instability). Additional interneurons such as the excitatory cholinergic interneurons in the striatum are found in some basal ganglia structures.

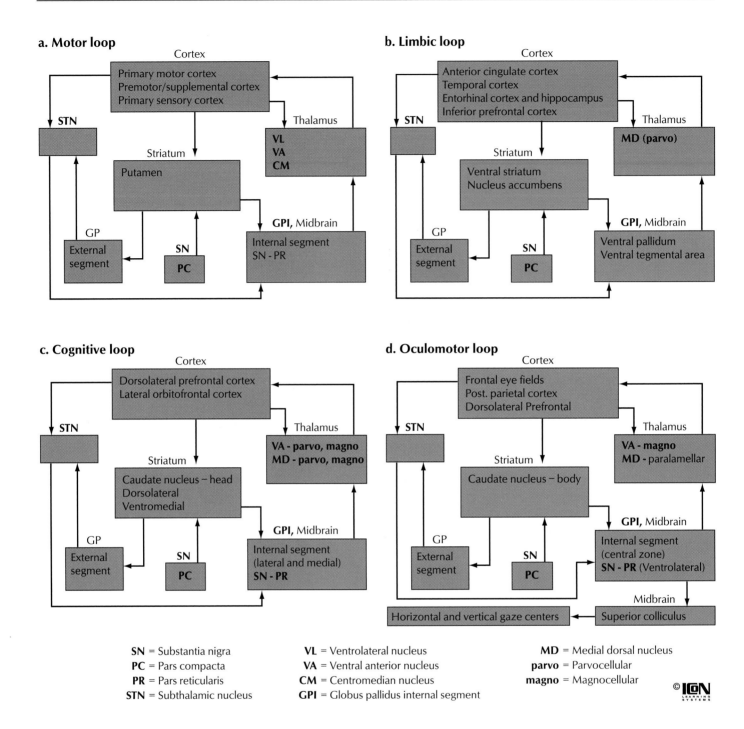

a. Motor loop

b. Limbic loop

c. Cognitive loop

d. Oculomotor loop

SN = Substantia nigra
PC = Pars compacta
PR = Pars reticularis
STN = Subthalamic nucleus

VL = Ventrolateral nucleus
VA = Ventral anterior nucleus
CM = Centromedian nucleus
GPI = Globus pallidus internal segment

MD = Medial dorsal nucleus
parvo = Parvocellular
magno = Magnocellular

FIGURE III.49: PARALLEL LOOPS OF CIRCUITRY THROUGH THE BASAL GANGLIA

The corticostriatal, striatopallidal, and pallidothalamic connections form parallel loops for motor, limbic, cognitive, and oculomotor circuitry. The motor circuitry is processed through the putamen, the limbic circuitry through the ventral pallidum and the nucleus accumbens, the cognitive circuitry through the head of the caudate nucleus, and the oculomotor circuitry through the body of the caudate nucleus. Connections through the GP and the SN pars reticulata or ventral tegmental area then project to appropriate regions of the thalamus to link back to the cortical neurons of origin for the initial corticostriatal projections. These parallel loops through the basal ganglia and the cortex modulate specific subroutines of cortical activity distinct to the appropriate function. The SN pars compacta may act as the principal interconnections among these parallel loops.

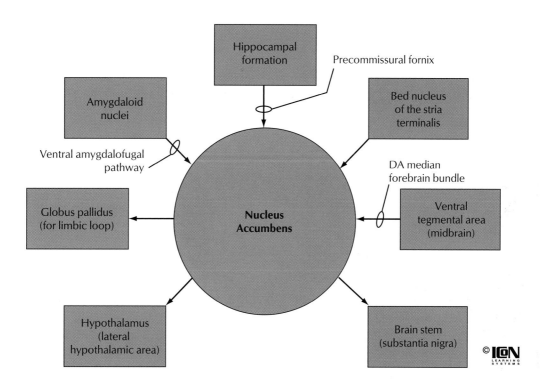

FIGURE III.50: CONNECTIONS OF THE NUCLEUS ACCUMBENS

The nucleus accumbens is located at the anterior end of the striatum in the interior of the ventral and rostral forebrain. Inputs are derived from limbic structures (amygdala, hippocampal formation, bed nucleus of the stria terminalis), and the ventral tegmental area, via a rich dopaminergic projection. The nucleus accumbens is central to motivational states and addictive behaviors. It also appears to be a principal region in brain reward circuits associated with joy, pleasure, and gratification. The involvement of the nucleus accumbens with a specific limbic basal ganglia loop helps to provide motor expression of emotional responses and accompanying gestures and behaviors.

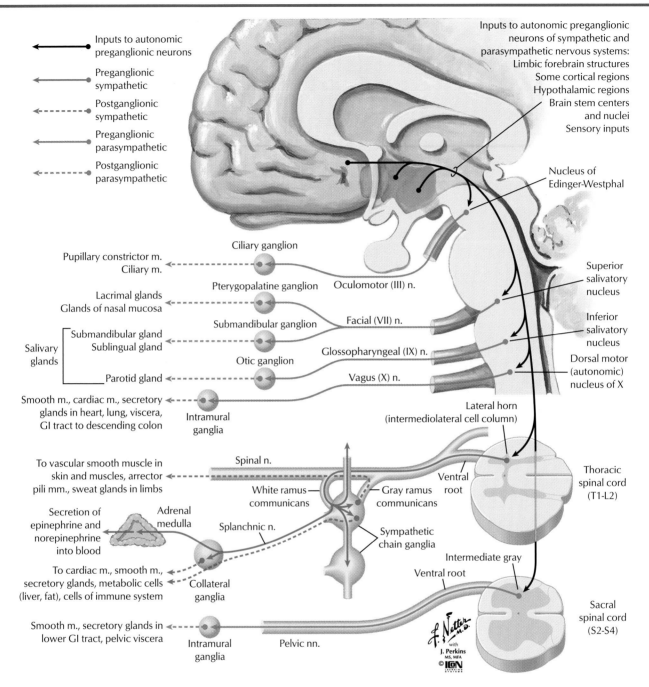

Inputs to autonomic
preganglionic neurons

Preganglionic
sympathetic

Postganglionic
sympathetic

Preganglionic
parasympathetic

Postganglionic
parasympathetic

Inputs to autonomic preganglionic
neurons of sympathetic and
parasympathetic nervous systems:
Limbic forebrain structures
Some cortical regions
Hypothalamic regions
Brain stem centers
and nuclei
Sensory inputs

Nucleus of
Edinger-Westphal

Ciliary ganglion

Pupillary constrictor m.
Ciliary m.

Oculomotor (III) n.

Superior
salivatory
nucleus

Pterygopalatine ganglion

Lacrimal glands
Glands of nasal mucosa

Submandibular ganglion

Facial (VII) n.

Inferior
salivatory
nucleus

Submandibular gland
Sublingual gland

Glossopharyngeal (IX) n.

Salivary
glands

Otic ganglion

Dorsal motor
(autonomic)
nucleus of X

Parotid gland

Vagus (X) n.

Smooth m., cardiac m., secretory
glands in heart, lung, viscera,
GI tract to descending colon

Intramural
ganglia

Lateral horn
(intermediolateral cell column)

To vascular smooth muscle in
skin and muscles, arrector
pili mm., sweat glands in limbs

Spinal n.

White ramus
communicans

Gray ramus
communicans

Ventral
root

Thoracic
spinal cord
(T1-L2)

Secretion of
epinephrine and
norepinephrine
into blood

Adrenal
medulla

Splanchnic n.

Sympathetic
chain ganglia

To cardiac m., smooth m.,
secretory glands, metabolic cells
(liver, fat), cells of immune system

Collateral
ganglia

Intermediate gray

Ventral root

Smooth m., secretory glands in
lower GI tract, pelvic viscera

Intramural
ganglia

Pelvic nn.

Sacral
spinal cord
(S2-S4)

FIGURE III.51: GENERAL ORGANIZATION OF THE AUTONOMIC NERVOUS SYSTEM

The autonomic nervous system is a 2-neuron chain connecting preganglionic neurons through ganglia to visceral target tissues (cardiac muscle, smooth muscle, secretory glands, metabolic cells, cells of the immune system). The sympathetic division (sympathetic nervous system [SNS]) is a thoracolumbar (T1-L2) system arising from the intermediolateral cell column of the lateral horn, acting through chain ganglia and collateral ganglia; it is a system for fight-or-flight, designed for reactions in an emergency. The parasympathetic division (parasympathetic nervous system [PsNS]) is a craniosacral system arising from brain stem nuclei associated with cranial nerves (CNs) III, VII, IX, and X and from the intermediate gray in the S2-S4 spinal cord. Connections from CNs III, VII, and IX act through cranial nerve ganglia; connections from CN X and S2-S4 act through intramural ganglia in or near the target tissue. The PsNS is a homeostatic reparative system. Central connections from the limbic forebrain, the hypothalamus, and the brain stem regulating SNS and PsNS outflow to the body act mainly through connections to vagal and sympathetic preganglionic neurons.

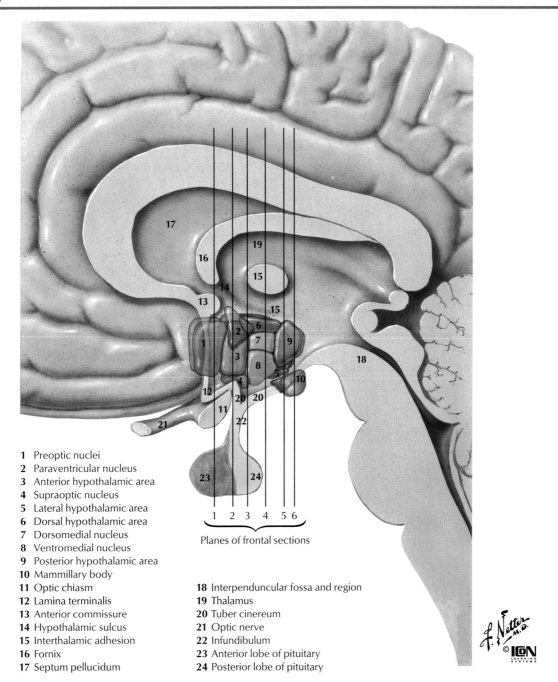

1 Preoptic nuclei
2 Paraventricular nucleus
3 Anterior hypothalamic area
4 Supraoptic nucleus
5 Lateral hypothalamic area
6 Dorsal hypothalamic area
7 Dorsomedial nucleus
8 Ventromedial nucleus
9 Posterior hypothalamic area
10 Mammillary body
11 Optic chiasm
12 Lamina terminalis
13 Anterior commissure
14 Hypothalamic sulcus
15 Interthalamic adhesion
16 Fornix
17 Septum pellucidum

18 Interpenduncular fossa and region
19 Thalamus
20 Tuber cinereum
21 Optic nerve
22 Infundibulum
23 Anterior lobe of pituitary
24 Posterior lobe of pituitary

Planes of frontal sections

FIGURE III.52: GENERAL ANATOMY OF THE HYPOTHALAMUS

The hypothalamus, a collection of nuclei and fiber tracts in the ventral diencephalon, regulates visceral autonomic functions and neuroendocrine function, particularly from the anterior and posterior pituitary. Many nuclei are found between the posterior boundary (mammillary bodies) and the anterior boundary (lamina terminalis, anterior commissure) of the hypothalamus; these nuclei are subdivided into 4 general hypothalamic zones: (1) preoptic, (2) anterior or supraoptic, (3) tuberal, and (4) mammillary or posterior. From the medial boundary at the CN III ventricle to the lateral boundary, the nuclei are subdivided into 3 general zones: (1) periventricular, (2) medial, and (3) lateral. The pituitary gland is attached at the base of the hypothalamus via the median eminence and the infundibulum (pituitary stalk). The median eminence is an important zone of neuroendocrine transduction.

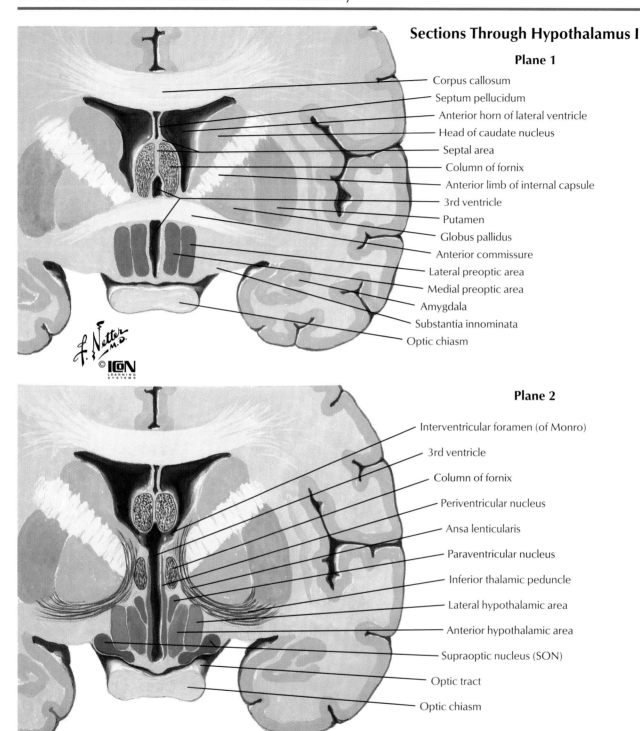

Sections Through Hypothalamus I

Plane 1

- Corpus callosum
- Septum pellucidum
- Anterior horn of lateral ventricle
- Head of caudate nucleus
- Septal area
- Column of fornix
- Anterior limb of internal capsule
- 3rd ventricle
- Putamen
- Globus pallidus
- Anterior commissure
- Lateral preoptic area
- Medial preoptic area
- Amygdala
- Substantia innominata
- Optic chiasm

Plane 2

- Interventricular foramen (of Monro)
- 3rd ventricle
- Column of fornix
- Periventricular nucleus
- Ansa lenticularis
- Paraventricular nucleus
- Inferior thalamic peduncle
- Lateral hypothalamic area
- Anterior hypothalamic area
- Supraoptic nucleus (SON)
- Optic tract
- Optic chiasm

FIGURE III.53: SECTIONS THROUGH THE HYPOTHALAMUS: PREOPTIC AND SUPRAOPTIC ZONES

The major nuclei in the preoptic zone include the medial and lateral preoptic areas. The organum vasculosum of the lamina terminalis (OVLT), a circumventricular organ, is present in this hypothalamic area. The major nuclei in the supraoptic (anterior) zone include the supraoptic nucleus (SON), the paraventricular nucleus (PVN), the suprachiasmatic nucleus, the anterior hypothalamic area, and the lateral hypothalamic area (LHA). Some nuclei, such as the PVN, have many subregions (magnocellular and parvocellular) that contain collections of chemically specific neurons with discrete projections and functions. These groups of neurons sometimes intermingle within one subregion of the nucleus.

Sections Through Hypothalamus II

Plane 3

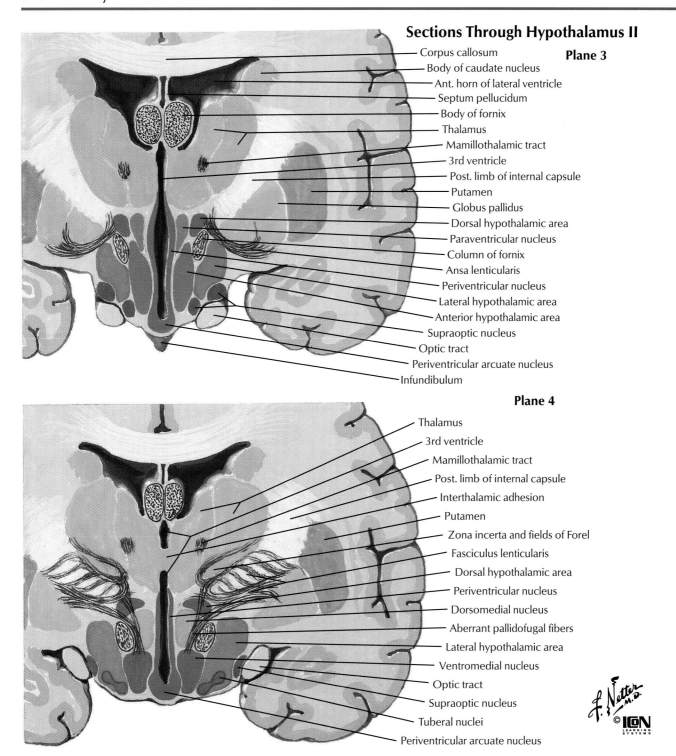

- Corpus callosum
- Body of caudate nucleus
- Ant. horn of lateral ventricle
- Septum pellucidum
- Body of fornix
- Thalamus
- Mamillothalamic tract
- 3rd ventricle
- Post. limb of internal capsule
- Putamen
- Globus pallidus
- Dorsal hypothalamic area
- Paraventricular nucleus
- Column of fornix
- Ansa lenticularis
- Periventricular nucleus
- Lateral hypothalamic area
- Anterior hypothalamic area
- Supraoptic nucleus
- Optic tract
- Periventricular arcuate nucleus
- Infundibulum

Plane 4

- Thalamus
- 3rd ventricle
- Mamillothalamic tract
- Post. limb of internal capsule
- Interthalamic adhesion
- Putamen
- Zona incerta and fields of Forel
- Fasciculus lenticularis
- Dorsal hypothalamic area
- Periventricular nucleus
- Dorsomedial nucleus
- Aberrant pallidofugal fibers
- Lateral hypothalamic area
- Ventromedial nucleus
- Optic tract
- Supraoptic nucleus
- Tuberal nuclei
- Periventricular arcuate nucleus

FIGURE III.54: SECTIONS THROUGH THE HYPOTHALAMUS: TUBERAL ZONE

The major nuclei in the tuberal zone include the dorsomedial (DM) nucleus, the ventromedial (VM) nucleus, the PVN, the arcuate nucleus, the periarcuate area (β-endorphin cells), the tuberal nuclei, the dorsal hypothalamic area, and the LHA. Some nuclei from the supraoptic zone (PVN, SON, LHA) extend caudally into the tuberal zone. The median eminence extends from this region, and axons from releasing-factor and inhibitory-factor neurons that control the release of anterior pituitary hormones funnel down to the contact zone, where they release these factors into the hypophysial portal system, which bathes the cells of the anterior pituitary.

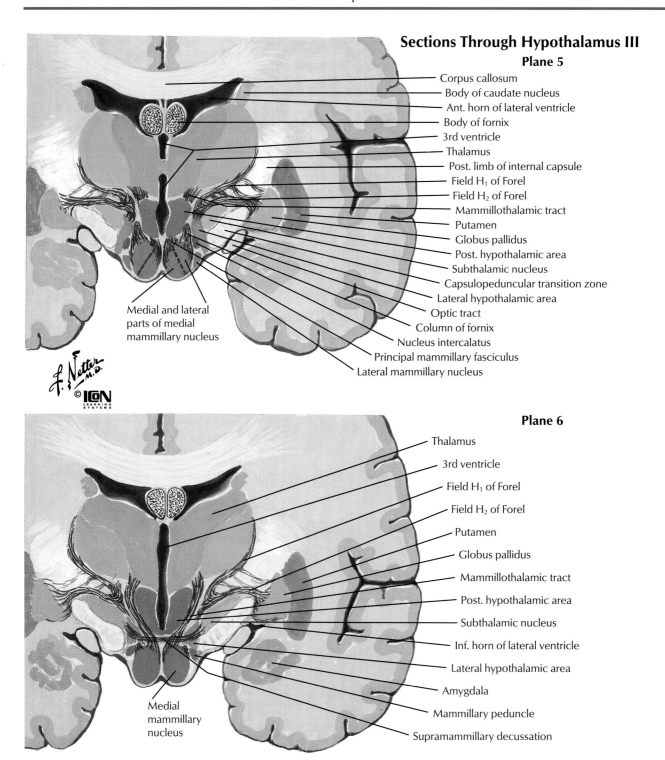

Sections Through Hypothalamus III

Plane 5

- Corpus callosum
- Body of caudate nucleus
- Ant. horn of lateral ventricle
- Body of fornix
- 3rd ventricle
- Thalamus
- Post. limb of internal capsule
- Field H₁ of Forel
- Field H₂ of Forel
- Mammillothalamic tract
- Putamen
- Globus pallidus
- Post. hypothalamic area
- Subthalamic nucleus
- Capsulopeduncular transition zone
- Lateral hypothalamic area
- Optic tract
- Column of fornix
- Nucleus intercalatus
- Principal mammillary fasciculus
- Lateral mammillary nucleus

Medial and lateral parts of medial mammillary nucleus

Plane 6

- Thalamus
- 3rd ventricle
- Field H₁ of Forel
- Field H₂ of Forel
- Putamen
- Globus pallidus
- Mammillothalamic tract
- Post. hypothalamic area
- Subthalamic nucleus
- Inf. horn of lateral ventricle
- Lateral hypothalamic area
- Amygdala
- Mammillary peduncle
- Supramammillary decussation

Medial mammillary nucleus

FIGURE III.55: SECTIONS THROUGH THE HYPOTHALAMUS: MAMMILLARY ZONE

The major nuclei in the mammillary zone include the medial and lateral mammillary nuclei, the posterior hypothalamic area, and the LHA. The LHA extends throughout most of the length of the hypothalamus and shows neuronal characteristics seen in the brain stem reticular formation.

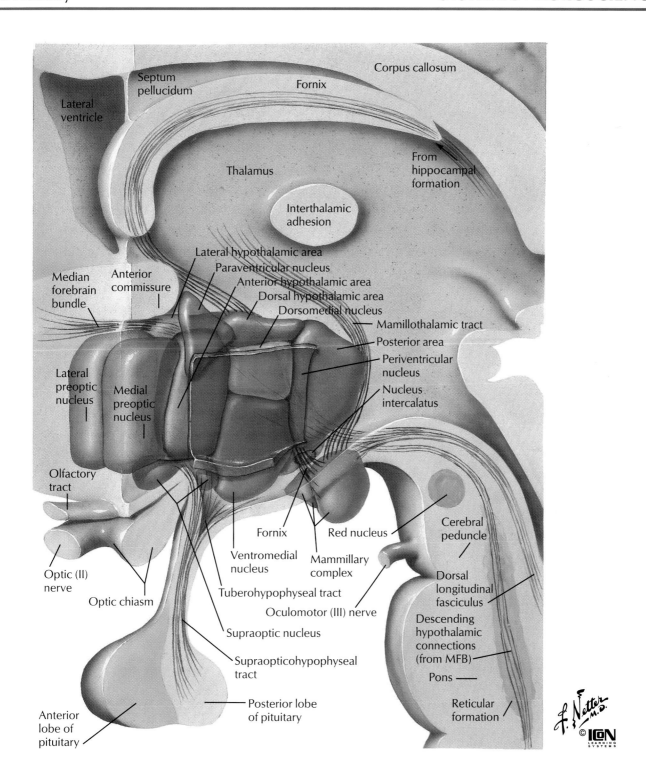

FIGURE III.56: SCHEMATIC RECONSTRUCTION OF THE HYPOTHALAMUS

A schematic 3-D reconstruction of the hypothalamus in sagittal section shows the nuclei, the areas, and the zones that occupy this small region of the diencephalon. Many pathways are represented, including the fornix, the mammillothalamic tract, the median forebrain bundle, the supraopticohypophysial tract, the tuberohypophysial (tuberoin-fundibular) tract, and brain stem connections with the hypothalamus, which include the dorsal longitudinal fasciculus, the descending median forebrain bundle, the mammillotegmental tract, and descending connections from the PVN to preganglionic autonomic nuclei.

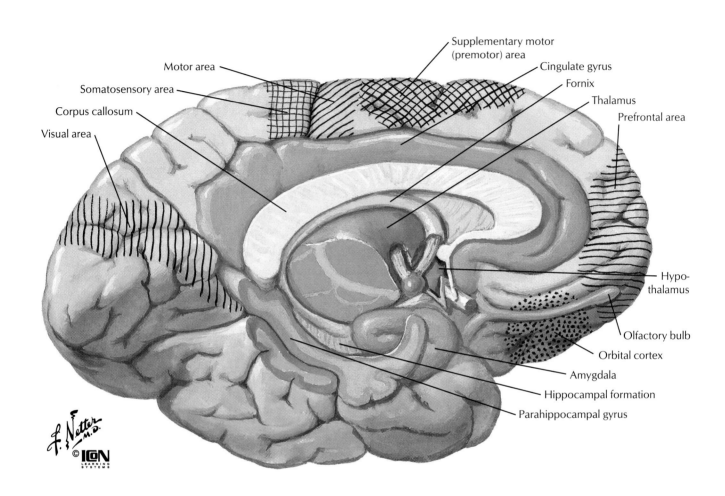

FIGURE III.57: FOREBRAIN REGIONS ASSOCIATED WITH THE HYPOTHALAMUS

A number of forebrain regions are intimately connected with the hypothalamus, some through direct fiber projections and some through indirect connections. Important cerebral cortex regions include the prefrontal cortex, the orbitofrontal (orbital) cortex, the cingulate cortex, the insular cortex, the parahippocampal cortex, and the periamygdaloid cortex. Important subcortical regions of the limbic forebrain include the hippocampus (a three-layered cortex), the amygdaloid nuclei, and the septal nuclei. Important thalamic connections include the medial dorsal and anterior nuclei. Important olfactory connections include the olfactory tract, nuclei, and cortex.

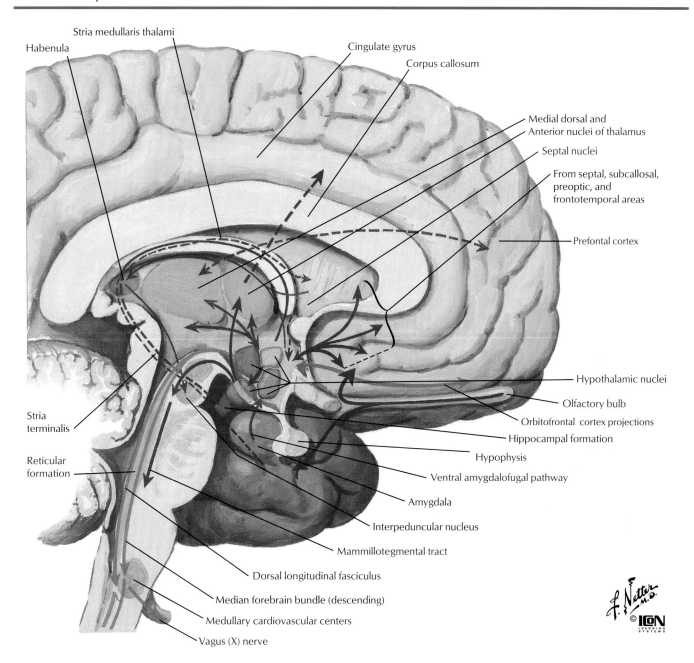

Stria medullaris thalami

Habenula

Cingulate gyrus

Corpus callosum

Medial dorsal and Anterior nuclei of thalamus

Septal nuclei

From septal, subcallosal, preoptic, and frontotemporal areas

Prefontal cortex

Stria terminalis

Reticular formation

Hypothalamic nuclei

Olfactory bulb

Orbitofrontal cortex projections

Hippocampal formation

Hypophysis

Ventral amygdalofugal pathway

Amygdala

Interpeduncular nucleus

Mammillotegmental tract

Dorsal longitudinal fasciculus

Median forebrain bundle (descending)

Medullary cardiovascular centers

Vagus (X) nerve

FIGURE III.58: AFFERENT AND EFFERENT PATHWAYS ASSOCIATED WITH THE HYPOTHALAMUS

Hypothalamic connections are numerous and complex. Some regions of the cerebral cortex (prefrontal, orbitofrontal) and the thalamus (anterior) send axonal projections directly to the hypothalamus. Diverse afferent pathways arise from the hippocampal formation and the subiculum (fornix), the amygdaloid nuclei (stria terminalis, ventral amygdalofugal pathway), and the habenula (fasciculus retroflexus). The retina sends direct retinohypothalamic fibers to the suprachiasmatic nucleus. Brain stem projections, some compact and some diffuse, ascend to the hypothalamus through multi-ple pathways (not shown here). Efferent connections from the hypothalamus include those to the median eminence (from multiple nuclei), the posterior pituitary (supraopticohypophysial tract), the septal nuclei and the anterior perforated substance (median forebrain bundle); those to the thalamus (mammillothalamic tract); and those to many brain stem and some spinal cord sites (dorsal longitudinal fasciculus, median forebrain bundle, mammillotegmental tract, direct connections from the PVN to preganglionic neurons, and others).

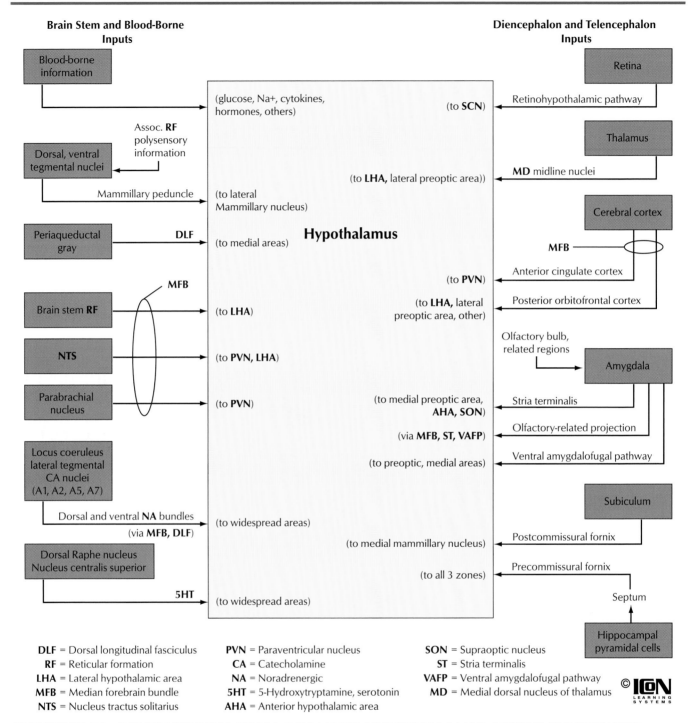

FIGURE III.59: SCHEMATIC DIAGRAM OF MAJOR HYPOTHALAMIC AFFERENT PATHWAYS

The hypothalamus receives extensive input from many regions of the CNS. Descending inputs arrive from limbic forebrain structures (hippocampal formation, subiculum, amygdala), the cerebral cortex (anterior cingulate, orbitofrontal, prefrontal), and the thalamus (medial dorsal). Ascending inputs arrive from extensive areas of the autonomic brain stem (tegmental nuclei, periaqueductal gray, parabrachial nuclei, nucleus tractus solitarius

[NTS]); the locus coeruleus and tegmental catecholamine nuclei; raphe serotonergic nuclei; and the brain stem reticular formation. The retina sends input directly to the suprachiasmatic nucleus, a portion of the hypothalamus that modulates diurnal rhythms. Blood-borne substances (cytokines, hormones, glucose, Na+, others) influence the hypothalamus via numerous routes and mechanisms.

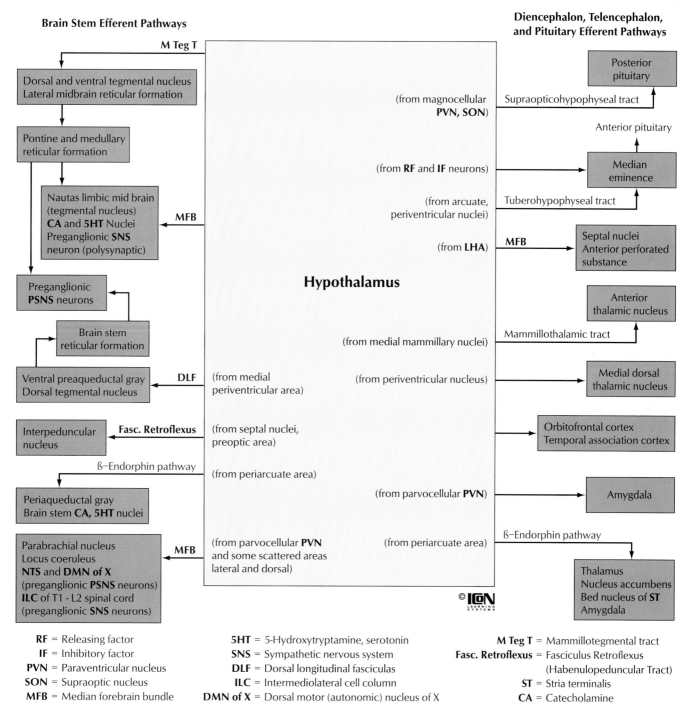

FIGURE III.60: SCHEMATIC DIAGRAM OF MAJOR HYPOTHALAMIC EFFERENT PATHWAYS

The hypothalamus gives rise to extensive efferent projections. Ascending efferents are sent to the limbic forebrain structures (amygdala, septal nuclei, anterior perforated substance), the cerebral cortex (orbitofrontal cortex and temporal association cortex), and the thalamus (medial dorsal, anterior). Extensive projections are sent to the median eminence (releasing and inhibitory factors for control of anterior pituitary hormones; dopamine projections from the arcuate nucleus and the PVN) and

to the posterior pituitary. Other efferent projections are sent directly and indirectly to the preganglionic neurons of the SNS and the PSNS (median forebrain bundle, dorsal longitudinal fasciculus, mammillotegmental tract, direct projections from the PVN), to widespread autonomic and visceral nuclei (noradrenergic neurons, serotonergic neurons, parabrachial nuclei, NTS, periaqueductal gray, tegmental nuclei, interpeduncular nucleus), and to the brain stem reticular formation.

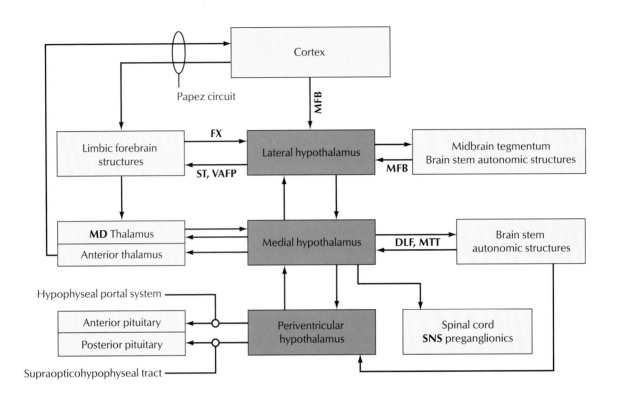

DLF = Dorsal longitudinal fasciculus
MFB = Median forebrain bundle
ST = Stria terminalis
VAFP = Ventral amygdalofugal pathway

MD = Medial dorsal nucleus of thalamus
FX = Fornix
MTT = Mammillothalamic tract
SNS = Sympathetic nervous system

FIGURE III.61: SUMMARY OF GENERAL HYPOTHALAMIC CONNECTIONS

The lateral, medial, and periventricular zones of the hypothalamus have specific connections with the cerebral cortex, the limbic forebrain structures, the thalamus, and widespread areas of the brain stem. Extensive efferent projections of the hypothalamus are directed toward regulation of pre-ganglionic sympathetic and parasympathetic neurons and toward release and regulation of hormones of the anterior and posterior pituitary. The anterior pituitary hormones regulate hormonal secretion and functional activities of many target structures throughout the body.

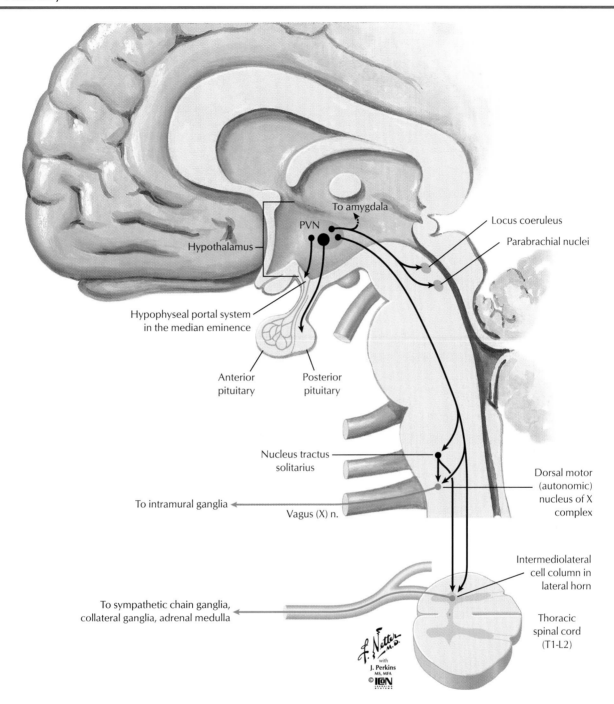

FIGURE III.62: PARAVENTRICULAR NUCLEUS OF THE HYPOTHALAMUS: REGULATION OF PITUITARY NEUROHORMONAL OUTFLOW, AUTONOMIC PREGANGLIONIC OUTFLOW, AND LIMBIC ACTIVITY

The PVN has many projections that help to coordinate pituitary neurohormonal outflow, autonomic preganglionic outflow, and limbic activity. Magnocellular neurons send axons to the posterior pituitary, releasing oxytocin and vasopressin into the general circulation. Corticotropin-releasing factor (CRF) neurons and some vasopressin neurons send axons to the median eminence; these axons release their hormones into the hypophyseal portal system, influencing the release of ACTH. PVN parvocellular neurons send direct descending projections to preganglionic neurons of the parasympathetics (dorsal motor nucleus of CN X) and the sympathetics (intermediolateral cell column in the T1-L2 lateral horn) and to the NTS. These neurons also send axons to several important limbic-related structures, such as the amygdala, the parabrachial nuclei, and the locus coeruleus.

275

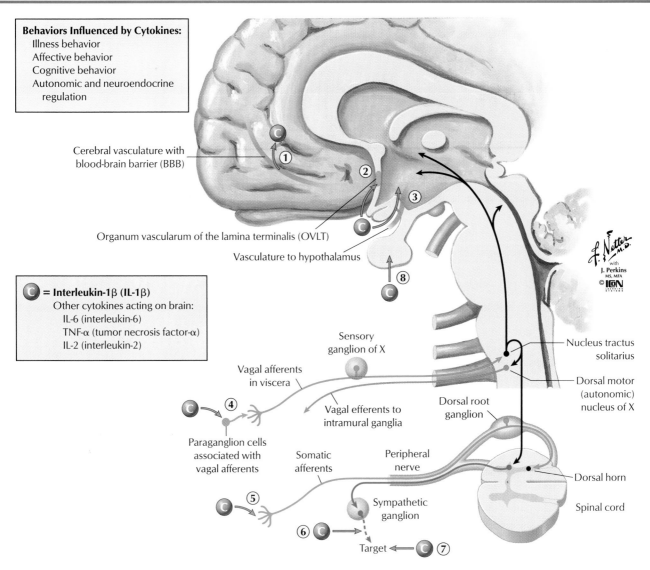

Behaviors Influenced by Cytokines:
Illness behavior
Affective behavior
Cognitive behavior
Autonomic and neuroendocrine
  regulation

Cerebral vasculature with
blood-brain barrier (BBB)

Organum vascularum of the lamina terminalis (OVLT)

Vasculature to hypothalamus

C = **Interleukin-1β (IL-1β)**
Other cytokines acting on brain:
IL-6 (interleukin-6)
TNF-α (tumor necrosis factor-α)
IL-2 (interleukin-2)

Sensory
ganglion of X

Vagal afferents
in viscera

Vagal efferents to
intramural ganglia

Dorsal root
ganglion

Nucleus tractus
solitarius

Dorsal motor
(autonomic)
nucleus of X

Paraganglion cells
associated with
vagal afferents

Somatic
afferents

Peripheral
nerve

Dorsal horn

Spinal cord

Sympathetic
ganglion

Target

(1) Cytokines transported directly across the BBB.

(2) Cytokines crossing into cerebrospinal fluid at OVLT, or acting on cells that release PGE_2 or neurons that project to visceral-autonomic structures.

(3) Cytokine-stimulated release of small molecules (such as NO) that directly cross into the brain and act as mediators.

(4) Cytokine stimulation of vagal afferents (through paraneurons) that modulate activity in nucleus tractus solitarius, influencing the multiple activities of the paraventricular nucleus and many other sites.

(5) Cytokine activation of other afferents that modulate dorsal horn sensory processing to many sites.

(6) Cytokine modulation of norepinephrine release from sympathetic nerve terminals.

(7) Cytokine modulation of neurotransmitter intracellular signaling in target cells.

(8) Cytokine modulation of pituitary hormone release.

FIGURE III.63: MECHANISMS OF CYTOKINE INFLUENCES ON THE HYPOTHALAMUS AND OTHER BRAIN REGIONS AND ON BEHAVIOR

Cytokines, including interleukin (IL)-1β, IL-6, tumor necrosis factor-α, and IL-2, can influence central neuronal activity and behavior. This diagram illustrates IL-1β access to the brain: (1) directly crossing the blood-brain barrier into the brain, (2) acting on circumventricular organs (OVLT), releasing small mediators such as PGE2, (3) acting on vascular endothelial cells, releasing nitric oxide (NO), which acts in the CNS, (4) activating vagal afferents into the NTS via paraganglion cells, and (5) activating other afferent nerve fibers. IL-1β can evoke illness behavior (fever, induction of slow-wave sleep, decreased appetite, lethargy, classic illness symptoms), influence autonomic and neuroendocrine regulation, and influence both affective and cognitive functions and behavior.

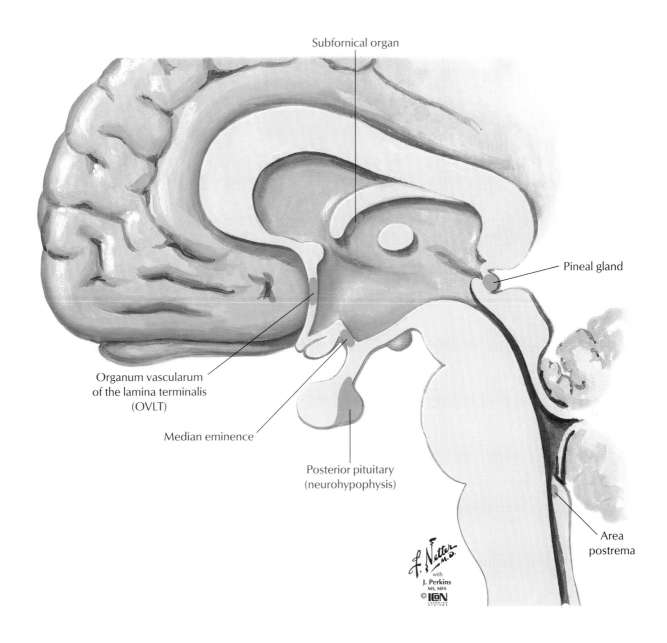

Subfornical organ

Pineal gland

Organum vascularum
of the lamina terminalis
(OVLT)

Median eminence

Posterior pituitary
(neurohypophysis)

Area
postrema

FIGURE III.64: CIRCUMVENTRICULAR ORGANS

Circumventricular organs are "windows on the brain" that are devoid of the usual tight-junction endothelial appositions and instead have fenestrated vasculature. Thus, the circumventricular organs have no blood-brain barrier. Some of these organs—the OVLT, the subfornical organ, and the area postrema—have associated neurons with projections to hypothalamic and other visceral structures. They also have cells that can release small molecules, such as PGE2, into the CSF, thus affecting target structures at a distance. The neuro-hypophysis is a site of axonal release (from PVN and SON magnocellular neurons) of oxytocin and arginine vasopressin into the general circulation. The median eminence is a zone of neuro-endocrine transduction for the secretion of releasing factors and inhibitory factors into the hypophyseal portal vasculature; these factors influence the release of anterior pituitary hormones. The pineal gland synthesizes and releases the hormone melatonin.

Blood Supply of Hypothalamus and Pituitary Gland

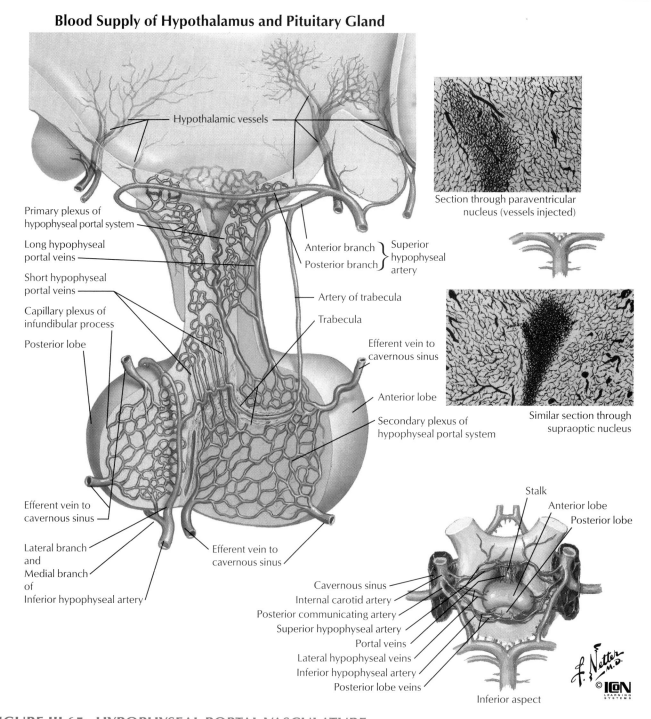

Hypothalamic vessels

Primary plexus of hypophyseal portal system

Long hypophyseal portal veins

Short hypophyseal portal veins

Capillary plexus of infundibular process

Posterior lobe

Anterior branch ⎫ Superior
Posterior branch ⎬ hypophyseal
⎭ artery

Artery of trabecula

Trabecula

Efferent vein to cavernous sinus

Anterior lobe

Secondary plexus of hypophyseal portal system

Efferent vein to cavernous sinus

Lateral branch and Medial branch of Inferior hypophyseal artery

Efferent vein to cavernous sinus

Section through paraventricular nucleus (vessels injected)

Similar section through supraoptic nucleus

Stalk
Anterior lobe
Posterior lobe

Cavernous sinus
Internal carotid artery
Posterior communicating artery
Superior hypophyseal artery
Portal veins
Lateral hypophyseal veins
Inferior hypophyseal artery
Posterior lobe veins

Inferior aspect

FIGURE III.65: HYPOPHYSEAL PORTAL VASCULATURE

The hypophyseal portal vascular system derives from arterioles that enter the median eminence at the base of the hypothalamus. The primary capillary plexus is a site where releasing and inhibitory factors that influence the secretion of anterior pituitary hormones are released from axons whose neurons reside in the hypothalamus and other CNS sites. These releasing and inhibitory factors then travel through venules into the secondary capillary plexus in very high concentrations and act directly on anterior pituitary cells, which synthesize and secrete the hormones of the anterior pituitary.

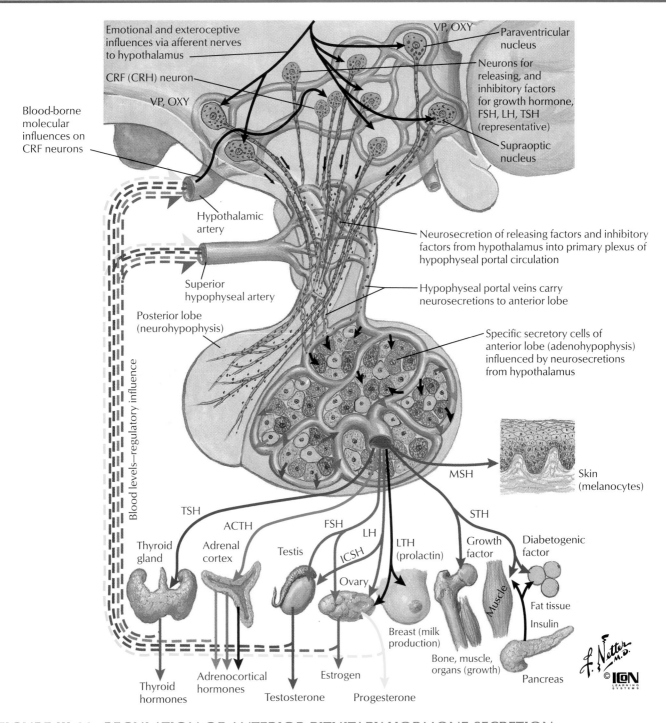

FIGURE III.66: REGULATION OF ANTERIOR PITUITARY HORMONE SECRETION

Neurons that synthesize releasing and inhibitory factors for control of anterior pituitary hormones send axons that terminate on the primary capillary plexus of the hypophyseal portal system (the zone of neuroendocrine transduction) and release these factors into the hypophyseal portal blood. These factors then flow into the secondary hypophyseal portal plexus and regulate the release of anterior pituitary hormones. These hormones act on target organs to affect the release of target organ hormones or to influence metabolic and functional activities. For example, CRF neurons release CRF into the hypophyseal portal blood, regulating the release of ACTH, which in turn regulates the release of cortisol from the adrenal cortex. Magnocellular neurons of the PVN and the SON send axons directly to the posterior pituitary; these axons release oxytocin and arginine vasopressin directly into the systemic circulation.

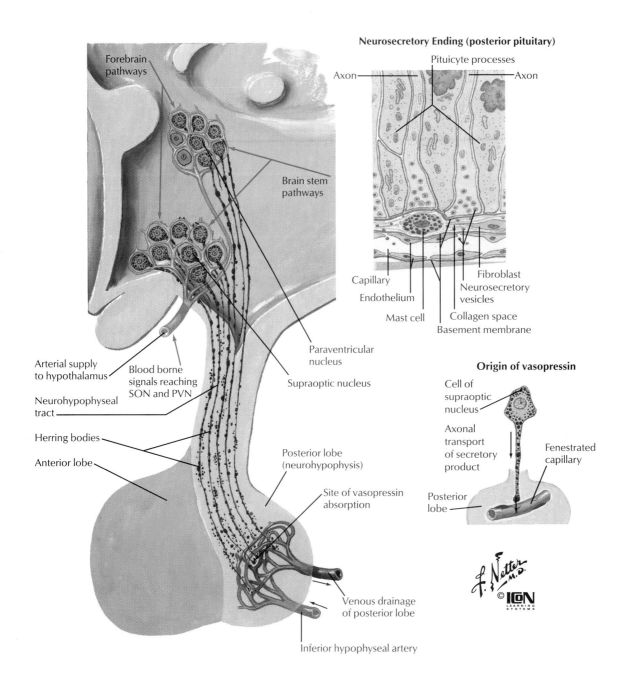

FIGURE III.67: POSTERIOR PITUITARY (NEUROHYPOPHYSEAL) HORMONES: OXYTOCIN AND VASOPRESSIN

Magnocellular neurons in the PVN and the SON send axons directly through the infundibular region and the pituitary stalk, to terminate on the vasculature in the posterior pituitary. Neurons from both nuclei synthesize and release oxytocin and arginine vasopressin into the systemic vasculature. Brain stem and forebrain pathways terminate on the magnocellular neurons and regulate their secretion of oxytocin and vasopressin. These magnocellular neurons possess extensive protein synthetic capacity and transport the vesicles in which their hormones are packaged to the axon terminals with very fast axoplasmic transport. The hormones are released from the terminals and diffuse through the fenestrated capillaries directly into the systemic vasculature (inset: Neurosecretory Efferent Endings From Magnocellular Neurons in PVN and SON).

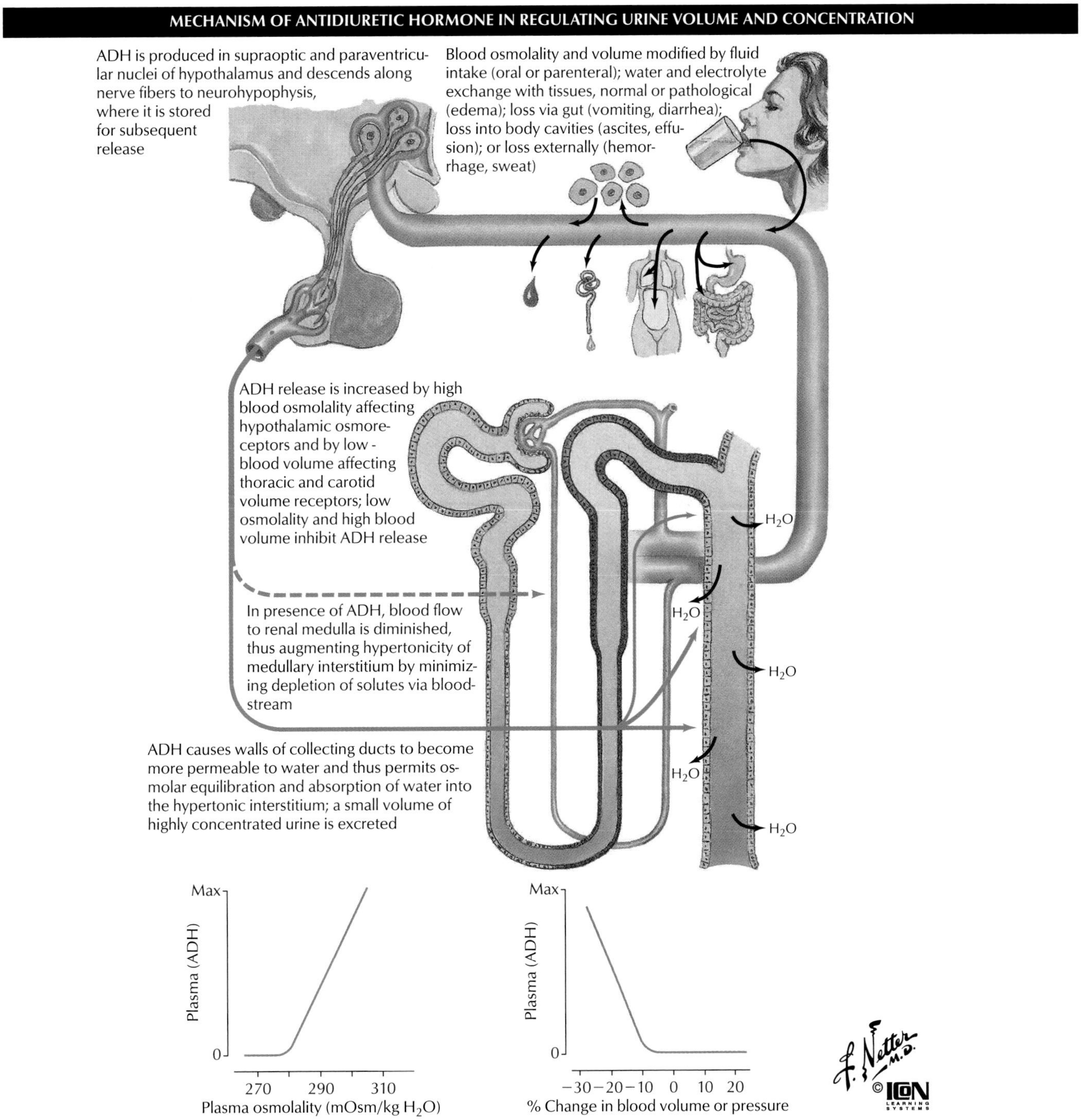

MECHANISM OF ANTIDIURETIC HORMONE IN REGULATING URINE VOLUME AND CONCENTRATION

ADH is produced in supraoptic and paraventricular nuclei of hypothalamus and descends along nerve fibers to neurohypophysis, where it is stored for subsequent release

Blood osmolality and volume modified by fluid intake (oral or parenteral); water and electrolyte exchange with tissues, normal or pathological (edema); loss via gut (vomiting, diarrhea); loss into body cavities (ascites, effusion); or loss externally (hemorrhage, sweat)

ADH release is increased by high blood osmolality affecting hypothalamic osmoreceptors and by low-blood volume affecting thoracic and carotid volume receptors; low osmolality and high blood volume inhibit ADH release

In presence of ADH, blood flow to renal medulla is diminished, thus augmenting hypertonicity of medullary interstitium by minimizing depletion of solutes via bloodstream

ADH causes walls of collecting ducts to become more permeable to water and thus permits osmolar equilibration and absorption of water into the hypertonic interstitium; a small volume of highly concentrated urine is excreted

H_2O

H_2O

H_2O

H_2O

H_2O

Max

Plasma (ADH)

0

270 290 310
Plasma osmolality (mOsm/kg H_2O)

Max

Plasma (ADH)

0

−30 −20 −10 0 10 20
% Change in blood volume or pressure

FIGURE III.68: VASOPRESSIN (ANTIDIURETIC HORMONE) REGULATION OF WATER BALANCE AND FLUID OSMOLALITY

Vasopressin regulates the volume of water secreted by the kidneys. Vasopressin secretion is regulated by the osmolality of body fluids and by blood volume and pressure. Changes in body fluid osmolality of a few percent are sufficient to significantly alter vasopressin secretion. Decreases in blood volume and pressure of 10% to 15% or more are needed to affect vasopressin secretion. The blood volume and pressure sensors are found in the pulmonary vessels, carotid sinus, and the aortic arch. These baroreceptors respond to stretch of the vessel wall, which is dependent on blood volume and pressure. The diagram shows the mechanisms of action of vasopressin on the kidney, with resultant effects on urine volume and concentration.

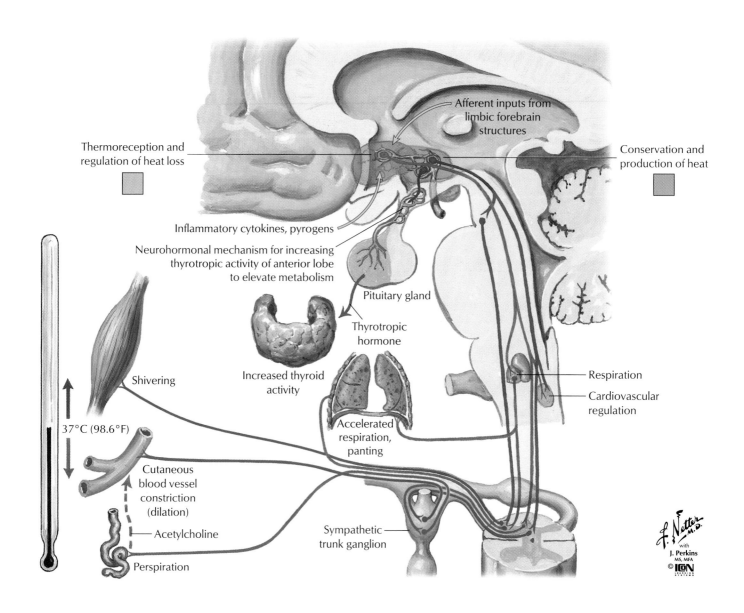

Thermoreception and regulation of heat loss

Conservation and production of heat

Afferent inputs from limbic forebrain structures

Inflammatory cytokines, pyrogens

Neurohormonal mechanism for increasing thyrotropic activity of anterior lobe to elevate metabolism

Pituitary gland

Thyrotropic hormone

Increased thyroid activity

Shivering

37°C (98.6°F)

Cutaneous blood vessel constriction (dilation)

Acetylcholine

Perspiration

Accelerated respiration, panting

Sympathetic trunk ganglion

Respiration

Cardiovascular regulation

FIGURE III.69: THE HYPOTHALAMUS AND THERMOREGULATION

The preoptic area of the hypothalamus contains warmth-sensitive neurons. The posterior hypothalamic area (PHA) contains cold-sensitive neurons. The preoptic area and the anterior hypothalamic area initiate neuronal responses for heat dissipation (parasympathetic); the PHA initiates neuronal responses for heat generation (sympathetic). Neuronal pathways arising from the brain stem and the limbic forebrain areas can modulate the activity of these thermoregulatory systems. The preoptic area is responsive to pyrogens and the inflammatory cytokine IL-1β; this area can generate an increased set-point for temperature regulation, thus initiating a disease-associated fever. Extensive hypothalamic connections with the brain stem and the spinal cord are used to initiate appropriate heat-dissipation or heat-generation responses. Appropriate behavioral responses also are initiated to optimize thermoregulation (e.g., going to a warmer or cooler location).

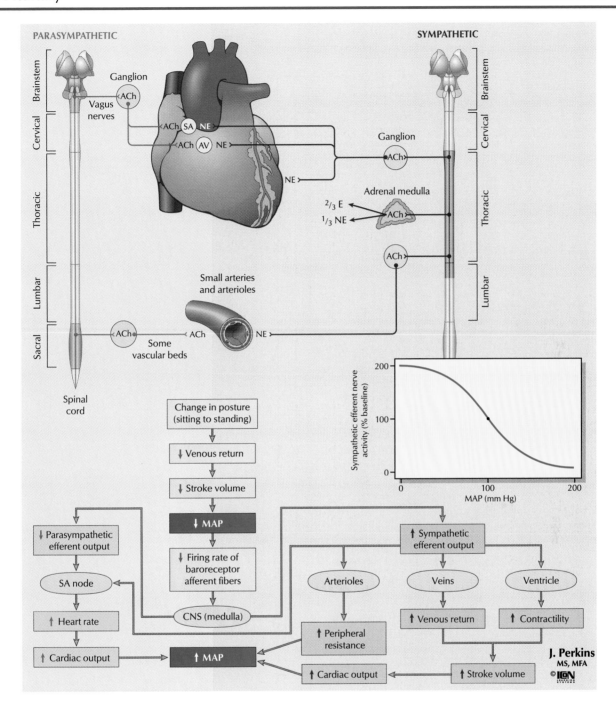

FIGURE III.70: SHORT-TERM REGULATION OF BLOOD PRESSURE

Both the sympathetic and parasympathetic divisions of the autonomic nervous system are involved in maintaining blood pressure on a second-by-second basis. Many descending pathways from the brain stem (including the NTS, tegmental catecholamine nuclei, the locus coeruleus, raphe nuclei, the rostral ventrolateral medulla, other medullary reticular regions, parabrachial nuclei, angiotensin II–containing neurons) and the hypothalamus regulate the autonomic preganglionic neurons associated with short-term blood pressure regulation. The hypothalamus and the NTS are the key sites integrating limbic forebrain and cortical influences over the brain stem regions that regulate blood pressure. These brain stem sites have extensive interconnections with each other. The example of blood pressure regulation in this plate is based on a change in posture. (ACh = acetylcholine, E = epinephrine, NE = norepinephrine, MAP = mean arterial pressure.)

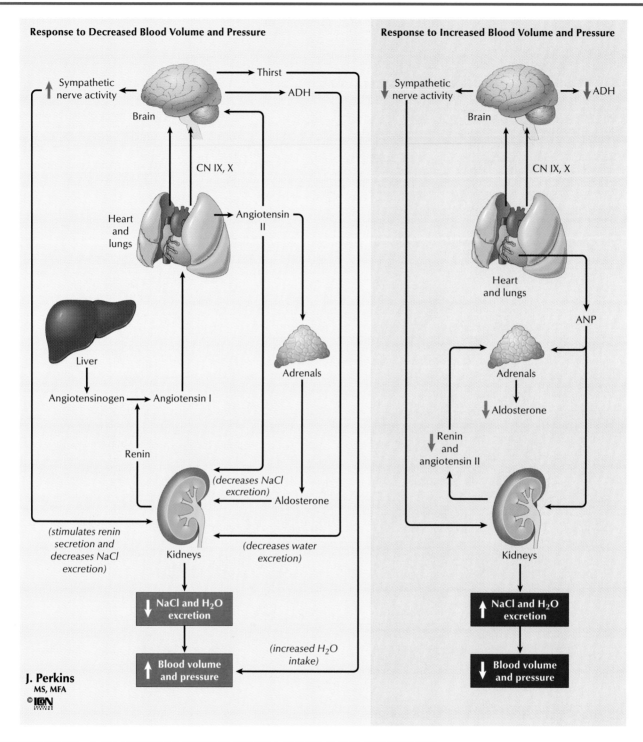

Response to Decreased Blood Volume and Pressure

Response to Increased Blood Volume and Pressure

J. Perkins
MS, MFA
©ICN

FIGURE III.71: LONG-TERM REGULATION OF BLOOD PRESSURE

When blood volume and blood pressure change, the kidneys respond by retaining or excreting NaCl and water in order to restore blood volume to its normal homeostatic state. With increased sympa- thetic activation, norepinephrine and epinephrine secretion from sympathetic nerve terminals and the adrenal medulla increase in the circulation and act on the kidney to reduce NaCl excretion.

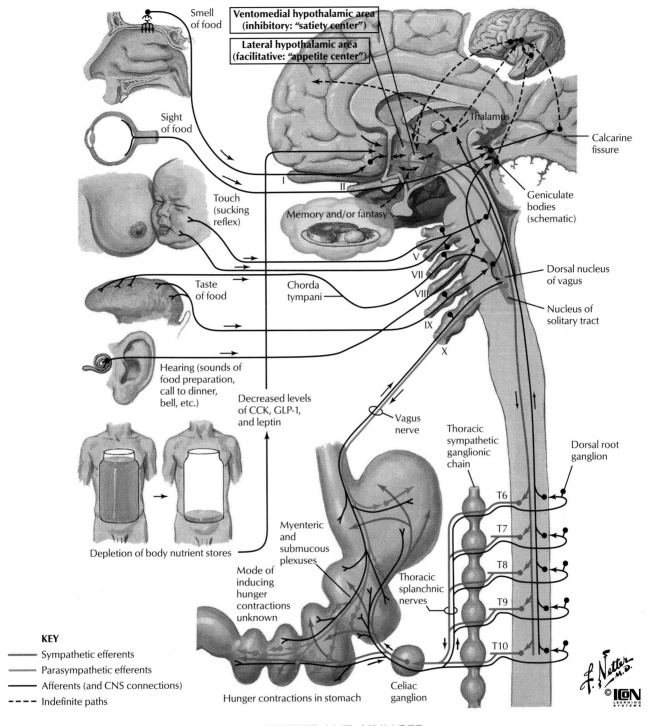

KEY
- ─── Sympathetic efferents
- ─── Parasympathetic efferents
- ─── Afferents (and CNS connections)
- - - - Indefinite paths

FIGURE III.72: NEURAL CONTROL OF APPETITE AND HUNGER

The sensations of hunger and satiety are complex and include multiple neural pathways and circulating hormones. Depicted here are pathways involved in the sensation of hunger. Although our understanding is incomplete, the hypothalamus is known to play a critical role in controlling appetite and food intake. When food is ingested, cholecystokinin and glucagon-like peptide-1 are released from neuroendocrine cells in the intestine. These hormones suppress appetite and give the sensation of satiety. In the absence of food, the levels of these hormones are low. Long-term regulation of food intake involves the hormone leptin, which is produced by fat cells. When fat stores are high, leptin is released and appears to act on the hypothalamus to suppress appetite. When body nutrient stores are depleted, leptin levels are lowered.

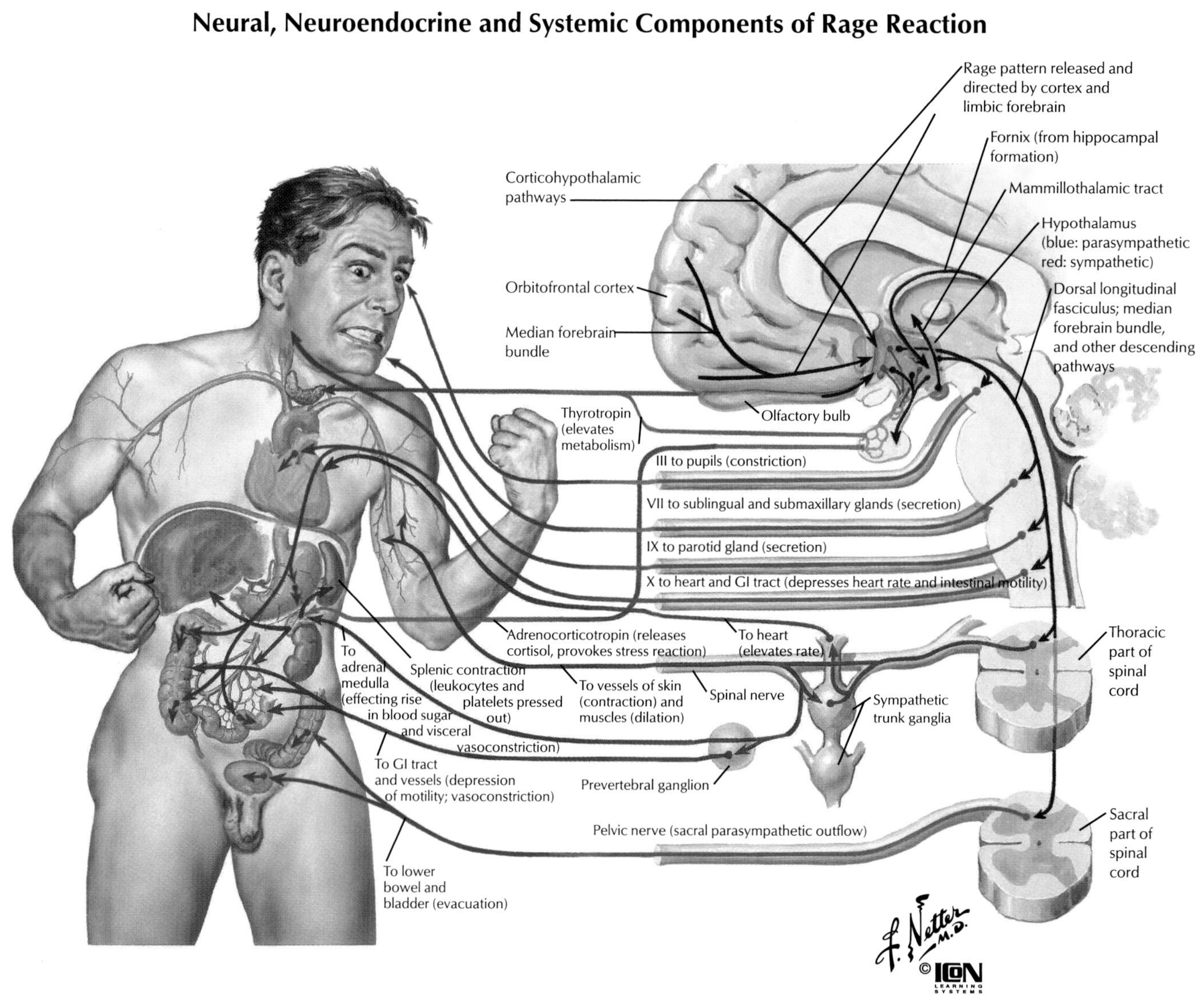

Neural, Neuroendocrine and Systemic Components of Rage Reaction

Rage pattern released and directed by cortex and limbic forebrain

Fornix (from hippocampal formation)

Mammillothalamic tract

Hypothalamus (blue: parasympathetic red: sympathetic)

Dorsal longitudinal fasciculus; median forebrain bundle, and other descending pathways

Corticohypothalamic pathways

Orbitofrontal cortex

Median forebrain bundle

Olfactory bulb

Thyrotropin (elevates metabolism)

III to pupils (constriction)

VII to sublingual and submaxillary glands (secretion)

IX to parotid gland (secretion)

X to heart and GI tract (depresses heart rate and intestinal motility)

Adrenocorticotropin (releases cortisol, provokes stress reaction)

To heart (elevates rate)

Thoracic part of spinal cord

To adrenal medulla (effecting rise in blood sugar and visceral vasoconstriction)

Splenic contraction (leukocytes and platelets pressed out)

To vessels of skin (contraction) and muscles (dilation)

Spinal nerve

Sympathetic trunk ganglia

To GI tract and vessels (depression of motility; vasoconstriction)

Prevertebral ganglion

Pelvic nerve (sacral parasympathetic outflow)

Sacral part of spinal cord

To lower bowel and bladder (evacuation)

FIGURE III.73: NEURAL AND NEUROENDOCRINE ROLES IN THE FIGHT-OR-FLIGHT RESPONSE

The classic sympathetic fight-or-flight response, shown here as a rage response, involves the secretion of neuroendocrine "stress hormones," which include cortisol from the hypothalamo-pituitary-adrenal (HPA) axis and norepinephrine and epinephrine from sympathetic nerve terminals and the adrenal medulla. Sympathetic connections with the viscera initiate physiological changes to support the integrated fight-or-flight response. These changes include diversion of blood from the viscera and the skin to the muscles, increased heart rate and cardiac output and contractility, bronchodilation, pupillary dilation, decreased gastrointestinal activation, decreased renal activity, and glycogenolysis from the liver. Inputs from the limbic forebrain, the cortex, and the brain stem regulate the hypothalamic control of neuroendocrine and autonomic outflow and are key in initiating the classic fight-or-flight response. In the fight-or-flight response, the brain stem parasympathetic neurons are inhibited.

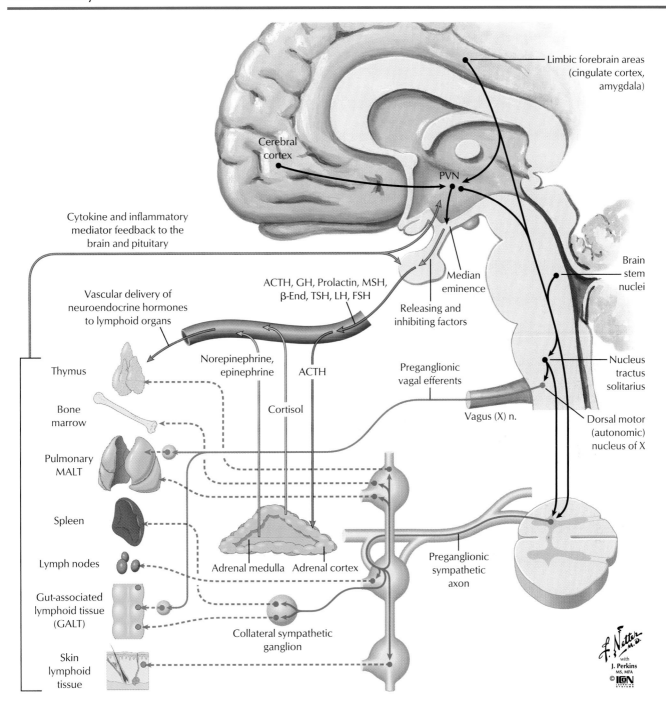

Limbic forebrain areas (cingulate cortex, amygdala)

Cerebral cortex

PVN

Cytokine and inflammatory mediator feedback to the brain and pituitary

Median eminence

Brain stem nuclei

ACTH, GH, Prolactin, MSH, β-End, TSH, LH, FSH

Releasing and inhibiting factors

Vascular delivery of neuroendocrine hormones to lymphoid organs

Nucleus tractus solitarius

Norepinephrine, epinephrine

ACTH

Preganglionic vagal efferents

Thymus

Dorsal motor (autonomic) nucleus of X

Bone marrow

Cortisol

Vagus (X) n.

Pulmonary MALT

Spleen

Lymph nodes

Adrenal medulla   Adrenal cortex

Preganglionic sympathetic axon

Gut-associated lymphoid tissue (GALT)

Collateral sympathetic ganglion

Skin lymphoid tissue

FIGURE III.74: NEUROIMMUNOMODULATION

Connections from the cerebral cortex, the limbic forebrain, the hypothalamus, and the brain stem exert extensive modulation over autonomic preganglionic outflow and neuroendocrine outflow. Neurohormones and neurotransmitters from this outflow target lymphoid organs and cells of the immune system. This circuitry provides the substrate for behavior, emotional responsiveness, chronic stressors, and positive complementary interventions to influence immune responses. Sympathetic postganglionic noradrenergic fibers directly innervate virtually all organs of the immune system. Vagal postganglionics innervate pulmonary and gut-associated lymphoid tissue. Pituitary hormones in the circulation, and their target organ hormones, modulate immune reactivity in all lymphoid organs. Cortisol, norepinephrine, and epinephrine are particularly important in mediating chronic stress responses related to immune reactivity. Circulating and local cytokines and inflammatory mediators act on the brain and the pituitary to provide immune-neural signaling.

Major Limbic Forebrain Structures

Anterior commissure
Cingulate gyrus
Interventricular foramen
Indusium griseum
Anterior nucleus of thalamus
Corpus callosum
Interthalamic adhesion
Septum pellucidum
Fornix
Precommissural fornix
Stria terminalis
Septal nuclei
Stria medullaris
Hypothalamus
Subcallosal area
Habenula
Paraterminal gyrus
Lamina terminalis
Calcarine sulcus (fissure)
Olfactory
medial stria
lateral stria
tract
bulb
Gyrus fasciolaris
Anterior perforated substance
Optic chiasm
Dentate gyrus
Postcommissural fornix
Fimbria of hippocampus
Mammillary body and mammillothalamic tract
Hippocampus
Medial forebrain bundle
Parahippocampal gyrus
Amygdaloid body (nuclei)
Descending connections to reticular and tegmental nuclei of brain stem (dorsal longitudinal fasciculus)
Uncus
Interpeduncular nucleus
Fasciculus retroflexus

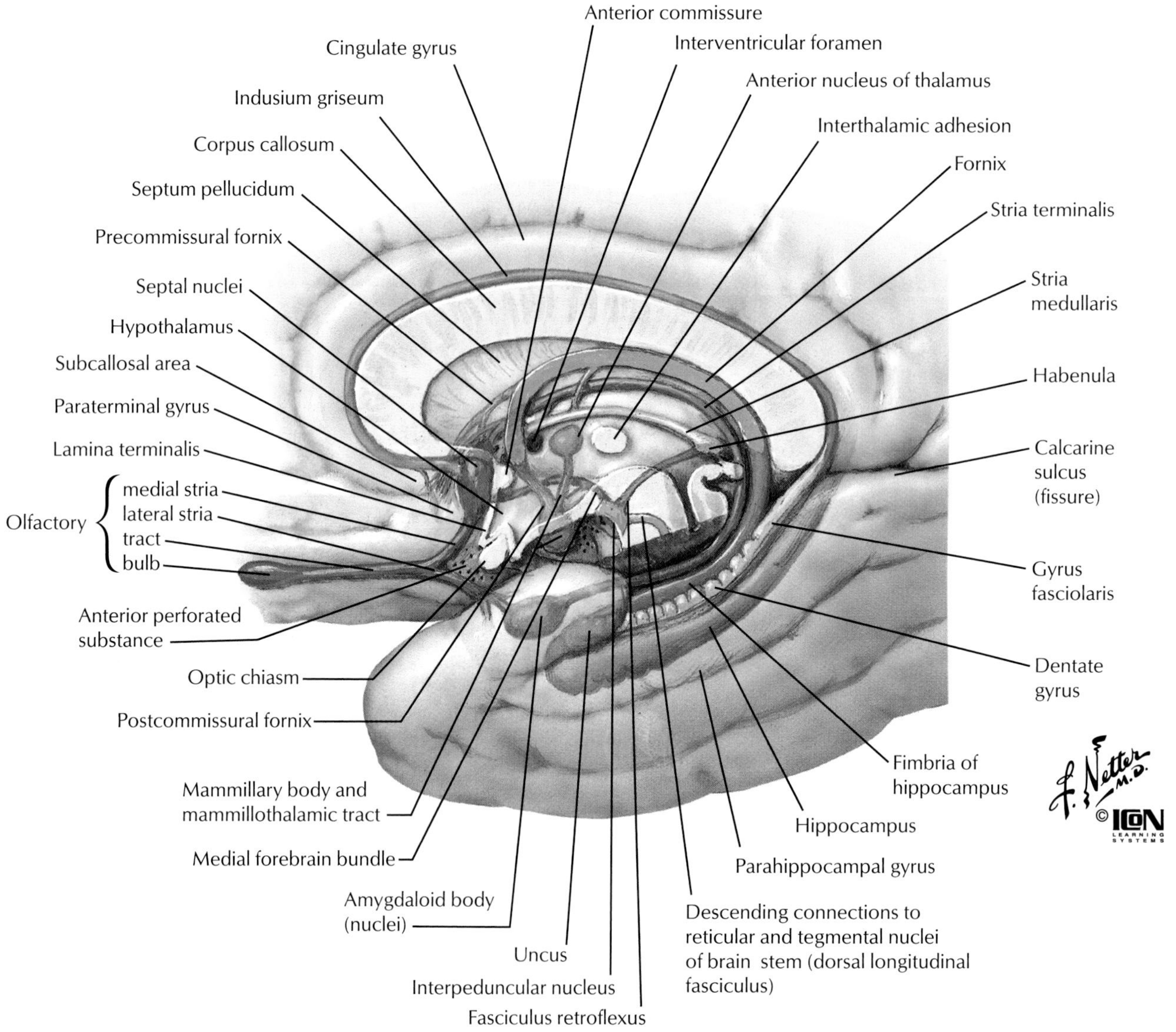

FIGURE III.75: ANATOMY OF THE LIMBIC FOREBRAIN

Structures of the limbic forebrain are found in a ring (limbus) that encircles the diencephalon. Two major temporal lobe structures, the hippocampal formation with its fornix and the amygdala with its stria terminalis, send C-shaped axonal projections through the cortex, around the diencephalon, and into the hypothalamus and the septal region. The amygdala also sends a more direct pathway (ventral amygdalofugal pathway) into the hypothalamus. The septal nuclei sit just rostral to the hypothalamus and send axons to the habenular nuclei via the stria medullaris thalami. The cingulate, prefrontal, orbitofrontal, entorhinal, and periamygdaloid areas of the cortex interconnect with subcortical and hippocampal components of the limbic forebrain and are often considered part of the limbic system. The limbic system is thought to be a major substrate for regulation of emotional responsiveness and behavior, for individualized reactivity to sensory stimuli, and for integrated memory tasks.

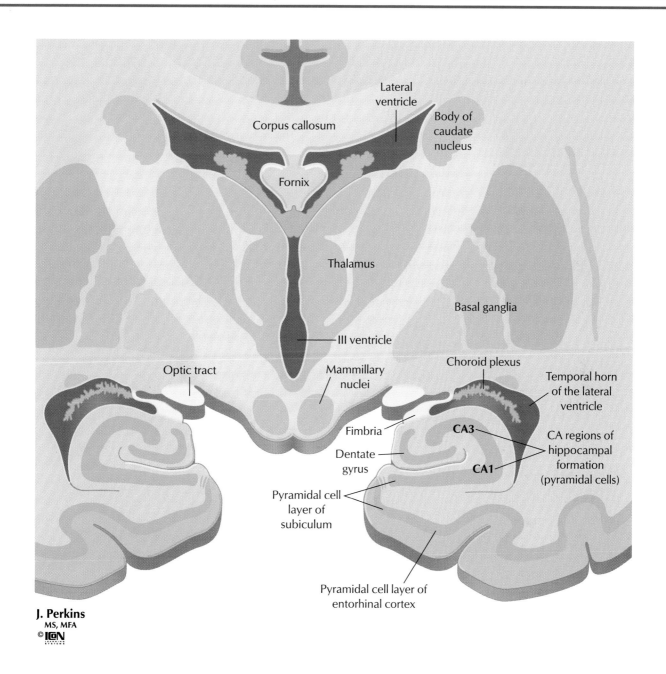

J. Perkins
MS, MFA
©ICN

FIGURE III.76: HIPPOCAMPAL FORMATION: GENERAL ANATOMY

The hippocampal formation consists of the dentate gyrus, the hippocampus proper (cornu ammonis [CA] regions), and the subiculum. These structures are intimately interconnected with the adjacent entorhinal cortex. The hippocampus is a seahorse-shaped structure found in the medial portion of the anterior temporal lobe. It bulges laterally into the temporal horn of the lateral ventricle. The hippocampus is divided into several zones of pyramidal cells, called CA regions (CA1-CA4). Granule cells populate the dentate gyrus. The dentate gyrus and the hippocampus are three-layered cortical regions. The hippocampal formation has extensive interconnections with cortical association areas and with limbic forebrain structures such as the septal nuclei and the cingulate gyrus. It is involved in consolidation of short-term memory into long-term traces, in conjunction with extensive regions of neocortex.

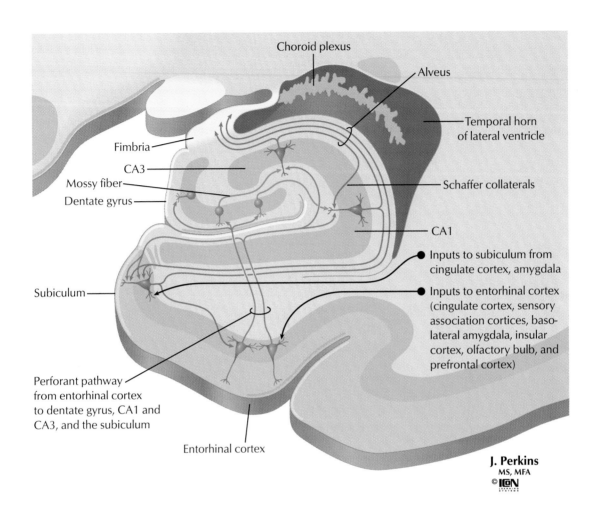

Choroid plexus

Alveus

Fimbria

CA3

Mossy fiber

Dentate gyrus

Temporal horn of lateral ventricle

Schaffer collaterals

CA1

Inputs to subiculum from cingulate cortex, amygdala

Inputs to entorhinal cortex (cingulate cortex, sensory association cortices, baso-lateral amygdala, insular cortex, olfactory bulb, and prefrontal cortex)

Subiculum

Perforant pathway from entorhinal cortex to dentate gyrus, CA1 and CA3, and the subiculum

Entorhinal cortex

J. Perkins
MS, MFA
©ICN

FIGURE III.77: NEURONAL CONNECTIONS IN THE HIPPOCAMPAL FORMATION

The hippocampal formation has an internal circuitry interconnected with the entorhinal cortex. Pyramidal neurons of the entorhinal cortex send axons to granule cell dendrites in the dentate gyrus. These granule cell axons (mossy fibers) synapse on pyramidal cell dendrites in CA3. Pyramidal cells in CA3 project to pyramidal cell dendrites in CA1 (Schaffer collaterals) and CA2. CA1 pyramidal axons project to pyramidal neurons in the subiculum. The subiculum sends axonal projections back to the pyramidal neurons of the entorhinal cortex. This information flow represents an internal circuit. Superimposed on this circuitry are a host of interconnections with association regions of neocortex and other limbic forebrain structures. Neurons of the subiculum and CA neurons of CA1 and CA3 send axons into the fornix as efferent projections to target structures. The subiculum also sends axons to the amygdala and the association areas of the temporal lobe.

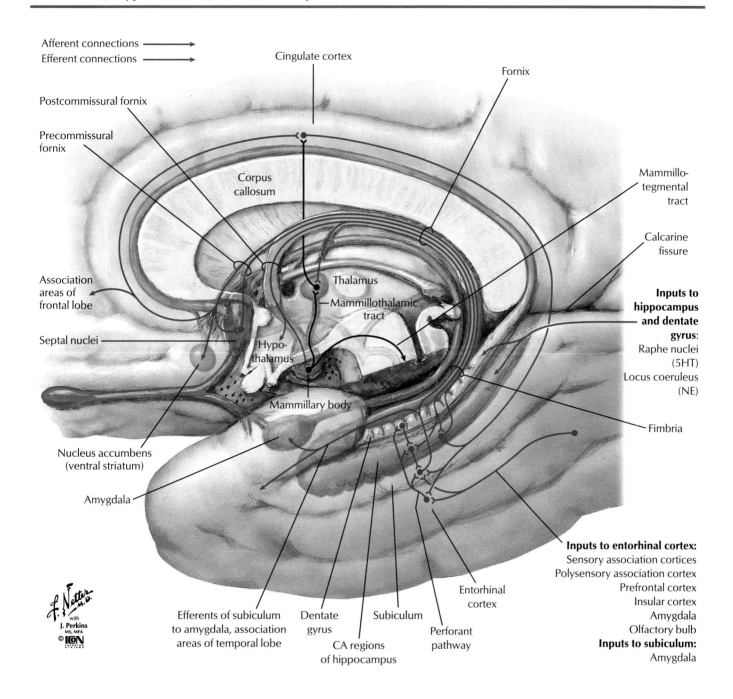

Afferent connections ⟶
Efferent connections ⟶

Cingulate cortex

Fornix

Postcommissural fornix

Precommissural fornix

Mammillo-tegmental tract

Corpus callosum

Calcarine fissure

Association areas of frontal lobe

Thalamus

Mammillothalamic tract

Inputs to hippocampus and dentate gyrus:
Raphe nuclei (5HT)
Locus coeruleus (NE)

Septal nuclei

Hypo-thalamus

Mammillary body

Fimbria

Nucleus accumbens (ventral striatum)

Amygdala

Entorhinal cortex

Inputs to entorhinal cortex:
Sensory association cortices
Polysensory association cortex
Prefrontal cortex
Insular cortex
Amygdala
Olfactory bulb
Inputs to subiculum:
Amygdala

Efferents of subiculum to amygdala, association areas of temporal lobe

Dentate gyrus

CA regions of hippocampus

Subiculum

Perforant pathway

FIGURE III.78: MAJOR AFFERENT AND EFFERENT CONNECTIONS OF THE HIPPOCAMPAL FORMATION

Pyramidal neurons in the subiculum and the hippocampal regions CA1 and CA3 give rise to the efferent fornix. The subiculum projects to hypothalamic nuclei (especially mammillary nuclei) and thalamic nuclei via the postcommissural fornix. CA1 and CA3 neurons send axons to the septal nuclei, the nucleus accumbens, the preoptic and anterior hypothalamic regions, the cingulate cortex, and the association areas of the frontal lobe. Afferent cholinergic axons from septal nuclei traverse the fornix to supply the dentate gyrus and the hippocampal CA regions. Massive inputs arrive in the hippocampal formation from sensory association cortices, polysensory association cortex, the prefrontal cortex, the insular cortex, amygdaloid nuclei, and the olfactory bulb via projections to the entorhinal cortex. The entorhinal cortex is fully integrated into the internal circuitry of the hippocampal formation. The subiculum is connected reciprocally with the amygdala and also sends axons to cortical association areas of the temporal lobe.

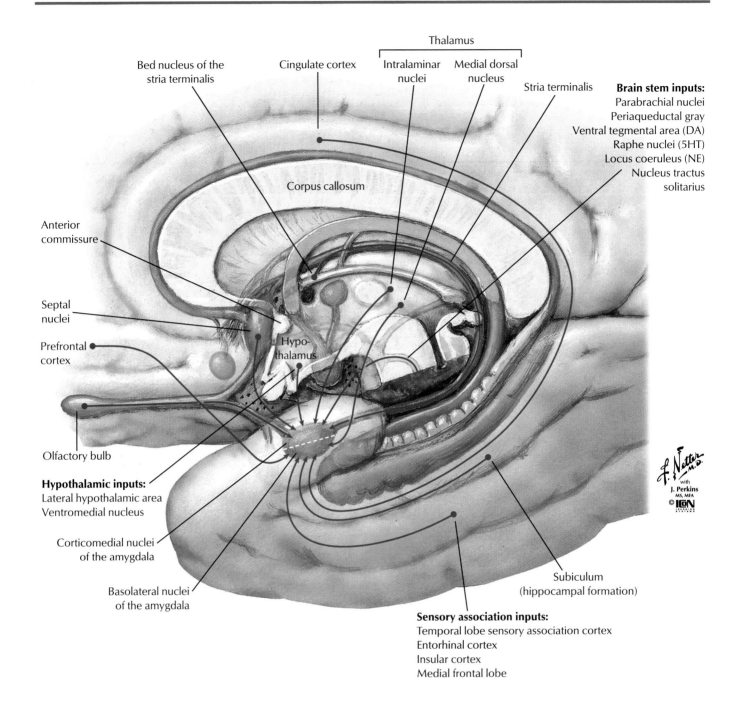

Thalamus

Bed nucleus of the
stria terminalis

Cingulate cortex

Intralaminar
nuclei

Medial dorsal
nucleus

Stria terminalis

Brain stem inputs:
Parabrachial nuclei
Periaqueductal gray
Ventral tegmental area (DA)
Raphe nuclei (5HT)
Locus coeruleus (NE)
Nucleus tractus
solitarius

Corpus callosum

Anterior
commissure

Septal
nuclei

Prefrontal
cortex

Hypo-
thalamus

Olfactory bulb

Hypothalamic inputs:
Lateral hypothalamic area
Ventromedial nucleus

Corticomedial nuclei
of the amygdala

Basolateral nuclei
of the amygdala

Subiculum
(hippocampal formation)

Sensory association inputs:
Temporal lobe sensory association cortex
Entorhinal cortex
Insular cortex
Medial frontal lobe

FIGURE III.79: MAJOR AFFERENT CONNECTIONS OF THE AMYGDALA

The amygdala is an almond-shaped collection of nuclei in the medial portion of the anterior temporal lobe. It is involved in the emotional interpretation of external sensory information and internal states. It provides individual-specific behavioral and emotional responses, particularly for fear and aversion. The amygdala is subdivided into corticomedial and basolateral nuclei and the central nucleus, which mainly provides efferent projections to the brain stem. Afferents to the corticomedial nuclei arrive mainly from subcortical limbic sources, including the olfactory bulb, septal nuclei, hypothalamic nuclei (VM, LHA), the thalamus (intralaminar nuclei), the bed nucleus of the stria terminalis, and extensive autonomic monoamine nuclei of the brain stem. Afferents to the basolateral nuclei arrive mainly from cortical areas, including extensive sensory association cortices, the prefrontal cortex, the cingulate cortex, and the subiculum.

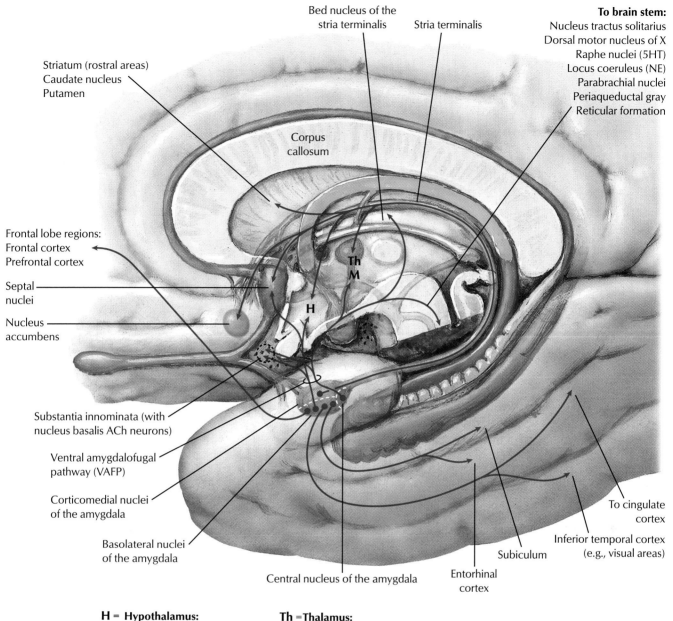

Bed nucleus of the stria terminalis

Stria terminalis

To brain stem:
Nucleus tractus solitarius
Dorsal motor nucleus of X
Raphe nuclei (5HT)
Locus coeruleus (NE)
Parabrachial nuclei
Periaqueductal gray
Reticular formation

Striatum (rostral areas)
Caudate nucleus
Putamen

Corpus callosum

Th
M

H

Frontal lobe regions:
Frontal cortex
Prefrontal cortex

Septal nuclei

Nucleus accumbens

Substantia innominata (with nucleus basalis ACh neurons)

Ventral amygdalofugal pathway (VAFP)

Corticomedial nuclei of the amygdala

Basolateral nuclei of the amygdala

Central nucleus of the amygdala

Entorhinal cortex

Subiculum

To cingulate cortex

Inferior temporal cortex (e.g., visual areas)

H = **Hypothalamus:**
Preoptic area
Anterior hypothalamic area
Ventromedial nucleus
Lateral hypothalamic area
Paraventricular nucleus

Th = **Thalamus:**
Medial dorsal nucleus

M = **Midline thalamic nuclei**

FIGURE III.80: MAJOR EFFERENT CONNECTIONS OF THE AMYGDALA

Efferents from the corticomedial nuclei project through the stria terminalis and are directed mainly toward subcortical nuclei such as septal nuclei, the MD (DM) nucleus of the thalamus, hypothalamic nuclei, the bed nucleus of the stria terminalis, the nucleus accumbens, and the rostral striatum. Efferents from the basolateral nuclei project through the ventral amygdalofugal pathway to extensive cortical regions, including the frontal cortex, the cingulate cortex, the inferior temporal cortex, the subiculum, and the entorhinal cortex; and to subcortical limbic regions, including hypothalamic nuclei, septal nuclei, and the cholinergic nucleus basalis in the substantia innominata. The central amygdaloid nucleus receives input mainly from internal amygdaloid connections and sends extensive efferents through the ventral amygdalofugal pathway to extensive autonomic nuclei and monoaminergic nuclei of the brain stem, midline thalamic nuclei, the bed nucleus of the stria terminalis, and the cholinergic nucleus basalis.

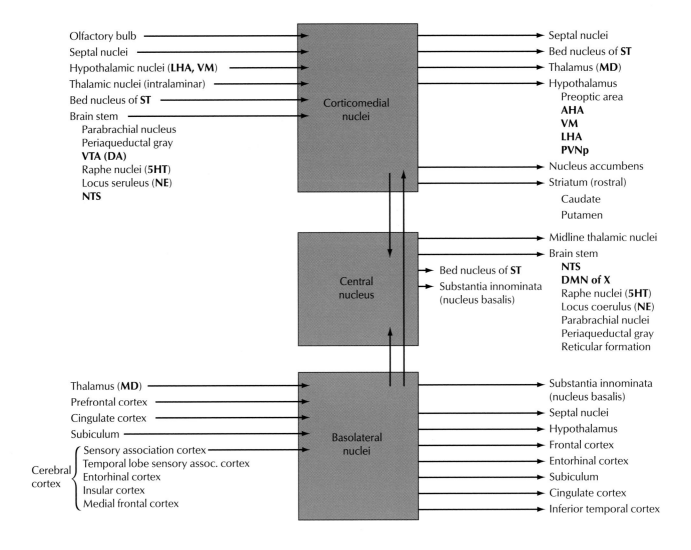

DA = Dopamine
5HT = 5-Hydroxytryptamine (serotonin)
NE = Norepinephrine
ST = Stria terminalis
VTA = Ventral tegmental area
NTS = Nucleus tractus solitarius

MD = Medial dorsal nucleus of thalamus
AHA = Anterior hypothalamic area
VM = Ventromedial
LHA = Lateral hypothalamic area
PVNp = Paraventricular nucleus, parvocellular
DMN of X = Dorsal motor (autonomic) nucleus of X

© ICN LEARNING SYSTEMS

FIGURE III.81: SUMMARY OF MAJOR AFFERENTS, EFFERENTS, AND INTERCONNECTIONS OF THE AMYGDALA

The corticomedial amygdala is connected reciprocally mainly with subcortical limbic forebrain structures, with extensive additional inputs from brain stem autonomic and monoaminergic nuclei. The basolateral amygdala is connected reciprocally with extensive regions of limbic and association cortex, with additional efferents to subcortical limbic forebrain regions. Both the corticomedial and the basolateral nuclei send axons to the central nucleus of the amygdala. The central nucleus has massive descending efferents to extensive autonomic and monoaminergic nuclei of the brain stem as well as to some subcortical limbic forebrain regions. These interconnections provide the integrated circuitry that permits analysis of both external and internal information, which provides an emotional and interpretative context for the initiation and control of appropriate behavioral and emotional responses.

AFFERENTS

Major afferents from:
Hippocampal CA pyramidal cells
Amygdaloid nuclei
    Corticomedial nuclei via stria terminalis
    Basolateral nuclei via ventral
        amygdalofugal pathway
Ventral tegmental area
Hypothalamus
    Preoptic area
    Anterior hypothalamic area
    Paraventricular nucleus
    Lateral hypothalamic area
Locus coeruleus (NE; not shown)

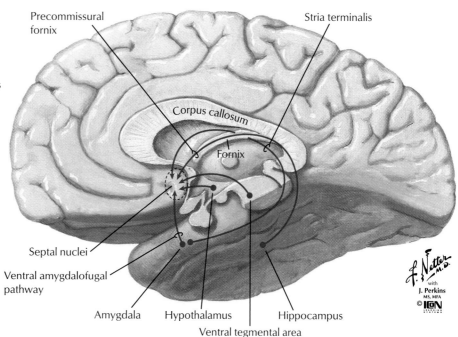

EFFERENTS

Major efferents to:
Hippocampal CA regions ⎱ Via fornix
Dentate gyrus (ACh path) ⎰
Habenular nuclei ⎱ Via stria
Medial dorsal nucleus ⎰ medullaris
    of the thalamus   thalami
Ventral tegmental area — Via median
Hypothalamus   forebrain bundle
    Preoptic area
    Anterior hypothalamic area
    Ventromedial nucleus
    Lateral hypothalamic area

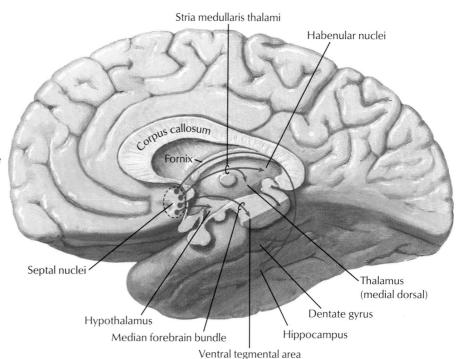

FIGURE III.82: MAJOR AFFERENT AND EFFERENT CONNECTIONS OF THE SEPTAL NUCLEI

The septal nuclei are subcortical nuclei implicated by early ablation and stimulation studies in the regulation of emotional responsiveness (such as rage behavior). In experimental studies, the septal nuclei appear to play a role in emotional behaviors, sexual behavior, aggressive behavior, modulation of autonomic functions, and attention and memory functions (from the cholinergic neurons). Afferents to the septal nuclei arrive mainly from the hippo-campus, the corticomedial and basolateral amygdala, the ventral tegmental area in the midbrain, and several hypothalamic nuclei. Efferents from the septal nuclei project mainly to the hippocampus and the dentate gyrus (via the fornix), the habenular nuclei and the MD (DM) nucleus of the thalamus (via the stria medullaris thalami), the ventral tegmental area (via the median forebrain bundle), and several hypothalamic nuclei.

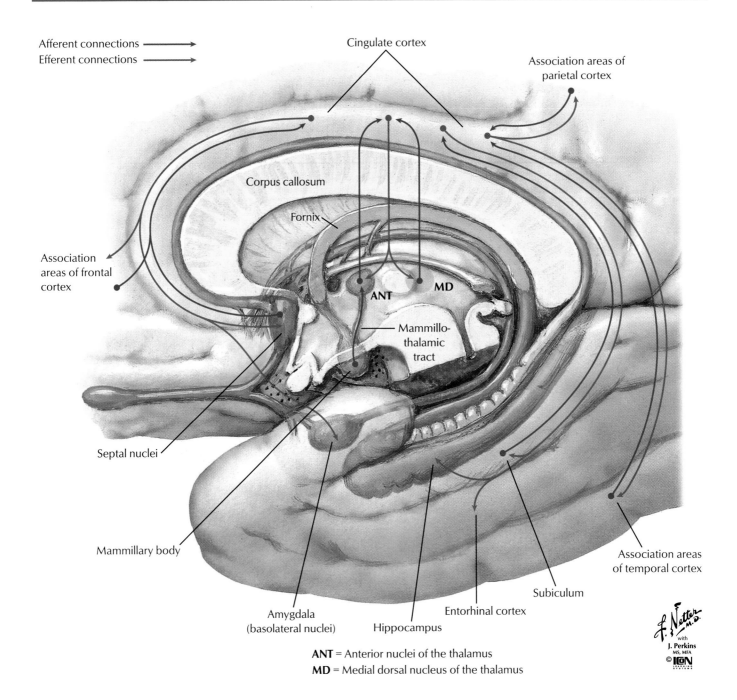

Afferent connections ⟶
Efferent connections ⟶

Cingulate cortex

Association areas of parietal cortex

Corpus callosum

Fornix

Association areas of frontal cortex

ANT

MD

Mammillo-thalamic tract

Septal nuclei

Mammillary body

Amygdala (basolateral nuclei)

Hippocampus

Entorhinal cortex

Subiculum

Association areas of temporal cortex

ANT = Anterior nuclei of the thalamus
MD = Medial dorsal nucleus of the thalamus

FIGURE III.83: MAJOR CONNECTIONS OF THE CINGULATE CORTEX

The cingulate cortex is located above the corpus callosum. This cortical region is involved in the regulation of autonomic functions (respiratory, digestive, cardiovascular, papillary), some somatic functions (motor tone, ongoing movements), and emotional responsiveness and behavior. Lesions of the cingulate cortex result in indifference to pain and other sensations with emotional connotation and social indifference. Afferents to the cingulate cortex arrive from association areas of the frontal, parietal, and temporal lobes, the subiculum, septal nuclei, and thalamic nuclei (MD, anterior). Efferents from cingulate cortex neurons project to association areas of the frontal, parietal, and temporal lobes and to limbic forebrain regions such as the hippocampus, the subiculum, the entorhinal cortex, the amygdala, and septal nuclei. These limbic forebrain regions send extensive projections to the hypothalamus for regulation of the autonomic and somatic regions of the brain stem and the spinal cord.

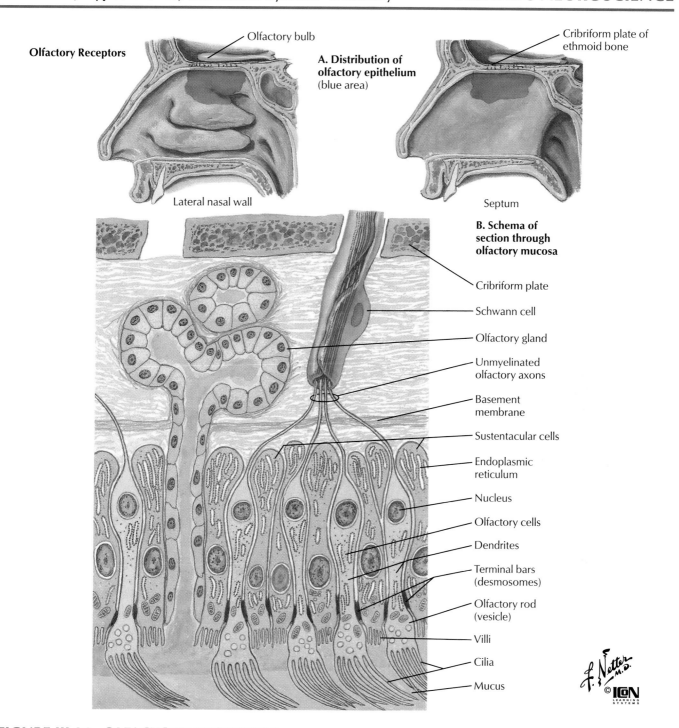

Olfactory Receptors

Olfactory bulb

A. Distribution of olfactory epithelium (blue area)

Lateral nasal wall

Cribriform plate of ethmoid bone

Septum

B. Schema of section through olfactory mucosa

Cribriform plate

Schwann cell

Olfactory gland

Unmyelinated olfactory axons

Basement membrane

Sustentacular cells

Endoplasmic reticulum

Nucleus

Olfactory cells

Dendrites

Terminal bars (desmosomes)

Olfactory rod (vesicle)

Villi

Cilia

Mucus

FIGURE III.84: OLFACTORY RECEPTORS

Olfactory receptors are found in a patch of olfactory epithelium that lines the medial and lateral walls of the roof of the nasal cavity. They are primitive specialized bipolar neurons whose nuclei are in the base of the epithelium. A dendritic process extends toward the epithelial surface, widening into a rod with 10 to 30 motile cilia that project into the mucous cover. Odorants act on receptors (G-protein–coupled) on these cilia and bring about a slow depolarizing generator potential. Odorant interaction with receptors is complex, often requiring odorant-binding proteins to carry the odorant through the mucosa. The bipolar neurons of the olfactory epithelium are CNS neurons; they are unusual because they undergo continuous replacement and turnover from basal stem cells in the epithelium. The UNM olfactory axons cluster together in groups (enwrapped by a Schwann cell) before passing through the cribriform plate. Injuries to the cribriform plate can result in anosmia.

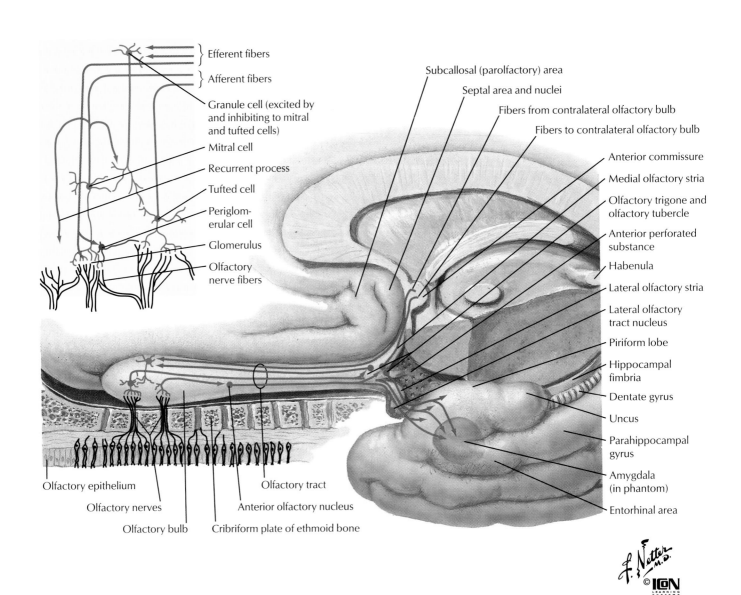

FIGURE III.85: OLFACTORY PATHWAYS

Primary sensory axons from bipolar neurons pass through the cribriform plate and synapse in the olfactory glomeruli in the glomerular layer of the olfactory bulb. The glomeruli are the functional units for processing specific odor information. The olfactory nerve fibers synapse on the dendrites of the tufted and mitral cells, the secondary sensory neurons that give rise to the olfactory tract projections. Periglomerular cells are interneurons that interconnect the glomeruli. Granule cells modulate excitability of tufted and mitral cells.

Centrifugal connections (from serotonergic raphe, noradrenergic locus coeruleus) modulate activity in the glomeruli and on periglomerular cells. The olfactory tract bypasses the thalamus and projects to the anterior olfactory nucleus, the nucleus accumbens, the primary olfactory cortex, the amygdala, the periamygdaloid cortex, and the lateral entorhinal cortex. The olfactory cortex has interconnections with the orbitofrontal cortex and the insular cortex, the hippocampus, and the lateral hypothalamus.

INDEX

INDEX